CRASH COURSE
Metabolism and Nutrition

Metabolism and Nutrition

Albert Clark, MD
Professor of Biochemistry and Pathology
Queen's University
Kingston, Ontario

UK edition authors
Jason O'Neale Roche and Sarah Benyon

UK series editor
Daniel Horton-Szar

ELSEVIER
MOSBY

ELSEVIER
MOSBY

1600 John F. Kennedy Blvd.
Ste 1800
Philadelphia, PA 19103-2899

CRASH COURSE: METABOLISM AND NUTRITION

ISBN-13: 978-1-4160-3117-8
ISBN-10: 1-4160-3117-0

Adapted from Crash Course Metabolism and Nutrition 2e by Jason O'Neale Roach, ISBN 0-7234-3297-X. © 2002, Elsevier Science Limited. All rights reserved.

The rights of Jason O'Neale Roach to be identified as the author of this work have been asserted by him in accordance with the Copyright, Designs and Patents Act, 1988.

Library of Congress Cataloging-in-Publication Data

Clark, Albert, MD
    Metabolism and nutrition / Albert Clark—1st U.S. ed.
        p. cm.—(Crash course)
    ISBN 1-4160-3117-0
    1. Nutrition.   2. Metabolism.   I. Title.   II. Series.

    QP141.C575 2006
    612.3′9—dc22

2005052249

Commissioning Editor: *Alex Stibbe*
Project Development Manager: *Stan Ward*
Project Manager: *David Saltzberg*
Designer: *Andy Chapman*
Cover Design: *Antbits Illustration*
Illustration Manager: *Mick Ruddy*

Printed in United States

Last digit is the print number:
9 8 7 6 5 4 3 2 1

Preface

Crash Course: Metabolism and Nutrition provides an integrated overview of metabolism and nutrition. The activities of the metabolic pathways in the various tissues are described, and the relationships and interactions between the pathways and the tissues are outlined. This approach allows, for example, the integration of the pathways in the chapter on glucose homeostasis and what happens when there is a problem in the regulation of the pathways in the common metabolic disease, diabetes. The biochemical defects in a range of metabolic and nutritional diseases are noted and related to clinical symptoms. Tests used to investigate and monitor patients with these diseases are described.

The contents of *Crash Course: Metabolism and Nutrition* makes it suitable for students studying medicine and related health sciences. It will be useful for medical students studying for board exams and for residents in general internal medicine as a reference for metabolic disorders.

Albert F Clark, PhD

Acknowledgments

Thanks to the authors of the UK edition, Jason O'Neale Roach and Saran Benyon, as well as the series editor, Daniel Horton-Szar.

Contents

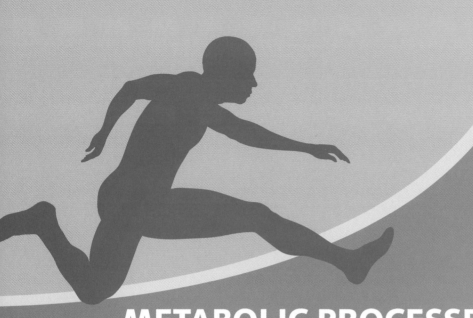

METABOLIC PROCESSES AND NUTRITION

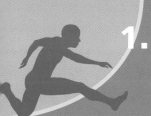

1. Overview of Metabolism

Metabolism

Metabolism involves an integrated set of chemical reactions occurring in the body. These reactions enable us to extract energy from the environment and use it to synthesize the building blocks used to make proteins, carbohydrates and fats. Some fundamental points to remember about metabolism:

- Each reaction does not occur in isolation but provides a substrate (the substance on which an enzyme acts) for the next.
- Pathways are built up in which the end product forms a substrate for other pathways, producing a continuous process.
- Many people compare metabolism to a map, in which the pathways are like roads with "stop-off points" (intermediates) along the way. These intermediates may be links to other pathways.
- Roads need traffic lights and speed humps (regulatory mechanisms) to control the amount and speed of traffic.
- Some of the roads are one way, meaning you have to travel a long way round to form some intermediates.
- Remember: when you make any journey, it is important to know where you are going, but you do not need to know the names of all the places you travel through.
- Remember also that pathways are linked, and alteration in the regulation of one pathway can influence the activity of other pathways.

Metabolic pathways can be classified as either catabolic or anabolic.

Catabolism

Catabolism is the breakdown (degradation) of energy-rich complex molecules such as protein, carbohydrate and fat to simpler ones, for example CO_2, H_2O and NH_3. The energy released is "captured" as adenosine triphosphate (ATP) and stored for use in synthetic, anabolic reactions.

Anabolism

Anabolism is the synthesis of complex molecules from simpler ones; for example, proteins from amino acids and glycogen from glucose. Synthetic reactions require energy that comes from the hydrolysis of ATP. Some examples of catabolic and anabolic pathways are shown in Fig. 1.1, and a scheme of overall metabolism is given in Fig. 1.2.

Metabolic pathways were not just invented to make the first year at medical school very dull! Do not get bogged down remembering every single step and enzyme in a pathway, as you will not be asked to regurgitate this sort of information in an exam. It is much more likely that you will have to discuss the overall functions of a cycle and the tissues in which they are particularly important.

The best way to revise metabolism is to draw simplified cycles of all the pathways, listing the six key criteria in Fig. 1.3 for each: purpose/function, location, site, reaction sequence, key steps and effect of inhibition.

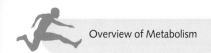

Examples of catabolic and anabolic pathways	
Catabolic pathways names end in "lysis" meaning "to break down"	**Anabolic pathways** names end in "genesis" meaning "to create"
glycogenolysis: glycogen breakdown proteolysis: protein breakdown lipolysis: trialglycerol breakdown glycolysis: glucose breakdown	glycogenesis: glycogen synthesis protein synthesis lipogenesis: fatty acid synthesis gluconeogenesis: glucose synthesis

Fig. 1.1 Examples of catabolic and anabolic pathways.

Regulation of pathways

Every metabolic pathway usually contains one reaction that is essentially irreversible and forms the rate-limiting reaction of the pathway. Enzymes catalyzing these reactions are subject to strict regulation to ensure that:

- The speed of the entire pathway is adapted to the cell's needs.
- For any molecule, its synthetic and breakdown pathways are not active at the same time, as this would lead to a "futile cycle."

Metabolic pathways may occur in different cell compartments, different cells, and different tissues of the body at the same time. The pathways are carefully regulated to ensure that the production of energy and intermediates meets the needs of the individual cell and to "fit in" with the requirements of the rest of the cells in the body. The control of metabolic pathways must also be flexible enough to enable adaptation to different conditions, such as the fed state as opposed to starvation, or periods of exercise. These control mechanisms coordinate the pathways in all cells of the body.

Mechanisms of control

There are three main mechanisms of control of metabolic pathways: supply of substrate, allosteric control, and hormonal control. Learn these now because they form the basis for control of all metabolic pathways.

Substrate supply

If the concentration of substrate is limiting, then the rate of the pathway decreases.

Allosteric control

Allosteric effectors bind to regulatory sites on an enzyme that are distinct from the catalytic (active) site. They may increase or decrease an enzyme's activity. Often, allosteric control is exerted by the end-product of a pathway; this may be positive (stimulate pathway) or negative (inhibit pathway).

Hormonal control

There are two possible mechanisms by which hormones such as insulin or glucagon can affect enzyme activity and thus the rate of metabolic pathways:

- Firstly, by reversible phosphorylation of enzymes, which may either increase or decrease their activity. For example, glucagon causes phosphorylation of both glycogen synthase and glycogen phosphorylase. Glycogen synthase is inhibited by phosphorylation whereas glycogen phosphorylase is activated. This ensures that glycogen synthesis and breakdown are not active at the same time and is discussed fully in Chapter 2.
- Secondly, hormones can affect the rate of a metabolic pathway by enzyme induction. Hormones can increase the amount of enzyme synthesized by stimulating the rate of transcription of its mRNA. Similarly, under certain conditions hormones can inhibit transcription and thus the synthesis of certain enzymes—this is called repression.

Basic principles of bioenergetics

Bioenergetics is the study of the energy changes accompanying biochemical reactions. It allows us to work out why some reactions occur (i.e., because they are energetically favorable) and why some do not. The direction and extent to which a chemical reaction occurs are determined by a combination of two factors:

- Enthalpy change, ΔH, which is the heat released or absorbed during a reaction.
- Entropy change, ΔS, a measure of the change in disorder or randomness in a reaction.

Neither enthalpy nor entropy change alone can predict whether a reaction can occur. Together they are used to calculate ΔG, the change in Gibbs free

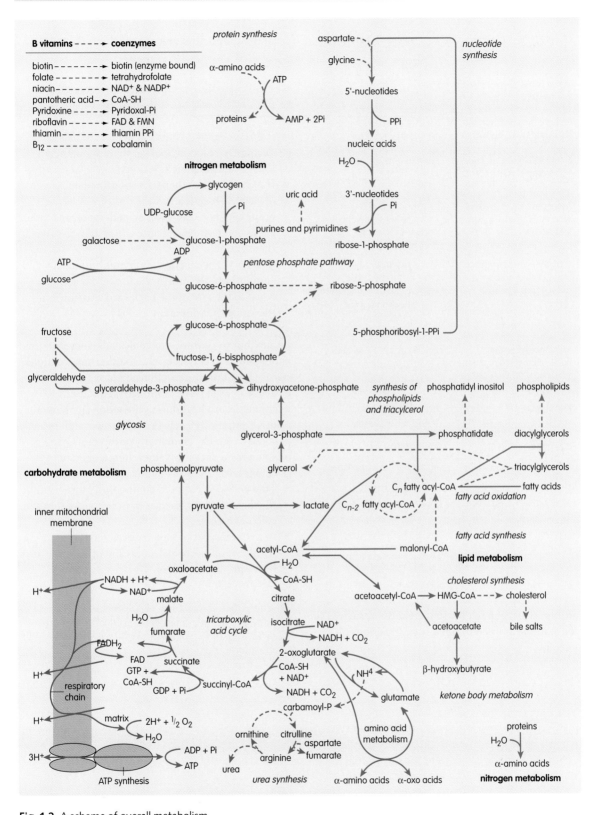

Fig. 1.2 A scheme of overall metabolism.

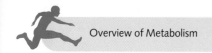

Key criteria for remembering a metabolic pathway	
Key criteria	**Example—glycolysis**
What is the purpose of the pathway? form a working definition of its function knowing: the substrates and products involved and any other key intermediates produced, for example, ATP or NADH	oxidation of glucose (substrate) to pyruvate (product) with the generation of energy in the form of ATP and NADH
Tissue location: particularly, tissues or cells in the body where the pathway is most important	glycolysis occurs in all cells of the body but in red blood cells it is the only energy-producing pathway
Cell site: where in the cell it occurs, for example cytosol, mitochondria or both	glycolysis occurs in the cell cytosol; pyruvate formed can be transported into mitochondria for further metabolism by the TCA cycle
Sequence of events know the overall reaction sequence and the number of stages and reactions	glycolysis has 10 reactions
Key steps: either those which form major control sites or those which are main "branch points"	hexokinase reaction phosphofructokinase reaction pyruvate kinase
Effect of inhibition of the cycle	increase in [intermediates] which arise before the site of inhibition decrease in [intermediates] formed after the block

Fig. 1.3 Key points for remembering a metabolic pathway.

energy of a reaction. It is ΔG that predicts favorability and direction of a reaction, since:

$$\Delta G = \Delta H - T \times \Delta S$$

where T = absolute temperature in degrees Kelvin (K) (°C + 273) and ΔG is the energy available to do work.

- If ΔG is negative, there is a net loss of energy during the reaction; making this a spontaneous, favorable, exergonic reaction.
- If ΔG is positive, there is a net gain of energy during the reaction and the reaction does not occur spontaneously; it is an endergonic reaction, as energy must be added to the system to drive the reaction.
- If ΔG is 0, the reaction is at equilibrium. At equilibrium, the rate of the forward reaction is equal to the rate of the backward reaction and there is no net direction.

Be sure not to confuse exergonic and exothermic and endergonic and endothermic. Exothermic reactions release heat during a reaction and have a negative enthalpy change ($-\Delta H$). Similarly, endothermic reactions absorb heat during a reaction and have a positive enthalpy change ($+\Delta H$). However, it is not possible to predict favorability or direction of a reaction from enthalpy values. Remember, only reactions with a negative ΔG occur spontaneously.

Free energy is required continuously for:
- Mechanical work, such as muscle contraction and cell movements.
- Active transport of molecules and ions.
- Synthesis of macromolecules and other molecules from simple precursors.

This energy is obtained in humans by the oxidation of foodstuffs. Some is transformed into a highly accessible form before use as the molecule adenosine triphosphate (see Chapter 2).

- Define catabolic and anabolic pathways (giving examples of each).
- What are the key points or criteria for learning metabolic pathways?
- Why are metabolic pathways regulated?
- What are the three main mechanisms of control in metabolic pathways?
- What are the principles behind predicting the direction of a reaction?

2. Carbohydrate and Energy Metabolism

Glycolysis and its regulation

An overview of glycolysis
Working definition
Glycolysis is the sequence of 10 reactions that break down one molecule of glucose (six carbons) to two three-carbon molecules of pyruvate. This sequence involves a net generation of two molecules of ATP and NADH (the reduced form of nicotinamide adenine dinucleotide). Glycolysis provides energy and intermediates for other metabolic pathways.

Location
All the cells of the body.

Site
Cell cytosol.

Aerobic and anaerobic respiration
Unlike other metabolic pathways, glycolysis can produce ATP under either aerobic or anaerobic conditions (see Fig. 2.2).
- Under aerobic conditions, the end-product, pyruvate, enters mitochondria. Here it is oxidized by the tricarboxylic acid (TCA) cycle and oxidative phosphorylation to CO_2 and H_2O. This produces large quantities of energy.
- Under anaerobic conditions, pyruvate is reduced by NADH to lactate in the cytosol. This results in regeneration of NAD^+, which is required for glycolysis, and thus allows the continued production of ATP in cells that lack mitochondria or are deprived of oxygen. This pathway produces a relatively small amount of energy.

Functions and importance of glycolysis
For many tissues glycolysis is an "emergency" energy-producing pathway when oxygen is the limiting factor. It is of the utmost importance in:

- Red blood cells (RBCs), because they lack mitochondria and therefore glycolysis is their only energy-producing pathway.
- Exercising skeletal muscle, when oxidative metabolism cannot keep up with increased energy demand.
- The brain, because glucose is its main fuel (it uses about 120 g/day).

Glycolysis also contributes to the synthesis of certain specialized intermediates; for example, 2,3-bisphosphoglycerate, an allosteric effector of hemoglobin. It also helps in the metabolism of other sugars, especially fructose and galactose (both of these topics are covered later in this chapter).

Glucose entry into cells
Glucose is not small enough to diffuse directly into the cell—it needs help. There are two transport mechanisms that exist specifically for glucose.

Facilitated diffusion
The first mechanism, facilitated diffusion, is mediated by a family of glucose transporters present in the cell membrane. At least five have been identified and are named GLUT-1 to GLUT-5; each has a different tissue distribution (Fig. 2.1).

The transporters are integral membrane proteins that bind glucose and transport it through the cell membrane into the cell. Glucose enters the cell down its concentration gradient from an area of high concentration outside the cell to an area of low concentration inside.

Sodium–glucose cotransporter
The second mechanism requires energy to transport glucose against its concentration gradient (i.e., from a low concentration outside the cell to a high concentration inside). This method of glucose transport occurs in the epithelial cells of the intestine (for the absorption of dietary glucose), renal tubules and the choroid plexus. The movement of glucose is

Examples of glucose transporters		
Transporter	Location	Function
GLUT-1	erythrocytes and most cell membranes	Provides basal glucose transport to cells at a relatively constant rate
GLUT-2	liver and β cells of pancreas	GLUT-2 transporters have a lower affinity for glucose than GLUT-1, therefore GLUT-2 are only active when there is a high blood glucose, that is, in the fed state
GLUT-4	muscle and fat cells	Insulin-dependent: muscle and fat cells "store" GLUT-4 transporters in intracellular vesicles. Insulin promotes glucose uptake by muscle and fat. In the presence of insulin, these vesicles fuse with the cell membrane, resulting in an increase in the number of GLUT-4 transporters in membrane

Fig. 2.1 Examples of glucose transporters.

coupled to the concentration gradient of sodium: sodium ions flow down their concentration gradient into the cell, providing the energy to transport glucose into the cell against its gradient.

Trapping glucose in the cell
Glucose may enter the cell but will not necessarily stay there. Glucose must undergo irreversible phosphorylation to be "trapped" inside the cell. Why? There are two reasons. First, phosphorylated glucose molecules cannot penetrate cell membranes because there are no carriers for them (glucose-6-phosphate is not a substrate for the glucose transporters). Secondly, converting glucose to glucose-6-phosphate keeps the concentration of free glucose inside the cell low compared with outside, maintaining the concentration gradient.

Stages of glycolysis
Glycolysis can be divided into two phases: an energy investment phase and an energy generating phase.

Energy investment phase (reactions 1–5 in Fig. 2.2)
Glucose is phosphorylated and cleaved into two molecules of glyceraldehyde-3-phosphate. This process uses two moles of ATP to activate and to increase the energy content of the intermediates (see Figs 2.2 and 2.3).

Energy generating phase (reactions 6–10)
Two molecules of glyceraldehyde-3-phosphate are converted into two molecules of pyruvate with the generation of four moles of ATP (see Figs 2.2 and 2.3).

The overall reaction can be written as:

$$Glucose + 2NAD^+ + 2ADP + 2Pi \rightarrow 2NADH + 2pyruvate + 2ATP + 2H_2O + 2H^+$$

The name of an enzyme can be easily worked out, if you forget it, by knowing the name of the substrate (or the product) and the type of reaction involved (Fig. 2.4). For example, pyruvate is phosphorylated by pyruvate kinase.

Synthesis of ATP
ATP can be synthesized from ADP by two processes: substrate-level phosphorylation and oxidative phosphorylation.

Substrate-level phosphorylation
Substrate-level phosphorylation is the formation of ATP by the direct phosphorylation of ADP, that is, the direct transfer of a phosphoryl group from a "high-energy" intermediate to ADP. It does not require oxygen and is therefore important for ATP generation in tissues short of oxygen, for example in exercising skeletal muscle. Reactions 7 and 10 of glycolysis (see Fig. 2.2) are both examples of substrate-level phosphorylation. Further examples are found in Fig. 2.25.

Oxidative phosphorylation
Oxidative phosphorylation requires oxygen and is the most important mechanism for the synthesis of ATP. It involves the oxidation of two nucleotides: NADH and the reduced form of flavin adenine

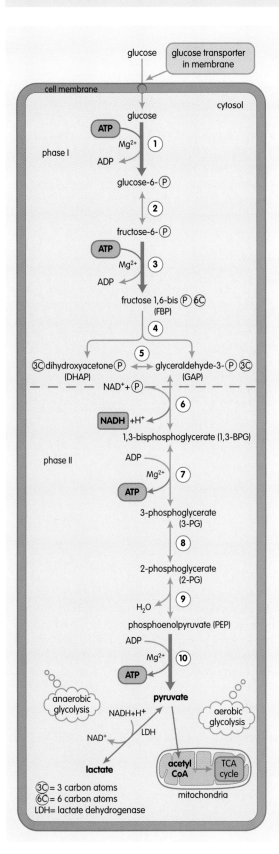

dinucleotide ($FADH_2$) by the electron transport chain.

Energy yield of glycolysis
Anaerobic glycolysis
The overall reaction can be written as:

$$Glucose + 2Pi + 2ADP \rightarrow 2lactate + 2ATP + 2H_2O$$

The net effect is the generation of two moles of ATP from the anaerobic oxidation of one mole of glucose (Fig. 2.5). There is no net production of NADH because it is used by lactate dehydrogenase to reduce pyruvate to lactate. It is important to remember that, although anaerobic glycolysis only produces a small amount of ATP, it is an extremely valuable energy source for cells when the oxygen supply is limited.

Aerobic glycolysis
The overall reaction can be written as:

$$Glucose + 2Pi + 2NAD^+ + 2ADP \rightarrow 2pyruvate$$
$$+ 2ATP + 2NADH + 2H^+ + H_2O$$

Two moles of NADH are generated from the oxidation of one mole of glucose; each NADH is oxidized by the electron transport chain to yield about 2.5 ATP. Therefore, the net effect of aerobic glycolysis is the generation of 7 ATP per mole of glucose (2 directly by substrate-level phosphorylation and about 5 indirectly by oxidative phosphorylation) (see Fig. 2.5).

Importance of NAD regeneration from NADH
NAD^+ is the primary oxidizing agent of glycolysis and an important cofactor for glyceraldehyde-3-phosphate dehydrogenase (reaction 6 in Fig. 2.2). However, only a limited amount of NAD+ is available. Therefore, a major problem is its regeneration from NADH, which is essential for glycolysis to continue. There are three possible mechanisms for the regeneration of NAD^+:
• Firstly, under anaerobic conditions, pyruvate is reduced to lactate by lactate dehydrogenase, with the simultaneous oxidation of NADH to NAD^+ in the cell cytosol (see Fig. 2.2). This is a reversible

Fig. 2.2 The glycolytic (Embden–Meyerhof) pathway. Glycolysis takes place in the cell cytosol and consists of two distinct phases—energy investment (1–5) and energy generation (6–10). The names of the enzymes catalyzing reactions 1 to 10 can be found in Fig. 2.3.

Stages of glycolysis		
Phase I: Energy investment phase		
Step	**Enzyme**	**Type of reaction**
1.	Hexokinase: most tissues (glucokinase in liver and β cells of pancreas)	phosphorylation **irreversible regulatory step**
2.	phosphoglucose isomerase	isomerization aldose → ketose
3.	phosphofructokinase-1 (PFK-1)	phosphorylation **irreversible rate-limiting step of glycolysis**
4.	aldolase	cleavage FBP (6C) → DHAP(3C) + GAP(3C)
5.	triose phosphate isomerase	isomerization Note that phase I produces two molecules of glyceraldehyde-3-phosphate (GAP)
Phase II: Energy generating phase each molecule of glyceraldehyde-3-phosphate undergoes the following reactions:		
6.	glyceraldehyde-3-phosphate dehydrogenase	oxidative phosphorylation 2 NADH are generated per molecule of glucose oxidized
7.	phosphoglycerate kinase	substrate-level phosphorylation
8.	phosphoglycerate mutase	transfer of phosphate group from C3 to C2
9.	enolase	dehydration
10.	pyruvate kinase N.B. All kinases require Mg^{2+} as a co-factor	substrate-level phosphorylation **irreversible regulatory step**

Fig. 2.3 Stages of glycolysis. Steps 1 to 10 refer to reactions 1 to 10 in Fig. 2.2.

Enzymes and the types of reactions they catalyze	
Enzyme	**Type of reaction**
kinase	phosphorylation
mutase	transfer of a functional group from one position to another in the same molecule
isomerase	conversion of one isomer into another (isomers are compounds with the same chemical formula, e.g. fructose and glucose are both $C_6H_{12}O_6$)
synthase	synthesis of molecule
carboxylase decarboxylase	addition of CO_2 removal of CO_2
dehydrogenase	oxidation–reduction reaction

Fig. 2.4 Enzymes and the types of reactions they catalyze.

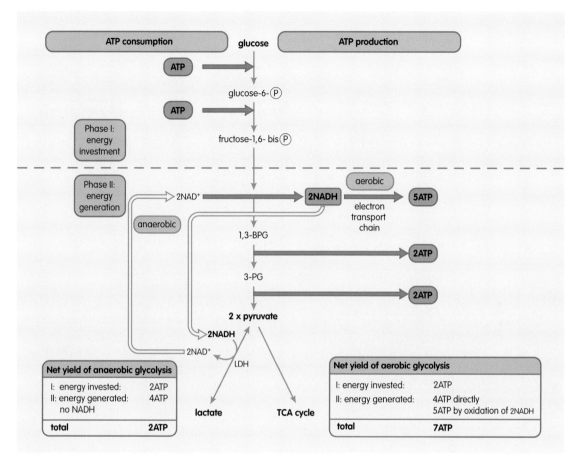

Fig. 2.5 ATP yield from aerobic and anaerobic glycolysis showing the two phases of energy investment and energy generation. (Refer to text for explanation of ATP yields.)

reaction in which the direction is determined by the ratio of NADH to NAD^+.

- Secondly, under aerobic conditions, NADH is oxidized to NAD^+ by the electron transport chain in mitochondria. NADH must first enter the mitochondria, either via the glycerol-3-phosphate shuttle or the malate–aspartate shuttle (Figs 2.6 and 2.7).
- Thirdly, under anaerobic conditions in yeast (alcoholic fermentation), pyruvate is decarboxylated to CO_2 and acetaldehyde, which is then reduced by NADH to yield NAD^+ and ethanol.

Relevance of a high concentration of lactate in the blood

If anaerobic glycolysis continues, lactate will accumulate. The concentration of lactate in the blood is normally about 1 mmol/L. A blood lactate concentration above this is called hyperlactatemia; increase in the lactate concentration (usually above 5 mmol/L) can cause lactic acidosis. During lactic acidosis the blood pH may decrease from the normal range (7.35–7.45). Mild lactic acidosis may be caused by intense exercise, such as sprinting, leading to increased lactate production and muscle cramps (this is covered later in Chapter 7). Severe lactic acidosis may be the result of tissue hypoxia, occurring, for example, because of circulatory collapse or shock, such as may happen after myocardial infarction or massive hemorrhage.

Functions of the malate–aspartate and glycerol-3-phosphate shuttles

NADH produced by glycolysis must enter the mitochondrial matrix before it can be oxidized by the

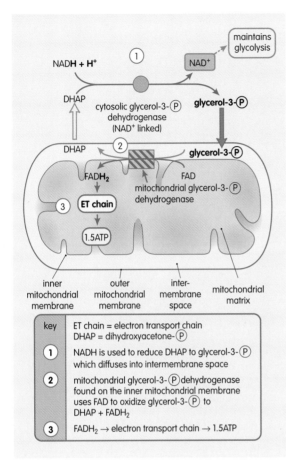

Fig. 2.6 The glycerol-3-phosphate shuttle, located mainly in brain and muscle cells.

The functions of the shuttles are therefore to:
- Transport electrons from NADH into mitochondria for ATP generation by the electron transport chain.
- Regenerate NAD to allow glycolysis to continue.

Main regulatory sites of glycolysis

Three reactions in glycolysis are essentially irreversible, namely steps 1, 3, and 10 (see Fig. 2.2). These constitute the main regulatory sites of glycolysis (ΔG is negative and exergonic for each reaction). The control of these steps and the enzymes catalyzing them are now discussed.

Step 1: Hexokinase (ΔG = −17 kJ/mol)
Hexokinase is controlled by product inhibition: high levels of glucose-6-phosphate allosterically inhibit it (see Fig. 2.11). Hexokinase is present in most cells and has a high affinity for glucose ($K_m = 0.1$ mM). The enzyme is therefore most active when the concentration of glucose in the blood is low or limiting; for example, following an overnight fast or in a muscle during exercise.

In the liver and beta cells of the pancreas, hexokinase is replaced by glucokinase, which has a lower affinity for glucose ($K_m = 10$ mM). Glucokinase is activated by high concentrations of glucose in the blood, and by insulin; therefore, it is active after a carbohydrate-rich meal. It is not inhibited by glucose-6-phosphate, which enables the liver to respond to high blood glucose levels. Therefore, dietary glucose goes to the liver to be dealt with by glucokinase before it enters the systemic circulation, preventing hyperglycemia (high blood glucose).

Step 3: Phosphofructokinase-1 (ΔG = −14 kJ/mol)
Phosphofructokinase-1 (PFK-1) is the most important regulatory enzyme because it catalyzes the rate-limiting step and is also the first reaction unique to glycolysis. It may be regulated in two ways:

Regulation of PFK-1 by energy levels
High ATP levels allosterically inhibit PFK-1 because they indicate an "energy-rich" cell; therefore, there is no need for further energy generation by glycolysis. Increased ATP level also lowers the affinity of PFK-1 for its substrate, fructose-6-phosphate.

Citrate enhances the inhibitory effect of ATP. This is because an increased citrate level indicates an abundance of products and metabolic intermediates

electron transport chain to make ATP. The inner mitochondrial membrane is impermeable to NADH and there is no carrier protein in the membrane to transport it across. Therefore, instead of transporting NADH itself across, its two "high energy" electrons are transported into mitochondria by shuttle mechanisms. In the glycerol-3-phosphate shuttle (located mainly in brain and muscle cells), electrons are transferred from NADH to FADH$_2$ (see Fig. 2.6). FADH$_2$, in turn, donates them to the electron transport chain to generate 1.5 ATP. In the malate–aspartate shuttle (located mainly in liver and heart cells), electrons of cytosolic NADH are transferred to mitochondrial NADH (see Fig. 2.7). They are then transferred to the electron transport chain to make about 2.5 moles of ATP.

Fig. 2.7 The malate–aspartate shuttle is located mainly in liver and heart cells. N.B. The outer mitochondrial membrane is not shown.

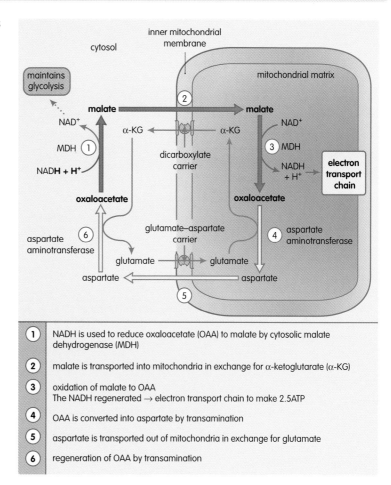

1	NADH is used to reduce oxaloacetate (OAA) to malate by cytosolic malate dehydrogenase (MDH)
2	malate is transported into mitochondria in exchange for α-ketoglutarate (α-KG)
3	oxidation of malate to OAA The NADH regenerated → electron transport chain to make 2.5ATP
4	OAA is converted into aspartate by transamination
5	aspartate is transported out of mitochondria in exchange for glutamate
6	regeneration of OAA by transamination

(e.g., pyruvate, acetyl CoA and oxaloacetate) and therefore there is no need to break down more glucose.

Increased levels of adenosine monophosphate (AMP) allosterically activate PFK-1 because they signal that energy stores are depleted.

Regulation of PFK-1 by fructose 2,6-bisphosphate

Fructose 2,6-bisphosphate (F2,6-BP) is formed by the phosphorylation of fructose-6-phosphate catalysed by phosphofructokinase-2 (PFK-2). It is converted back again by fructose 2,6-bisphosphatase (Figs. 2.8 and 2.9).

The properties and actions of F2,6-BP are:

- It is the most potent allosteric activator of PFK-1 and glycolysis (see Fig. 2.8).
- Specifically it increases the affinity of PFK-1 for its substrate, fructose-6-phosphate and it relieves inhibition of PFK-1 by ATP.
- In the liver, it inhibits fructose 1,6-

bisphosphatase, an enzyme of gluconeogenesis (the pathway responsible for making glucose which is unique to the liver; see Fig. 5.17).

Therefore, the reciprocal action of F2,6-BP ensures that the glycolytic (glucose breakdown) and gluconeogenic (glucose forming) pathways are not active at the same time (see Fig. 2.8).

Regulation of fructose 2,6-bisphosphate

Since F2,6-BP is such an important allosteric activator of glycolysis, its concentration must be carefully regulated. Its concentration is controlled by hormone-dependent reversible phosphorylation of PFK-2 and fructose 2,6-bisphosphatase, the enzymes responsible for its synthesis and breakdown (see Fig. 2.9).

In the liver, an increase in the ratio of insulin to glucagon (e.g., following a meal) leads to dephosphorylation and activation of PFK-2. This results in an increase in the synthesis of F2,6-BP and

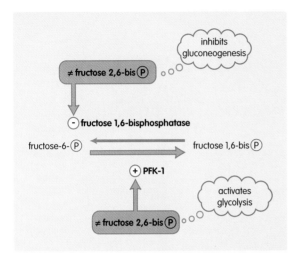

Fig. 2.8 Activation of phosphofructokinase-1 (PFK-1) and glycolysis by fructose 2,6-bisphosphate.

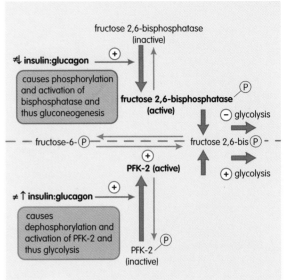

Fig. 2.9 Control of fructose 2,6-bisphosphate production by hormone-dependent reversible phosphorylation of phosphofructokinase-2 (PFK-2) and fructose 2,6-bisphosphatase.

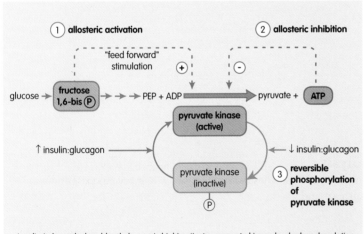

• insulin (released when blood glucose is high) activates pyruvate kinase by dephosphorylation
• glucagon (present when blood glucose is low) inactivates pyruvate kinase by phosphorylation

Fig. 2.10 Pyruvate kinase is regulated by allosteric activation and inhibition and also by hormone-dependent reversible phosphorylation of the enzyme.

thus in the rate of glycolysis. A decrease in the ratio of insulin to glucagon, such as occurs during starvation, leads to phosphorylation and activation of fructose 2,6-bisphosphatase. This decreases the amount of F2,6-BP and the rate of glycolysis.

Step 10: Pyruvate kinase ($\Delta G = -31\,kJ/mol$)

Pyruvate kinase catalyzes the final step of glycolysis and is subject to both allosteric regulation and hormone-dependent reversible phosphorylation. Fig 2.10 illustrates the regulation of pyruvate kinase.

Pyruvate kinase deficiency

This is a rare, autosomal recessive disorder. In homozygotes, pyruvate kinase activity in RBCs is about 5–20% of normal. Because RBCs lack mitochondria, they rely on glycolysis for ATP production. ATP is necessary for the maintenance of RBC membrane flexibility and shape, enabling their passage through small vessels. The RBC also maintains osmotic equilibrium via ATP-dependent pumps in its membrane. Pyruvate kinase deficiency is the most common glycolytic enzyme defect and causes a chronic hemolytic anemia.

Pathogenesis   In pyruvate kinase deficiency the rate of glycolysis and production of ATP is inadequate to maintain the energy requirements of the cell and the membrane structure. Alteration in cell shape creates distorted "prickle-shaped" cells, which are rigid and more sensitive to phagocytosis by cells of the reticuloendothelial system, mostly macrophages. Therefore, RBCs have a shorter life span, leading to increased hemolysis. Inhibition of pyruvate kinase leads to an accumulation of earlier glycolytic intermediates, especially 2,3-bisphosphoglycerate (2,3-BPG). 2,3-BPG decreases the affinity of hemoglobin for oxygen, allowing greater unloading of oxygen to the tissues, which therefore decreases the severity of the hypoxia. A diagnosis is based on:

- Presence of anemia.
- Blood film showing prickle cells and an increased number of reticulocytes (red cell precursors).
- Pyruvate kinase activity.

Hormonal regulation of glycolysis

Insulin, released after the consumption of a carbohydrate-rich meal, increases the synthesis and thus the amount of the enzymes glucokinase, PFK-1 and pyruvate kinase; this is known as induction. The increased synthesis of all three enzymes leads overall to an increase in the rate of glycolysis. When glucagon levels are high (e.g., in starvation or diabetes), there is a decrease in the synthesis of these enzymes (repression) and therefore a decrease in the rate of glycolysis.

The overall regulation of glycolysis is mapped out in Fig. 2.11.

The branch points of glycolysis, that is where it leads into other pathways, are shown in Fig. 2.12. This figure also illustrates how a number of glycolytic

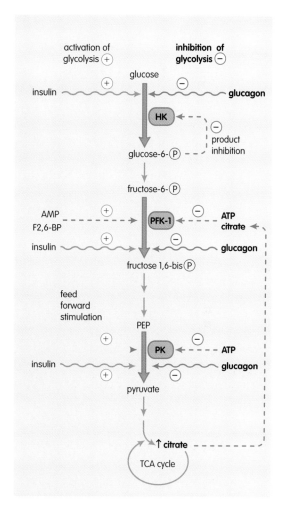

Fig. 2.11 Overall regulation of glycolysis. Remember, although this looks very complicated, the regulation of glycolysis can be divided into the allosteric control and the hormonal control. Refer to Chapter 1 for a summary of the mechanisms of control if necessary (F2,6-BP, fructose 2,6-bisphosphate; HK, hexokinase; PFK-1, phosphofructokinase-1; PK, pyruvate kinase).

intermediates serve as "entry points" for other sugars or substrates into glycolysis.

Central role of acetyl CoA

Structure of acetyl CoA

Acetyl CoA (Fig. 2.13) is formed from coenzyme A (abbreviated to CoA or CoASH). CoA is a large organic compound containing:

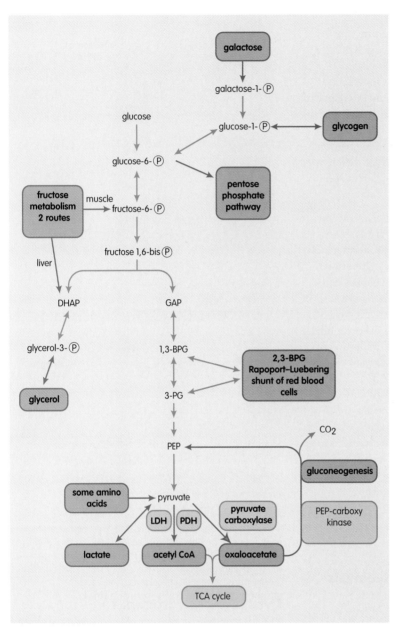

Fig. 2.12 The branch points of glycolysis, which lead off to many other pathways. All these pathways are covered later in the book (LDH, lactate dehydrogenase; PDH, pyruvate dehydrogenase; GAP, glyceraldehyde phosphate; PEP, phosphoenol pyruvate; 1,3-BPG, 1,3-bisphosphoglycerate; 3-PG, 3-phosphoglycerate.)

- An adenine group.
- A ribose sugar.
- Pantothenic acid (a B vitamin).
- A sulphydryl or thiol group (–SH), the active group.

The thiol group (–SH) of CoA reacts with carboxyl groups (–COOH) to form acyl CoA molecules. If the carboxyl group is an acetyl group (CH_3COO^-), acetyl CoA will be formed.

Acetyl CoA is a high-energy compound, which enables it to serve as a donor of acetyl groups; for example, in fatty acid synthesis and the TCA cycle. It is a carrier of acetyl groups just as ATP is a carrier of phosphate groups.

Fig. 2.13 The structure of acetyl CoA. Acetyl CoA is made by the formation of a high-energy thioester bond between the thiol group of CoA and the —COOH group of acetic acid.

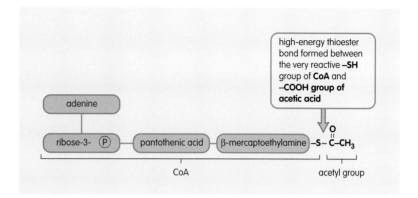

Formation of acetyl CoA from pyruvate
Working definition
Pyruvate dehydrogenase (PDH) catalyzes the irreversible, oxidative decarboxylation of pyruvate to acetyl CoA.

Location
Mitochondrial matrix.

Significance
The formation of acetyl CoA is completely irreversible; $\Delta G = -33.4\,kJ/mol$. Therefore, pyruvate cannot be formed from acetyl CoA; that is, carbohydrates can be converted to fats but not vice versa. This reaction is a key point in metabolism because it means there can be no net synthesis of glucose from fatty acids (Fig. 2.15).

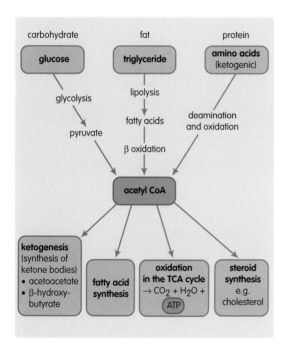

Fig. 2.14 The central role that acetyl CoA plays in metabolism. The main pathways that produce and utilize acetyl CoA.

Role of acetyl CoA in metabolism
Acetyl CoA plays a central role in metabolism. In fact, most energy-generating metabolic pathways of the cell eventually produce it. It can be formed from carbohydrate, fat, and protein. It is also the starting point for the synthesis of fats, steroids, and ketone bodies. Its oxidation provides energy for many tissues (Fig. 2.14).

Pyruvate dehydrogenase
PDH is a multi-enzyme complex consisting of three enzymes E1, E2, and E3. A multi-enzyme complex is a group of enzymes that catalyze two or more sequential steps in a metabolic pathway. As the enzymes are physically associated, the reactions occur in sequence without the release of intermediates; this minimizes side reactions. PDH requires the presence of five coenzymes (Fig. 2.16).

The mechanism of action of PDH is a complex, five-step pathway, and it is not necessary to know it in detail. Basically, pyruvate is decarboxylated, and then an acetyl group is transferred first to lipoate and

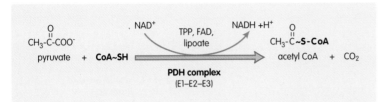

Components of the pyruvate dehydrogenase complex		
Enzyme	Name of enzyme	Coenzymes
E1	pyruvate decarboxylase	TPP
E2	dihydrolipoyl transacetylase	lipoic acid CoA
E3	dihydrolipoyl dehydrogenase	FAD NAD$^+$

Fig. 2.16 Components of the pyruvate dehydrogenase (PDH) complex.

then to CoA to form acetyl CoA. Thiamine pyrophosphate (TPP) and CoA are involved in the transfer of the two-carbon acetyl group. NAD$^+$, FAD, and lipoic acid are involved in the oxidation–reduction reactions. The NADH formed can be oxidized by the electron transport chain to generate 2.5 moles of ATP.

The control of pyruvate dehydrogenase

PDH is controlled by two mechanisms: allosteric control and reversible phosphorylation (see Fig. 2.17).

1. Allosteric control—product inhibition

NADH and acetyl CoA compete with NAD$^+$ and CoA for binding sites on the enzymes. NADH specifically inhibits E3, and acetyl CoA specifically inhibits E2.

2. Regulation by reversible phosphorylation of PDH

The PDH complex can exist in two forms: an active nonphosphorylated form and an inactive phosphorylated form (see Fig. 2.17). Associated with the PDH complex are two enzymes, PDH kinase and PDH phosphatase, which have important regulatory roles.

PDH kinase catalyzes the phosphorylation and thus inactivation of PDH. PDH kinase is activated by the products NADH and acetyl CoA, resulting in inactivation of PDH; this is in addition to their direct, allosteric effect on the PDH complex. PDH kinase is also activated by an increase in the ATP to ADP ratio, since this signifies an energy-rich cell and thus a decreased need for energy production by the TCA cycle.

PDH phosphatase dephosphorylates and thus activates PDH. It is activated by insulin and Ca^{2+}, which lead to an increase in the formation of acetyl CoA.

Deficiency of thiamin

A dietary deficiency of thiamin (vitamin B$_1$) leads to a deficiency of the coenzyme thiamine pyrophosphate. This results in a decrease in the activity of PDH and an accumulation of pyruvate. The excess pyruvate is converted into lactate, which may build up in the blood, leading to lactic acidosis. Vitamin B$_1$ deficiency can lead to:

• Beriberi, a neurological and cardiovascular disorder.
• Wernicke's syndrome, which is seen in nutritionally deprived alcoholics, and also in people with poor diet who are thiamin deficient. It may progress to Korsakoff's psychosis, which is an irreversible amnesic syndrome characterized by impairment of short-term memory (this is discussed further in Chapter 8).

Inherited PDH deficiency is very rare and presents with a similar lactic acidosis. The build-up of lactate may lead to severe neurologic defects.

Fig. 2.17 The control of PDH complex by product inhibition and reversible phosphorylation (numbers refer to the text above).

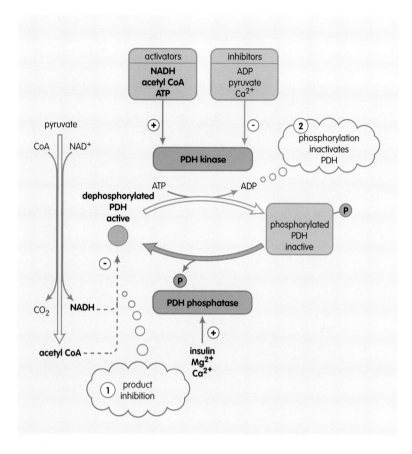

Working definition

A cyclical series of eight reactions that oxidize one molecule of acetyl CoA completely to two molecules of CO_2, generating energy, either directly as ATP or in the form of reducing equivalents (NADH or $FADH_2$). The cycle is aerobic; the absence or a deficiency of oxygen leads to total or partial inhibition of the cycle.

Location

All mammalian cells that contain mitochondria (i.e., not red blood cells).

Site

All the enzymes are found free in the mitochondrial matrix, except succinate dehydrogenase, which is found on the inner face of the inner mitochondrial membrane.

Functions

- The TCA cycle provides a final common pathway for the oxidation of carbohydrate, fat,

You should know thoroughly the role of acetyl CoA in metabolism because it is a common essay question. Be able to discuss briefly the pathways that produce and utilize acetyl CoA (see Fig. 2.14) and the conditions under which they are particularly active. For example, ketogenesis is active at low levels most of the time, but during prolonged starvation it becomes very important!

The tricarboxylic acid cycle

The tricarboxylic acid (TCA) cycle is also known as the citric acid cycle or the Krebs cycle.

and protein, since glucose, fatty acids, and many amino acids are all metabolized to acetyl CoA or to other intermediates of the cycle (see Fig. 2.23).

- The main function of the cycle is the production of energy, either directly as ATP or as the reducing equivalents NADH or $FADH_2$, which are oxidized by the electron transport chain. Each turn of the cycle produces 10 molecules of ATP; it is therefore the main pathway for energy generation in mammals.
- The cycle provides substrates for the electron transport chain.
- The cycle is also a source of biosynthetic precursors. For example, porphyrin is synthesized from succinyl CoA, and amino acids are synthesized from oxaloacetate and α-ketoglutarate.
- Some of the cycle intermediates also exert regulatory effects on other pathways; for example, citrate inhibits PFK-1 in glycolysis.

In summary, the cycle occupies a pivotal role in metabolism and is considered to be an amphibolic pathway; that is, it operates both catabolically (oxidation of substrates) and anabolically (synthetic reactions).

Stages of the TCA cycle

The cycle can be subdivided into three stages based on the role oxaloacetate plays as a carrier of acetyl CoA (Figs 2.18 and 2.19).

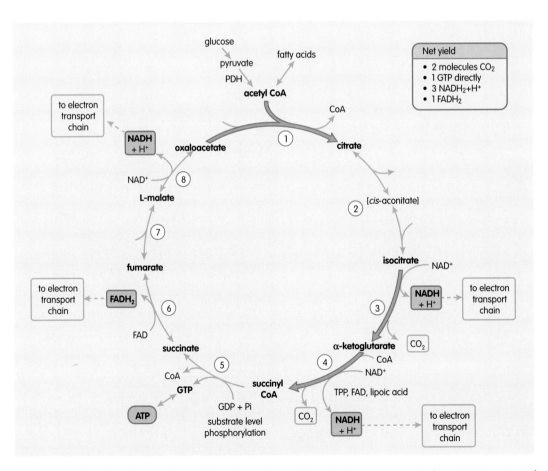

Fig. 2.18 The tricarboxylic acid cycle. Steps 1, 3, and 4 are irreversible, rate-limiting steps. Numbers 1 to 8 correspond to Fig. 2.19 (PDH, pyruvate dehydrogenase).

The stages of the TCA cycle	
Types of reaction	**Enzyme**
stage I: 1. condensation: 2C + 4C = 6C	citrate synthase
stage II: 2. isomerization: two steps: dehydration then rehydration	aconitase
3. oxidative decarboxylation: 6C → 5C	isocitrate dehydrogenase
4. oxidative decarboxylation: 5C → 4C	α-ketoglutarate dehydrogenase complex requires coenzymes TPP, FAD, lipoic acid, NAD⁺, and CoA (like PDH)
5. substrate-level phosphorylation	succinyl CoA synthetase nucleoside diphosphate kinase catalyzes GTP → ATP
stage III: 6. oxidation 7. hydration 8. oxidation	succinate dehydrogenase fumarase malate dehydrogenase

Fig. 2.19 The stages of the tricarboxylic acid (TCA) cycle (numbers 1–8 refer to Fig. 2.18).

- Stage I: the attachment of acetyl CoA to the oxaloacetate carrier (reaction 1).
- Stage II: the break-up of the carrier (reactions 2 to 5).
- Stage III: the regeneration of the carrier (reactions 6 to 8).

It is important to know that:
- Steps 1, 3, and 4 are irreversible rate-limiting steps.
- The last three steps of the TCA cycle, which convert succinate to oxaloacetate, involve a characteristic sequence of reactions—oxidation, hydration and oxidation—also found in the β-oxidation of fatty acids. The reverse of this is found in fatty acid synthesis, so be aware of it.
- In reaction 6, FAD is the electron acceptor because the reducing power of succinate is not sufficient to reduce NAD. FAD is covalently bound to succinate dehydrogenase.

Energetics and yield of the TCA cycle

The overall reaction may be written as:

$$\text{Acetyl CoA} + 3\text{NAD} + \text{FAD} + \text{GDP} + \text{Pi} + 2\text{H}_2\text{O}$$
$$\rightarrow \text{CoA} + 2\text{CO}_2 + 3\text{NADH} + \text{FADH}_2 + \text{GTP} + 3\text{H}^+$$

To learn the intermediates of the TCA cycle, it is best to use a mnemonic: A Certificate In Kama Sutra Should Further My Orgasm!

Two carbon atoms enter the cycle as acetyl CoA and two carbon atoms leave it as CO_2 (but they are not the same carbon atoms). There is no net consumption or production of oxaloacetate or any other intermediates of the cycle.

One molecule of ATP is generated directly by substrate-level phosphorylation, reaction 5, from guanosine triphosphate (GTP). Three molecules of NADH and one of $FADH_2$ are produced for each molecule of acetyl CoA oxidized by the cycle (reactions 3, 4, 6, and 8). They are then oxidized by the electron transport chain on the inner mitochondrial membrane, generating ATP by oxidative phosphorylation. Remember, the oxidation of NADH by the electron transport chain yields 2.5 ATP and the oxidation of $FADH_2$ yields 1.5 ATP, since it joins the chain further down, bypassing the first oxidative phosphorylation site (see Fig. 2.26).

Therefore, the ATP yield for each molecule of acetyl CoA oxidized (i.e., per turn of cycle) is:
- 1 ATP directly by substrate-level phosphorylation.
- 9 ATP indirectly by the oxidative phosphorylation of three NADH (3×2.5 ATP) and one $FADH_2$ (1×1.5 ATP) by the electron transport chain; giving a total of 10 ATP.

Fig. 2.20 illustrates the ATP yield from the oxidation of one molecule of glucose under aerobic and anaerobic conditions. Under aerobic conditions, the total yield depends upon the shuttle mechanism employed to transport the NADH generated during glycolysis into the mitochondria (see Figs 2.6 and 2.7). Therefore oxidation of 1 molecule of glucose produces:

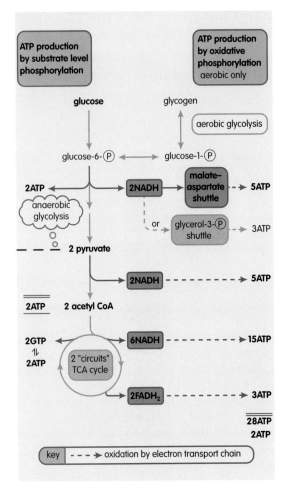

Fig. 2.20 The ATP yield from the oxidation of one molecule of glucose under aerobic and anaerobic conditions. Interestingly, the oxidation of one molecule of glycogen "saves" an ATP molecule. The extra ATP comes from the fact glycogen is broken down into glucose-1-phosphate, bypassing the need for the first phosphorylation step of glycolysis.

- Under anaerobic conditions: 2 ATP.
- Under aerobic conditions: approximately 32 ATP if the malate–aspartate shuttle is used or 30 ATP if the glycerol-3-phosphate shuttle is used.

Oxidation of 1 molecule of glycogen produces per glucose unit:
- Under anaerobic conditions: 3 ATP.
- Under aerobic conditions: 33 ATP if the malate–aspartate shuttle is used and 31 ATP if the glycerol-3-phosphate shuttle is used.

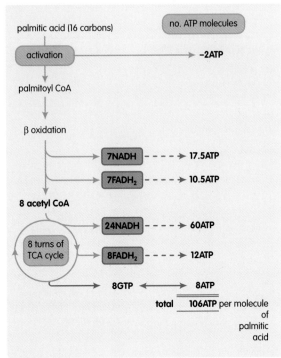

Fig. 2.21 The ATP yield from the oxidation of palmitic acid to acetyl CoA.

Fig. 2.21 shows the ATP yield from the oxidation of a fatty acid: it is easy to see that oxidation of a fatty acid yields far more energy than does glucose.

Please note that the exact ATP yields for these processes are still a matter of debate amongst biochemists. However, it is not so much the exact values that are important but rather the concepts involved.

Regulation of the TCA cycle

The TCA cycle is a central pathway of metabolism; it oxidizes acetyl CoA derived from carbohydrate, fat, and protein and provides substrates for a number of synthetic reactions. Its regulation must therefore be coordinated to satisfy the demands of other pathways in a number of tissues. PDH (see Fig. 2.15) determines whether or not pyruvate enters the TCA cycle; that is, it "guards the door" to the cycle.

The control of the cycle itself can be considered at two levels; allosteric regulation and respiratory control.

Regulation at the level of the cycle: allosteric regulation of enzyme activities

There are three key enzymes, all of which catalyze irreversible reactions:

- Citrate synthase.
- Isocitrate dehydrogenase.
- α-Ketoglutarate dehydrogenase.

All three enzymes are activated by Ca^{2+}. The levels of Ca^{2+} are increased, for example, during muscular contraction, thus increasing the rate of the cycle and ATP generation to cope with the increased energy demand of the muscle. The enzymes are also regulated by the ATP and NADH requirements of the cell. An increase in ATP, NADH, or the concentration of products indicates a high energy status of the cell. Due to a reduced need for energy production, these conditions inhibit the TCA cycle (see Fig. 2.22).

Respiratory control

The overriding control of the TCA cycle is by respiratory control. This is governed by the activity of the electron transport chain (which oxidizes NADH and $FADH_2$) and the rate of oxidative phosphorylation (ATP synthesis).

How does this occur?

- The activity of the TCA cycle is dependent on a continuous supply of NAD^+ and FAD, cofactors for the dehydrogenases.
- The electron transport chain is responsible for oxidizing any NADH and $FADH_2$ formed during glycolysis and the TCA cycle back to their oxidized forms, i.e., NAD^+ and FAD.
- As the activity of the electron transport chain is tightly coupled to the generation of ATP by oxidative phosphorylation (see Fig. 2.26), the TCA cycle is also dependent on the ADP:ATP ratio.

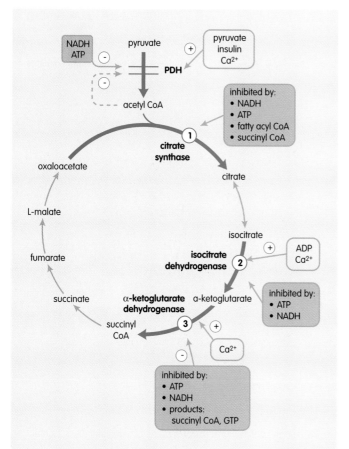

Fig. 2.22 Regulation of the tricarboxylic acid (TCA) cycle. The three rate-limiting reactions (numbered) of the TCA cycle are all inhibited by ATP and NADH.

- Therefore, anything affecting the supply of substrates, namely oxygen, ADP, or the source of reducing equivalents (NAD+ or FAD), may inhibit the cycle.

The TCA cycle is a source of intermediates for biosynthesis

The TCA cycle, as well as being a degradative pathway for the generation of ATP, has most of its intermediates as substrates for biosynthetic pathways (remember: an amphibolic pathway). The main synthetic pathways that use TCA cycle intermediates are:

- Lipid synthesis: both fatty acids and cholesterol are made from acetyl CoA in the cytosol. Acetyl CoA formed in the mitochondria cannot cross the inner mitochondrial membrane but citrate can. Cytosolic acetyl CoA is recovered from the breakdown of citrate by ATP–citrate lyase (see Fig. 2.23).
- Amino acid synthesis: for example, aspartate from oxaloacetate and glutamate from α-ketoglutarate (see Chapter 5).

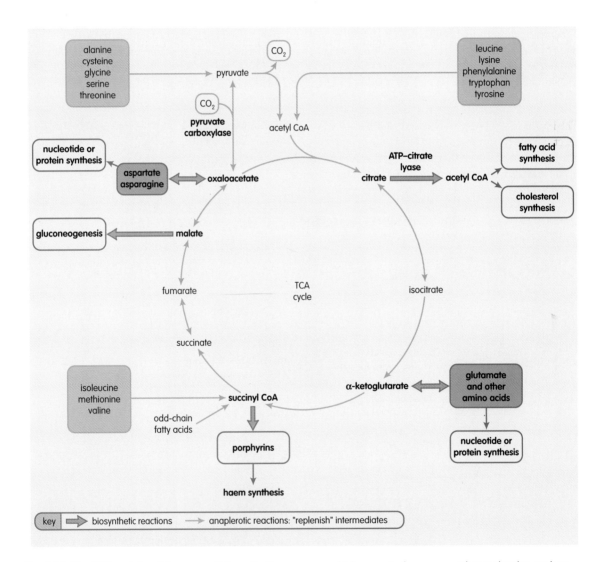

Fig. 2.23 The TCA cycle is a rich source of biosynthetic precursors which go on to form many other molecules, such as porphyrins, amino acids and fatty acids.

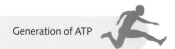

- Porphyrin biosynthesis: from succinyl CoA (see Chapter 6).
- Gluconeogenesis (glucose synthesis): this occurs in the cell cytosol from oxaloacetate.

However, oxaloacetate cannot cross the inner mitochondrial membrane but malate can. Malate is reconverted to oxaloacetate in the cytosol (see Fig. 5.17).

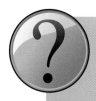

Remember the principle of respiratory control says that:

The rate of oxidative phosphorylation is proportional to $\dfrac{[ADP][Pi]}{[ATP]}$

For example:

- A low concentration of ADP or phosphate (i.e., less substrate available) leads to a decrease in the rate of ATP formation. As electron transport and ATP synthesis are coupled, electron transport and thus NADH and $FADH_2$ oxidation will also decrease. Therefore, high ATP:ADP or NADH:NAD^+ inhibits the TCA cycle.
- Secondly, if the concentration of ADP increases, the production of ATP increases until it matches the rate of consumption by energy-requiring reactions such as muscle contraction or biosynthetic reactions.

The intermediates that are used for synthetic reactions must be replaced for the TCA cycle to be able to continue. For example, if oxaloacetate is used to make amino acids for protein synthesis, it must be reformed. The carboxylation of pyruvate by pyruvate carboxylase reforms the oxaloacetate:

$$\text{Pyruvate} + \text{ATP} + CO_2 + H_2O \leftrightarrow \text{oxaloacetate} + \text{ADP} + \text{Pi}$$

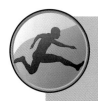

The role of the tricarboxylic acid (TCA) cycle as a source of biosynthetic precursors is a common essay question, so learn it well.

This is an example of an anaplerotic reaction, that is, it replenishes or fills up the intermediates of the cycle. Others include (see Fig. 2.23):

- The oxidation of odd-chain fatty acids to succinyl CoA.
- The breakdown of various amino acids.
- The transamination and deamination of amino acids to oxaloacetate and α-ketoglutarate.

Generation of ATP

ATP is the universal currency of energy in the cell

The body requires a continual supply of energy for its functions, such as:

- Muscle contraction.
- Biosynthesis of proteins, carbohydrates and fats.
- Active transport of molecules and ions across cell membranes.

The oxidation of metabolic fuels (protein, carbohydrate and fat) yields energy in the form of ATP. Adenosine triphosphate (Fig. 2.24) is a nucleotide containing:

- The purine base, adenine.
- A five-carbon sugar, ribose.
- Three phosphate units, forming a triphosphate.

ATP is an energy-rich molecule as it contains two phosphoanhydride bonds. When ATP is hydrolyzed to ADP, one of these bonds is broken, releasing a large amount of free energy:

$$\text{ATP} + H_2O \rightarrow \text{ADP} + \text{Pi}$$

$\Delta G = -30.66\,\text{kJ/mol}$ (i.e., a spontaneous, favorable reaction)

The energy liberated is used to drive metabolic reactions and other processes. For example, in

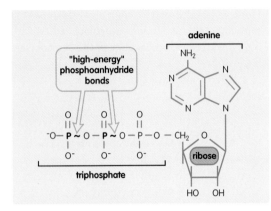

Fig. 2.24 The structure of adenosine triphosphate (ATP). ATP is made up of the purine adenine, the five-carbon sugar ribose, and three phosphate units linked by high-energy phosphoanhydride bonds.

Examples of substrate-level phosphorylation		
Example	Reaction	Enzyme
glycolysis	1,3-BPG + ADP ↔ 3-PG + ATP	phosphoglycerate kinase
	PEP + ADP → pyruvate + ATP	pyruvate kinase
TCA cycle	succinyl-CoA + GDP ↔ succinate + GTP	succinyl-CoA synthetase

Fig. 2.25 Examples of substrate-level phosphorylation.

glycolysis, the hydrolysis of ATP is coupled to the formation of high-energy phosphorylated intermediates such as 1,3-bisphosphoglycerate or phosphoenolpyruvate (see Fig. 2.2). ATP can also be hydrolyzed to AMP, releasing pyrophosphate (PPi), which undergoes further spontaneous hydrolysis to two molecules of inorganic phosphate ($2 \times$ Pi), therefore breaking both phosphoanhydride bonds.

Synthesis of ATP

ATP is synthesized from ADP by two processes: substrate-level phosphorylation and oxidative phosphorylation.

Substrate-level phosphorylation

Substrate-level phosphorylation is defined as the formation of ATP by direct phosphorylation of ADP. It occurs because some reactions have enough free energy to produce ATP directly from the metabolic pathway. The reaction does not require oxygen, making it important for generating ATP in tissues short of oxygen, for example, contracting skeletal muscle. Examples are found in glycolysis and the TCA cycle (Fig. 2.25).

Oxidative phosphorylation

Most ATP is generated by oxidative phosphorylation, which requires oxygen.

Definition

A process in which ATP is formed as electrons are transferred from NADH and FADH$_2$ to molecular oxygen via a series of electron carriers that make up the electron transport chain.

Location

The inner surface of the inner mitochondrial membrane in all cells that contain mitochondria.

Pyruvate from glycolysis, fatty acids via β-oxidation and some amino acids through transamination reactions provide acetyl CoA, which is oxidized by the TCA cycle to CO_2 and H_2O. During these processes high-energy electrons are donated from metabolic intermediates to the coenzymes NAD and FAD, to form the energy-rich reduced forms NADH and FADH$_2$. Therefore, energy is conserved as these reducing equivalents.

Origin of the reduced intermediates NADH and FADH$_2$

NADH is formed via glycolysis in the cytosol and via the TCA cycle and β-oxidation in mitochondria. FADH$_2$ comes from both the TCA cycle and β-oxidation in the mitochondria. NADH and FADH$_2$ donate their electrons, one at a time, to the electron transport chain. As each high-energy electron is passed down the chain, it loses most of its free energy. Part of this energy is captured and used to produce ATP from ADP and inorganic phosphate.

How does this occur?

- The transport of electrons down the electron transport chain is coupled to the transport of protons across the inner mitochondrial membrane, from the mitochondrial matrix into the inner mitochondrial space (Fig. 2.26).
- This occurs at three specific proton-pumping sites and thus creates an electrochemical gradient across the membrane.

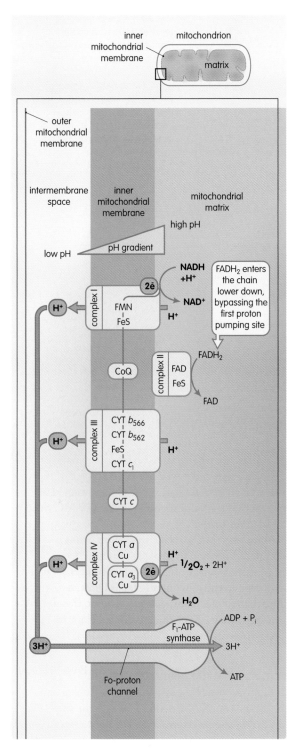

Fig. 2.26 An overview of oxidative phosphorylation, showing components of the electron transport chain (refer also to Fig. 2.27).

- The protons are only allowed back into the mitochondrial matrix via an enzyme, ATP synthase, present in the inner mitochondrial membrane.
- The movement of protons activates ATP synthase to catalyze ATP synthesis.
- Any energy not trapped as ATP is released as heat.

Therefore, the oxidation of NADH and $FADH_2$ by the electron transport chain is coupled to the generation of ATP (phosphorylation) by creating a proton gradient across the inner mitochondrial membrane (the electron transport chain is sometimes called the respiratory chain because it only works in the presence of oxygen).

The electron transport chain
Components of the electron transport chain
The chain consists of four protein complexes (see Fig. 2.26). These are integral membrane proteins present in the inner mitochondrial membrane, through which electrons pass (Fig. 2.27). The electron-carrying groups within these complexes are either flavins, iron–sulphur proteins, heme groups, or copper ions. The complexes are arranged in order of increasing standard redox potential (measured in volts) and increasing electron affinity.

The standard redox potential (E_o) is a measure of the tendency of a particular redox pair (e.g., NAD^+ and NADH or FAD and $FADH_2$) to lose electrons. The more negative the E_o value, the greater the tendency to lose electrons (i.e., lower electron affinity), whereas the more positive the E_o value, the more likely the redox pair is to accept electrons (higher electron affinity). Therefore, electrons flow from electron carriers with more negative E_o values to carriers with more positive E_o values, until they are passed to molecular oxygen, which has the highest E_o value.

The complexes are linked by two soluble membrane proteins: ubiquinone (coenzyme Q) and cytochrome c, which diffuse easily through the membrane.

The reactions within the chain
1. The oxidation of NADH or $FADH_2$ initiates electron transport down the chain.
2. Electrons of NADH are passed to complex I, whereas electrons of $FADH_2$ go directly to complex II. This is because $FADH_2$ is produced by succinate dehydrogenase, a TCA cycle enzyme,

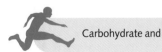
Components of the electron transport chain		
Electron carrier	**Components**	**Function**
complex I: NADH ubiquinone reductase	two types of redox proteins: • flavin mononucleotide (FMN) reduced by NADH → $FMNH_2$ • 1–5 iron–sulphur proteins (FeS) reduced by NADH → Fe^{3+}	enzyme catalyzes the oxidation of NADH **proton pumping site**
complex II: succinate ubiquinone reductase	TCA cycle enzyme succinate dehydrogenase FAD 1–3 iron–sulphur proteins	catalyzes the oxidation of $FADH_2$ by CoQ
CoQ (ubiquinone)	quinone derivative	shuttles electrons from complexes I and II to III
complex III: CoQ–cytochrome *c* reductase	*b* cytochromes (b_{562} and b_{566}) ubiquinol–cytochrome c_1 iron–sulphur proteins	catalyzes the oxidation of CoQ by cytochrome *c* **proton pumping site**
cytochrome *c*	cytochrome *c*	shuttles electrons between complexes III and IV
complex IV: cytochrome *c* oxidase	cytochromes *a* and a_3 two copper atoms	catalyzes the four-electron reduction of oxygen to H_2O **proton pumping site**

Fig. 2.27 Components of the electron transport chain. Complexes III, IV and cytochrome *c* are all cytochromes and contain a heme prosthetic group. The iron atom of the heme group is reversibly oxidized and reduced, that is, it alternates between Fe^{2+} and Fe^{3+} as part of its normal function as an electron carrier.

which is actually part of complex II (see Fig. 2.27).

3. Each component of the chain is alternately oxidized and reduced as electrons pass down the chain.

4. Finally, electrons are donated to molecular O2, reducing it to water.

Why use a chain of electron carriers instead of one reaction?

The oxidation of NADH leads to the pumping of protons at three sites across the membrane. When protons re-enter the matrix via ATP synthase, ATP is generated. Oxidation of NADH generates 2.5 molecules of ATP. If only a single reaction were employed, a lot of energy would be wasted, since there would be fewer proton pumping sites and thus less energy generation.

The oxidation of $FADH_2$ leads to the pumping of protons at only two sites across the membrane, bypassing the first site. This leads to only about 1.5 molecules of ATP being produced.

It is useful to note that until fairly recently it was thought that oxidation of NADH by the electron transport chain generated 3 ATP and oxidation of $FADH_2$ produced 2 ATP. However, recent studies on the ATP yield of oxidative phosphorylation have shown that the values are about 2.5 ATP for NADH and 1.5 for $FADH_2$. The reasons for the difference are complex, but basically the lower values compensate for additional protons used for phosphate transport into the mitochondrial matrix and the exchange of mitochondrial ATP for cytosolic ADP by ATP–ADP translocase.

The values 2.5 ATP for NADH and 1.5 for $FADH_2$ are used throughout this book.

Inhibitors of the respiratory chain

Inhibitors bind to a component of the chain and block the transfer of electrons at specific sites (Fig. 2.28). All the electron carriers of the chain before the block are reduced, whereas those after the block remain oxidized. As the electron transport chain and oxidative phosphorylation are tightly coupled, inhibition leads to a decrease in ATP synthesis.

Tetramethyl-*p*-phenyldiamine (TMPD) is an artificial electron donor: it transfers electrons

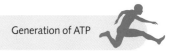

directly to cytochrome *c*. Vitamin C (ascorbate) is required to reduce TMPD, and they are both often used in combination to study the chain.

Generation of ATP via a proton gradient

The mechanism can be explained by the chemiosmotic or Mitchell's hypothesis. The flow of electrons down the electron transport chain does not lead directly to ATP synthesis. Instead, electron transport is coupled to pumping of protons across the inner mitochondrial membrane into the

Inhibitors of the electron transport chain	
Inhibitor	**Action**
rotenone and amytal	inhibit electron transfer within NADH dehydrogenase (complex I)
antimycin A	inhibits electron flow from reduced cytochrome b_{562} to cytochrome c_1 (complex III), therefore preventing proton pumping
cyanide, carbon monoxide, or azide	inhibit electron transfer in cytochrome oxidase (complex IV)
oligomycin and dicyclohexylcarbodiimide (DCCD)	block the proton channel part (Fo) of ATP synthase, decreasing ATP synthesis

Fig. 2.28 Inhibitors of the electron transport chain.

intermembrane space at complexes I, III and IV. Proton translocation creates an electrochemical gradient across the membrane (both electrical and pH components). Energy stored in this proton gradient is used to make ATP by ATP synthase.

Structure of ATP synthase

ATP synthase consists of two subunits (see Fig. 2.26): F_0, a proton channel, and F_1, the enzyme, ATP synthase. Protons re-enter the mitochondrial matrix normally only through the F_0 proton channel. The movement of these protons activates ATP synthesis by the F_1 subunit. A flow of approximately 3 protons through ATP synthase is required to make each ATP. Therefore, electron transport and phosphorylation are coupled by the proton gradient.

Uncoupling of the electron transport chain from phosphorylation

Any substance that increases the permeability of the inner mitochondrial membrane to protons, so that they can re-enter the mitochondrial matrix at sites other than ATP synthase, causes uncoupling. As a result the re-entry of protons dissipates the proton gradient without ATP production.

Uncouplers

2,4-Dinitrophenol (DNP) is a lipophilic (lipid-soluble) proton carrier that can diffuse freely across the inner mitochondrial membrane (see Fig. 2.29). It carries protons across the membrane, dissipating the proton gradient. This results in a decreased flow of protons through ATP synthase and thus decreased

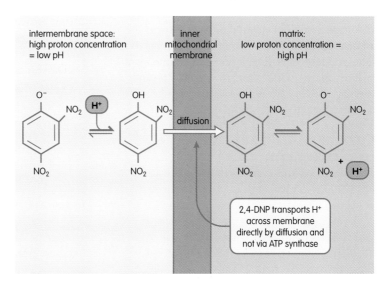

Fig. 2.29 The action of the uncoupler, 2,4-dinitrophenol (2,4-DNP) is to transport protons across the mitochondrial membrane without the production of ATP, dissipating the proton gradient.

Fig. 2.30 Comparison of the roles of liver and muscle glycogen.

Comparison of the roles of liver and muscle glycogen		
	Liver glycogen	Muscle glycogen
Main function	**maintenance of blood glucose concentration**, particularly between meals and early stages of fasting	**fuel reserve for muscle contraction**
Other roles	**used as a fuel by any tissue** liver contains glucose-6-phosphatase, which removes the phosphate group from glucose-6-phosphate, allowing glucose to leave the liver	none: **cannot leave muscle** muscle lacks glucose-6-phosphatase therefore glucose-6-phosphate cannot leave the cell; it enters glycolysis to generate energy instead
Size of stores	approximately 10% wet weight of liver; **stores last only about 12–24 h during a fast**	approximately 1–2% wet weight of muscle (however, humans have much more muscle than liver glycogen; and therefore about twice as much muscle glycogen as liver glycogen)
Hormonal control	glucagon and adrenaline promote glycogen breakdown insulin promotes synthesis	adrenaline promotes glycogen breakdown insulin promotes synthesis

ATP production (it short-circuits ATP synthase). Therefore, electron transport occurs normally but with no consequent ATP production. The energy produced by electron transport is released as heat. Another uncoupling agent is trifluorocarbonylcyanide methoxyphenylhydrazone (FCCP).

Uncoupling occurs physiologically in brown adipose tissue. Newborn babies and hibernating mammals contain brown fat, usually in their neck and upper back. The mitochondria of brown fat contain the uncoupling protein thermogenin in their inner mitochondrial membrane. This acts as a proton channel and allows the dissipation of the proton gradient and thus the release of energy as heat, enabling them to keep warm.

Control of ATP generation: respiratory control

The principle of respiratory control is discussed on pp. 22–23 and it would be useful to recap on this now.

A supply of ADP (substrate) is necessary for ATP synthesis; a low concentration of ADP will result in decreased production of ATP. Since electron transport and ATP synthesis are tightly coupled, electron transport and thus oxidation of NADH and $FADH_2$ will also be inhibited.

Glycogen metabolism

Role of glycogen

Excess dietary glucose is stored as glycogen. Glucose can be rapidly and easily mobilized from glycogen when the need arises; for example, between meals or during exercise. A constant supply of glucose is essential for life because it is the main fuel of the brain and the only energy source that can be used by cells lacking mitochondria or by contracting skeletal muscle (during anaerobic glycolysis). Glycogen is therefore an excellent short-term storage material that can provide energy immediately.

Glycogen stores

The main stores of glycogen are in muscle and in the liver, where they have different functions (Fig. 2.30). Remember that muscle glycogen cannot leave muscle and therefore cannot contribute to the concentration of glucose in the blood. Fig. 2.31 is a graph showing

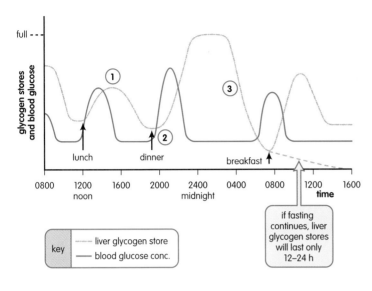

Fig. 2.31 A graph showing the approximate variation of liver glycogen stores and blood glucose against the time of day.
1. After a meal glycogen stores rise; between meals glycogen stores fall as glucose is released from liver glycogen to help maintain the concentration of glucose in the blood.
2. After a meal there is an increase in blood glucose; between meals it stabilizes.
3. Overnight glycogen stores are mobilized to help maintain blood glucose concentration.

the variation in liver glycogen stores and blood glucose plotted against the time of day.

Structure of glycogen
Glycogen is a large, highly branched polymer of glucose molecules. There are two types of linkages found between the glucose molecules (see Fig. 2.32A):
• Most are joined by an α-1,4 linkage to make straight chains.
• An α-1,6 linkage occurs every 8 to 12 glucose residues to make branch points.

Glycogen is present in the cytosol as granules (the diameter varies between 100 and 400Å). As well as glycogen, the granules contain the enzymes that catalyze glycogen synthesis and degradation, and also some of the enzymes that regulate these processes.

Why is it an advantage to have a branched structure?
A branched structure creates a large number of exposed, terminal glucose molecules (i.e., many ends) that are easily accessible to the enzymes of glycogen breakdown. This enables rapid degradation and glucose release when necessary (e.g., a "fight-or-flight" response). Branching therefore increases the rate of glycogen synthesis and degradation. It also increases the solubility of glycogen.

Glycogen synthesis: glycogenesis
Glycogen synthesis takes place in the cell cytosol. The process requires:
• Three enzymes: uridine diphosphate (UDP)-glucose pyrophosphorylase, glycogen synthase and the branching enzyme, amylo(1,4 → 1,6)transglycosylase.
• The glucose donor, UDP-glucose.
• A primer to initiate glycogen synthesis if there is no pre-existing glycogen molecule.
• Energy.

There are three stages to glycogenesis (Fig. 2.32B).

Stage I: Initiation—formation of glucose donor
UDP-glucose pyrophosphorylase catalyzes the synthesis of UDP-glucose (an activated form of glucose) from glucose-1-phosphate and UTP (see Fig. 2.32B). The reaction is reversible but is driven forward by the rapid hydrolysis of pyrophosphate by pyrophosphatase. In fact, many biosynthetic reactions are driven by the hydrolysis of pyrophosphate—remember DNA synthesis.

Stage II: Elongation of the glycogen chain
Glycogen synthase transfers glucose from UDP-glucose to the C4 position of an existing glycogen chain to form an α-1,4 glycosidic linkage. The

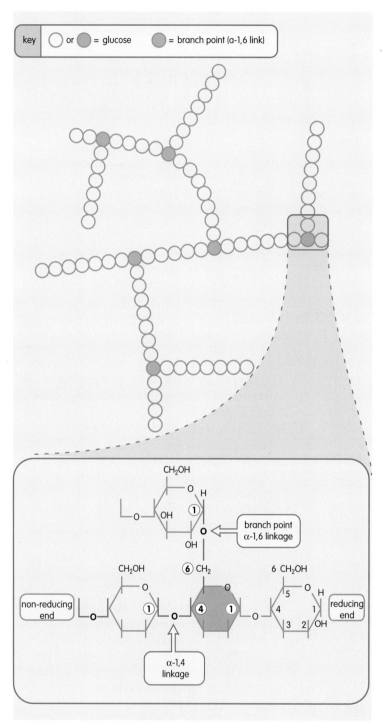

Fig. 2.32A The branched structure of glycogen, showing the two types of linkages found between glucose molecules. Most glucose molecules are joined by α-1,4 linkages to make straight chains. α-1,6 linkages occur about every 8–12 glucose residues and enable branch points to be formed. Numbers refer to the appropriate carbon atoms in the component glucose molecules.

Fig. 2.32B Glycogen synthesis consists of three stages, starting with the formation of UDP-glucose, which then takes part in the elongation of the glycogen molecule. When the growing glycogen chain is long enough, a polysaccharide of between five and eight units is broken off and transferred to a neighboring chain to form a branch chain.

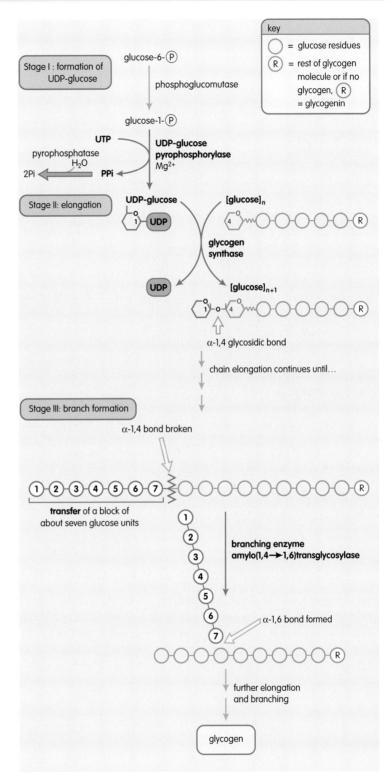

enzyme can only add glucose molecules to a chain already containing at least four glucose residues; that is, it cannot initiate chain synthesis: it requires a primer for this. The primer can either be a glycogen fragment or, in the absence of this, the protein glycogenin can be used.

Stage III: Formation of glycogen branches

Glycogen synthase only forms linear, straight-chain glycogen molecules. A specific branching enzyme called amylo$(1,4\rightarrow1,6)$transglycosylase is required to form branches. When the growing chain contains 11 or more residues, this enzyme transfers a number of them, usually seven, from the nonreducing end of the glycogen chain to a neighbouring chain, establishing a branch point. Therefore an α-1,4 link is broken, but an α-1,6 linkage is formed. The branching enzyme is very specific with regard to the length of chain it transfers (usually between five and eight residues). The new branch point must be at least four residues away from an existing branch.

Glycogen degradation: glycogenolysis

Glycogen degradation or, as it is otherwise known, glycogenolysis, takes place in the cell cytosol. There are two stages to glycogenolysis (Fig. 2.33).

Stage I: Shortening of the glycogen chain

Glycogen phosphorylase catalyzes the sequential removal of glucose residues from the non-reducing end of glycogen. The enzyme requires pyridoxal phosphate (PLP) as a cofactor. Phosphorylase cleaves the terminal α-1,4 glycosidic link to release glucose-1-phosphate. This process is known as phosphorolysis, which is similar to hydrolysis but uses phosphate instead of water to split the bond. The glucose-1-phosphate produced can be converted to glucose-6-phosphate by phosphoglucomutase, and can either enter glycolysis or, in the liver, is converted to glucose by glucose-6-phosphatase. Phosphorylase continues to degrade glycogen until it reaches a residue four molecules away from a branch point, where it stops.

Stage II: Removal of branches

This involves two enzymes: a transferase ([α-1,4$\rightarrow$ α-1,4] glucan transferase) that transfers the terminal three glucose residues (a trisaccharide) from one outer branch to another, "exposing" the α-1,6 branch point; and a debranching enzyme, amylo-α-1,6-glucosidase, which hydrolyzes the α-1,6 link to release free glucose. Together, the two enzymes convert the branched structure into a linear one. Glycogen phosphorylase can now continue until four units away from the next branch point.

A small amount of glycogen breakdown occurs in lysosomes via the enzyme α-1,4 glucosidase (maltase). Deficiency of this enzyme can lead to a fatal glycogen storage disorder, Pompe's disease (see Fig. 2.36).

Regulation of glycogen metabolism

The regulation of glycogen synthesis and degradation is very complex and not fully understood. Basically, it can be considered on two levels: hormonal regulation and allosteric control.

Hormonal regulation

Glycogen synthase and phosphorylase are regulated by hormone-dependent reversible phosphorylation. Glycogen phosphorylase exists in two forms:

- Phosphorylase a, the active, phosphorylated form.
- Phosphorylase b, the inactive, dephosphorylated form.

Adrenaline (in muscle and liver) and glucagon (liver only) stimulate glycogen breakdown. They activate cAMP-dependent protein kinase A which, via the reaction cascade shown in Fig. 2.34, causes the phosphorylation of glycogen phosphorylase, thereby activating this enzyme.

Glycogen synthase also exists in two forms:

- Glycogen synthase a, the active dephosphorylated form.
- Glycogen synthase b, the inactive phosphorylated form.

Adrenaline and glucagon are both catabolic hormones and therefore inhibit glycogen synthesis. Again, they activate the cAMP-dependent protein kinase A, which phosphorylates glycogen synthase, inactivating it (remember, the opposite happens to glycogen phosphorylase [i.e., it is activated], which ensures that both pathways are not active at the same time). Therefore, glycogen synthase and phosphorylase are reciprocally regulated.

Phosphorylation of both glycogen synthase and phosphorylase is reversed by protein phosphatase-1, which removes the phosphate groups by hydrolysis. The actions of adrenaline and glucagon in glycogen metabolism are shown in Fig. 2.34.

Fig. 2.33 Degradation of a glycogen molecule, showing the two stages necessary for its catabolism to monosaccharide units. Shortening of the glycogen chain releases glucose-1-phosphate, while hydrolysis of a branch point releases free glucose.

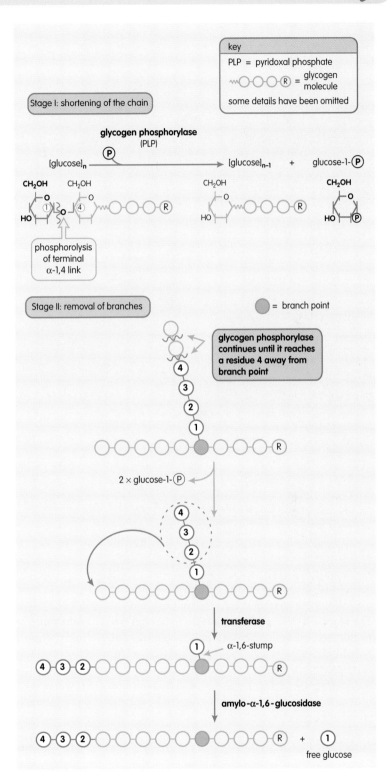

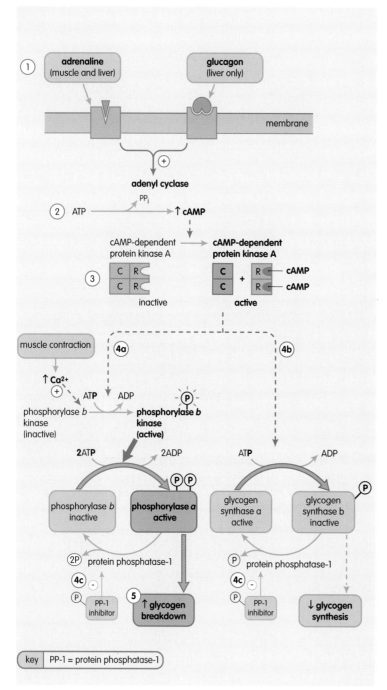

Fig. 2.34 The action of adrenaline and glucagon on glycogen metabolism. The mechanism of action is as follows:
1. The binding of adrenaline or glucagon activates adenyl cyclase via a G-protein-coupled pathway (not shown).
2. Adenyl cyclase catalyzes the formation of cAMP, which activates a cAMP-dependent protein kinase (protein kinase A).
3. This enzyme contains two regulatory (R) and two catalytic (C) subunits. cAMP binds to the regulatory subunits, allowing the active catalytic subunits to dissociate.
4. cAMP-dependent protein kinase catalyzes phosphorylation of:
    a. phosphorylase b kinase, activating it;
    b. glycogen synthase, inhibiting it;
    c. protein phosphatase-inhibitor-1, activating it, thus enabling it to inhibit protein phosphatase-1 (Ca^{2+} released by contracting muscle also helps activate phosphorylase b kinase).
5. Phosphorylation and activation of glycogen phosphorylase by phosphorylase b kinase activates glycogen breakdown.

The action of insulin

The exact mechanism of action of insulin remains unclear; however, it is an anabolic hormone and therefore stimulates glycogen synthesis and inhibits breakdown. How does this occur? Research suggests that the insulin receptor complex is activated by conformational changes and autophosphorylation of tyrosine residues in the cytoplasm. This activates tyrosine kinase within the cell and a series of further phosphorylations. One suggestion is that insulin then activates the enzyme phosphodiesterase, which catalyzes the breakdown of cAMP to AMP. A fall in cAMP levels leads to decreased activity of protein kinase A (the enzyme that normally inactivates glycogen synthase). This results in dephosphorylation of both glycogen phosphorylase (inactivating it) and glycogen synthase (activating it). There are also other proposed mechanisms for the action of insulin, but they are less well defined.

The mechanism of action of adrenaline and glucagon in glycogen metabolism shown in Fig. 2.34 is an example of an amplification pathway, in which the large number of steps involved amplifies the hormonal signal, allowing the rapid release of glucose. Only one or two molecules of hormone bind to their receptors, but they each cause the activation of a number of protein kinase molecules (100), which in turn activate many phosphorylase b kinase molecules (1000). This produces large numbers of active glycogen phosphorylase molecules (10,000) to degrade glycogen. If the binding of adrenaline directly activated glycogen phosphorylase it would require huge quantities of hormone for the same response.

Allosteric control
Liver glycogen phosphorylase
Glucose allosterically inhibits liver glycogen phosphorylase a. Phosphorylase a (phosphorylated, active form) contains two binding sites for glucose. The binding of glucose causes a conformational change; this exposes the phosphate groups, enabling their removal by protein phosphatase-1, thus converting it to phosphorylase b (the inactive form). Therefore, the product, glucose, inhibits glycogen breakdown. Glucose-6-phosphate also inhibits phosphorylase but activates glycogen synthase (Fig. 2.35).

Muscle glycogen phosphorylase
The main allosteric control is effected by 5′ AMP and Ca^{2+}. Calcium ions released during muscle contraction bind to calmodulin, a subunit of phosphorylase b kinase, activating it. For maximal activation, the enzyme also requires phosphorylation (see Fig. 2.34).

AMP is an indicator of the energy status of the cell. High levels of AMP signal a low energy status (i.e., low ATP), for example, during intense exercise. Therefore, AMP allosterically activates phosphorylase b; this increases glycogen breakdown in order to provide energy for muscle contraction.

Glycogen storage diseases
This group of inherited diseases is caused by a defect in an enzyme required for either glycogen synthesis or degradation; they are very rare. They are all inherited as autosomal recessive disorders, except for type VIII, which is sex-linked. The diseases either result in the production of an abnormal amount or an abnormal type of glycogen. The main glycogen storage diseases are summarized in Fig. 2.36.

Type I: von Gierke's disease
von Gierke's disease affects mainly the liver and the kidneys. It is caused by a deficiency of glucose-6-phosphatase, the gluconeogenic enzyme that catalyzes the hydrolysis of glucose-6-phosphate in the liver, releasing free glucose into the blood.

The deficiency leads to an increased concentration of glucose-6-phosphate in the liver

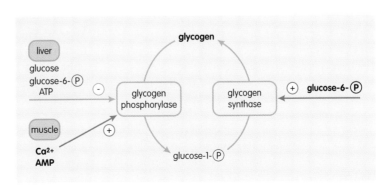

Fig. 2.35 Allosteric control of glycogen metabolism by glucose, glucose-6-phosphate, calcium ions, AMP and ATP.

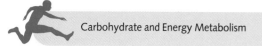
The main glycogen storage diseases				
Type	Name	Enzyme deficiency	Glycogen structure and amount	Tissues affected
I	von Gierke's disease	glucose-6-phosphatase	normal structure, ↑ amount	liver and kidney are loaded with glycogen; results in hypoglycemia since glucose cannot leave the liver
II	Pompe's disease	lysosomal a-1,4-glucosidase	normal structure, ↑↑↑ amount	accumulation of glycogen in lysosomes in all organs; prominent cardiomyopathy
III	Corl's disease	amylo-1,6-glucosidase (debranching enzyme)	outer chains missing or very short, ↑ amount	accumulation of branched polysaccharide in liver and muscle; like type I but milder
IV	Andersen's disease	branching enzyme	very long unbranched chains, normal amount	liver failure causes death in the first year of life
V	McArdle's disease	glycogen phosphorylase	normal structure, ↑ amount	muscle has abnormally high glycogen content (2.5–4.1%); diminished exercise tolerance
VI	Hers' disease	glycogen phosphorylase	normal structure, ↑ amount	↑ liver glycogen; tendency towards hypoglycemia
VII	Tarui's disease	phosphofructokinase	normal structure, ↑ amount	muscle as for type V

Fig. 2.36 The main glycogen storage diseases. They either result in the production of an abnormal amount or an abnormal type of glycogen.

and kidneys, which in turn results in an increased amount of normal glycogen stored. It also means that the liver is unable to release glucose between meals to regulate and maintain the blood glucose in response to glucagon, leading to a fasting hypoglycemia.

The main clinical features are liver enlargement, severe fasting hypoglycemia, failure to thrive, and ketosis as the body tries to use other fuels.

Type V: McArdle's syndrome

McArdle's syndrome affects muscle. It is a deficiency of muscle glycogen phosphorylase; the liver enzyme is normal. Therefore, the muscle has a high level of normal glycogen because it cannot break it down. During exercise, the decreased level of muscle phosphorylase means that glycogen stores cannot be used as fuel. Increased blood lactate is not seen after exercise because of insufficient glycolysis. Therefore, these patients have a decreased exercise tolerance:

they tire easily on intense exercise. Otherwise, they have a normal life span and development.

Role of 2,3-bisphosphoglycerate

The Rapoport–Luebering shunt
Location
In red blood cells (RBCs), glycolysis is modified by the Rapoport–Luebering shunt, otherwise known as the 2,3-bisphosphoglycerate (2,3-BPG) shunt.

Pathway
There are two steps in the shunt (Fig. 2.37):
1. Bisphosphoglycerate mutase converts 1,3-BPG into 2,3-BPG.
2. 2,3-BPG is hydrolyzed to 3-phosphoglycerate by 2,3-bisphosphoglycerate phosphatase.

ATP yield
Glycolysis is important to RBCs because it is their only energy source (they have no mitochondria and therefore must rely on anaerobic glycolysis).

However, the shunt bypasses the energy-generating reaction, meaning, therefore, that there is effectively no net production of ATP.

Regulation of the shunt
Both reactions of the shunt are nearly irreversible. 3-Phosphoglycerate stimulates bisphosphoglycerate mutase and therefore increases 2,3-BPG production. 2,3-BPG is a potent inhibitor of its own formation (i.e. negative feedback by the product).

Role of 2,3-BPG in hemoglobin function
Hemoglobin (Hb) is the oxygen-carrying protein found in RBCs. It has a high affinity for binding oxygen and therefore transports oxygen from the lungs to the tissues where it is needed. When Hb gets to the tissues, it has to release or "unload" the oxygen. A low pH (acid; high hydrogen ion concentration) or an increased CO_2 concentration in the tissue favors unloading, as both decrease the affinity of hemoglobin for oxygen; this is known as the Bohr effect.

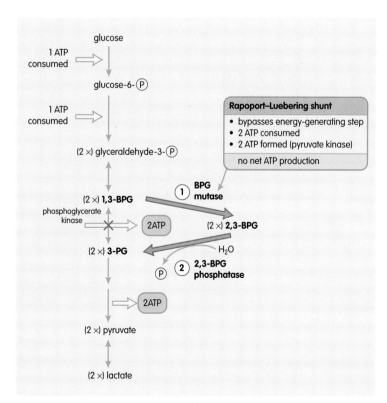

Fig. 2.37 The Rapoport–Luebering shunt in RBCs produces 2,3-bisphosphoglycerate (2,3-BPG) with no net energy production.

2,3-BPG present in high concentration in RBCs also helps unload oxygen from hemoglobin. Specifically, it is an allosteric effector that binds to and stabilizes deoxyhemoglobin, reducing its affinity for oxygen, therefore favoring the release of oxygen. 2,3-BPG fits in a "pocket" between the two β chains of hemoglobin, but only in the deoxygenated configuration. This pocket contains positively charged amino acids that form salt bridges with the negatively charged phosphate groups of 2,3-BPG, resulting in cross-linking of the β chains. 2,3-BPG cannot bind to oxyhemoglobin as the gap between the β chains is too small in the presence of oxygen. The reaction may be written as follows:

$$HbO_2 + 2,3\text{-}BPG \rightarrow Hb\text{-}2,3\text{-}BPG + O_2$$

Oxyhemoglobin   Deoxyhemoglobin

The oxygen is therefore released for use by the tissues.

Main physiologic effects of 2,3-BPG
Fetal hemoglobin
Fetal hemoglobin (HbF) contains two α chains and two γ chains ($\alpha_2\gamma_2$) and is the major type of hemoglobin found in the fetus and in the newborn. HbF has a lower affinity for 2,3-BPG than normal adult hemoglobin (HbA); therefore, it has a higher affinity for oxygen (i.e., holds on to its oxygen). Why? HbF only binds 2,3-BPG weakly as its two γ chains lack some of the positively charged amino acids found in the β chains of HbA. As 2,3-BPG reduces the affinity of hemoglobin for oxygen, the weak interaction between HbF and 2,3-BPG means that HbF has a higher oxygen affinity than normal HbA. This enables placental oxygen exchange from the mother's circulation to the fetus.

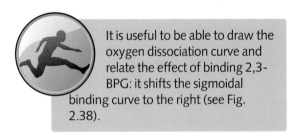

It is useful to be able to draw the oxygen dissociation curve and relate the effect of binding 2,3-BPG: it shifts the sigmoidal binding curve to the right (see Fig. 2.38).

Altitude acclimatization
The body responds to the chronic hypoxia observed at high altitude by increasing the concentration of 2,3-BPG in RBCs. This adaptation takes a few days. High levels of 2,3-BPG decrease the affinity of hemoglobin for oxygen, allowing greater unloading of oxygen to the tissues so that they receive enough oxygen, despite its decreased availability. On return to low altitude, the concentration of 2,3-BPG returns to normal quite quickly. Similarly, high concentrations of 2,3-BPG are observed in patients with chronic obstructive airways disease (COAD).

Clinical significance of 2,3-BPG
Blood transfusions
Storing blood in an acid–citrate–glucose medium leads to a decrease in the concentration of 2,3-BPG to low levels in about 1–2 weeks. The resulting blood has an abnormally high affinity for oxygen and, if given to a patient, it will not be able to unload oxygen to the tissues. The loss of 2,3-BPG can now be prevented by addition of substrates, e.g. inosine, to the storage medium. Inosine enters the RBC where it can be metabolized to 2,3-BPG by the pentose phosphate pathway (see Chapter 3).

Red cell glycolytic enzyme deficiencies
This group of inherited diseases occurs due to the deficiency of a glycolytic enzyme (e.g., hexokinase, phosphofructokinase, pyruvate kinase). The effect on both glycolysis and the concentration of 2,3-BPG depends on the site of the enzyme deficiency, i.e. either before or after the 2,3-BPG shunt, or a deficiency of one of the shunt enzymes. An abnormal concentration of 2,3-BPG affects the ability of the hemoglobin to transport and unload oxygen normally. Usually, this results in a hemolytic anemia due to the decreased rate of glycolysis and thus ATP production, leading to increased hemolysis of red cells (see Chapter 9).

Causes of a raised concentration of 2,3-BPG
The main causes are:
- Over the long-term, smoking is known to cause an increase in the concentration of 2,3-BPG. This partly compensates for a decreased oxygen supply caused by the exposure to carbon monoxide.
- Chronic anemia, which results in a decrease in the number of RBCs or the amount of hemoglobin, leading to decreased oxygen supply to the tissues. A compensatory increase in 2,3-BPG allows for greater unloading of oxygen to the tissues.
- Altitude acclimatization (see above).

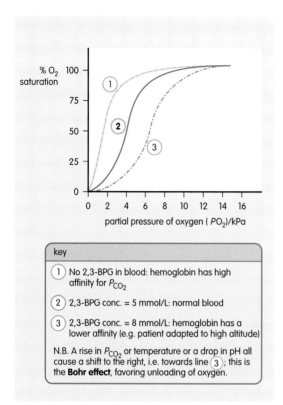

key

1. No 2,3-BPG in blood: hemoglobin has high affinity for P_{CO_2}

2. 2,3-BPG conc. = 5 mmol/L: normal blood

3. 2,3-BPG conc. = 8 mmol/L: hemoglobin has a lower affinity (e.g. patient adapted to high altitude)

N.B. A rise in P_{CO_2} or temperature or a drop in pH all cause a shift to the right, i.e. towards line (3); this is the **Bohr effect**, favoring unloading of oxygen.

Fig. 2.38 The effect of 2,3-BPG on hemoglobin is to decrease its affinity for oxygen, causing a shift to the right in the oxygen saturation curve.

Fructose, galactose, ethanol and sorbitol

Fructose metabolism

The main dietary source of fructose is the disaccharide sucrose, which is hydrolyzed by sucrase in the small intestine to fructose and glucose; fructose is also found in fruit and honey. Unlike glucose, fructose can enter cells without the help of insulin. There are two pathways for fructose metabolism, one in muscle, the other in liver, due to the presence of different enzymes in each tissue (see Fig. 2.39).

- In the liver, fructose is phosphorylated by the enzyme fructokinase to fructose-1-phosphate, which is then further metabolized to glyceraldehyde-3-phosphate to enter glycolysis or gluconeogenesis. Most dietary fructose is metabolized by the liver, such that little is left for metabolism by the muscle.

- In muscle, fructose is converted to fructose-6-phosphate by hexokinase to enter glycolysis after only one reaction.

Risks of excessive fructose ingestion

Fructose is metabolized rapidly compared with glucose. This is because it enters glycolysis as glyceraldehyde-3-phosphate, bypassing the rate-limiting step catalyzed by phosphofructokinase, the key control point of glycolysis (see Fig. 2.2). Also, fructose entry into cells is independent of insulin.

As the rate-limiting step of glycolysis is bypassed, if fructose ingestion becomes too high it can result in an unregulated accumulation of glycolytic intermediates. For example, fructose-1-phosphate may accumulate, which will deplete the liver stores of phosphate and thus limit ATP production. A decrease in the concentration of ATP further activates glycolysis, leading to the increased production of lactic acid. If this continues, it can lead to a potentially fatal lactic acidosis. For these reasons, intravenous fructose is no longer recommended for parenteral nutrition.

Errors of fructose metabolism

Errors of fructose metabolism are genetic (autosomal recessive) disorders that are due to a deficiency in one of the key enzymes involved in fructose metabolism; they are shown in Fig. 2.40.

Fructokinase deficiency: essential fructosuria

This is a benign, asymptomatic condition caused by an absence of fructokinase. All the fructose has to be metabolized by the hexokinase pathway, leading to a high concentration of fructose in the blood and fructose accumulation in the urine.

Fructose-1-phosphate aldolase deficiency: hereditary fructose intolerance

Fructose-1-phosphate aldolase (aldolase B) cleaves fructose-1-phosphate to dihydroxyacetone phosphate and glyceraldehyde, allowing the entry of fructose into glycolysis or gluconeogenesis (see Fig. 2.40). Deficiency leads to the accumulation of fructose-1-phosphate in the tissues, that is, phosphate is trapped in fructose-1-phosphate, leading to a decrease in available phosphate.

This leads to the inhibition of both glycogen phosphorylase (glycogenolysis) and aldolase A (glycolysis and gluconeogenesis) because they are normally activated by phosphorylation. This causes

41

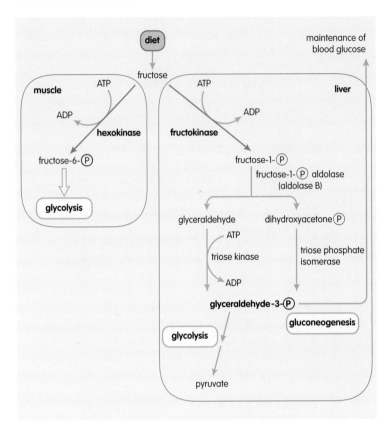

Fig. 2.39 The metabolism of fructose by liver and muscle cells leads to the production of intermediates that can then enter glycolysis.

the inhibition of glucose production, leading to hypoglycemia.

Clinically, fructose-1-phosphate aldolase deficiency presents as soon as a baby is weaned on to fructose-containing foods. Features include hypoglycemia, vomiting, and eventually liver failure. Treatment is by the removal of fructose and sucrose from the diet.

Galactose metabolism

The major dietary source of galactose is lactose in milk and milk products. Lactose is hydrolyzed in the small intestine by lactase to galactose and glucose. The entry of galactose into cells is independent of insulin.

Metabolism of galactose

The metabolism of galactose has four steps (Fig. 2.41):
1. Phosphorylation to galactose-1-phosphate by galactokinase.

2. Galactose-1-phosphate uridyl transferase catalyzes the transfer of the uridyl group of UDP-glucose to galactose-1-phosphate to make UDP-galactose and glucose-1-phosphate.
3. Glucose-1-phosphate can be converted to the glycolytic intermediate glucose-6-phosphate and thus enter glycolysis.
4. UDP-galactose is converted back to UDP-glucose by UDP-hexose-4-epimerase.

Galactosemia—an error of galactose metabolism

Galactosemia is a rare, autosomal recessive disorder, arising because of a deficiency in the enzyme galactose-1-phosphate uridyl transferase (see Fig. 2.41). Occasionally, it is caused by deficiency in galactokinase or UDP-hexose-4-epimerase. The formation of UDP-galactose is prevented, meaning that galactose cannot be converted into glucose-6-phosphate.

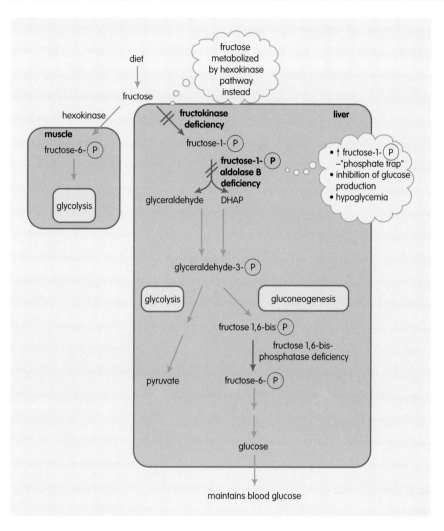

Fig. 2.40 Some errors of fructose metabolism.

The disease presents in neonates when lactose-containing milk feeds are introduced. As galactose cannot be converted into glucose, the babies become hypoglycemic. This results in galactosemia, galactosuria, and a build-up of toxic metabolic byproducts. This can lead to a high concentration of galactose in the lens of the eye, where it is reduced by aldose reductase to galactitol, which is thought to facilitate cataract formation. An accumulation of galactitol also occurs in nerve tissue, liver and kidneys, leading to liver damage and mental retardation.

The clinical features are poor feeding, vomiting, jaundice, hypoglycemia and hepatosplenomegaly. Eventually, liver failure, cataracts and severe mental retardation occur if the condition is left untreated. The treatment is a lactose- and galactose-free diet.

Catabolism of ethanol

In the liver, three enzyme systems exist for the catabolism of ethanol (Fig. 2.42):

1. Cytosolic alcohol dehydrogenase pathway, probably the main route for the oxidation of ethanol. The activity of this enzyme is largely governed by

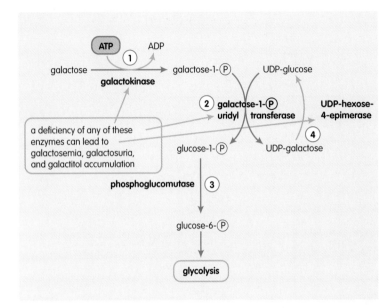

Fig. 2.41 The metabolism of galactose; a four-step pathway that converts galactose to glucose-6-phosphate. Glucose-6-phosphate then enters glycolysis (numbers refer to text.)

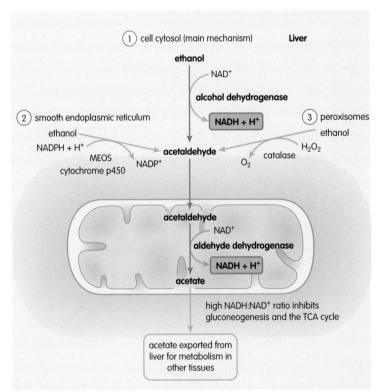

Fig. 2.42 The metabolism of ethanol. Three enzyme systems are responsible for the metabolism of ethanol in the liver: cytosolic alcohol dehydrogenase (main mechanism), microsomal ethanol oxidizing system (MEOS) in the smooth endoplasmic reticulum, and catalase in peroxisomes. The product, acetaldehyde, is then taken into the mitochondria for further metabolism to acetate (numbers refer to text.)

the availability of NAD⁺, which is required as a cofactor.

2. Microsomal ethanol oxidizing system (MEOS), which uses a cytochrome P450 enzyme system.
3. The peroxisome system, which uses the enzyme catalase.

The product of all three systems is acetaldehyde, which then enters mitochondria for further oxidation by aldehyde dehydrogenase to acetate. Certain ethnic groups, in particular the Chinese, are genetically deficient in aldehyde dehydrogenase and consequently have a lower alcohol tolerance.

Metabolic effects of ethanol

The fate of acetate depends on the ratio of NADH to NAD⁺. Both alcohol dehydrogenase and aldehyde dehydrogenase consume NAD⁺, contributing to a high NADH:NAD⁺, ratio resulting in:

- Inhibition of the TCA cycle. A high NADH:NAD⁺ ratio inhibits isocitrate dehydrogenase, α-ketoglutarate dehydrogenase and citrate synthase (see Fig. 2.22).
- Inhibition of gluconeogenesis. A high NADH:NAD⁺ ratio affects the dehydrogenase reactions, displacing the equilibrium in favor of the reduced compounds, such that oxaloacetate is converted to malate and pyruvate to lactate (see Fig. 5.17). Therefore, less pyruvate and oxaloacetate (substrates) are available for gluconeogenesis by the liver. Acetate is therefore exported out of the liver for metabolism by other tissues.

Clinical significance of excessive ethanol ingestion

High levels of alcohol can lead to hyperlactatemia (i.e., favors conversion of pyruvate to lactate, see above). Since both lactate and urate share the same mechanism for renal tubular secretion, the more lactate produced the more urate will be retained. Urate may crystallize out in the joints, especially in the toes, leading to gout.

Hypoglycemia can develop in malnourished or fasting individuals after a heavy drinking session. The inhibition of gluconeogenesis leads to this hypoglycemia; medical students beware!

Alcohol can induce the cytochrome P450 enzymes that are responsible for the metabolism of many drugs, for example, barbiturates. Therefore, for an alcoholic patient on medication, the metabolism and effects of the drugs may be altered.

Sorbitol metabolism (polyol pathway)
Synthesis

Sorbitol is a sugar alcohol that can be synthesized endogenously from glucose by a number of tissues, such as the lens and retina of the eye, the liver, kidney and Schwann cells (the cells of the peripheral nervous system that make myelin).

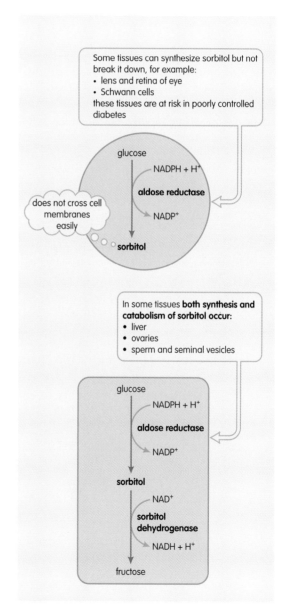

Fig. 2.43 The metabolism of sorbitol from glucose by aldose reductase. Some tissues contain sorbitol dehydrogenase, which oxidizes sorbitol to fructose.

Sorbitol synthesis requires the enzyme aldose reductase which reduces glucose to sorbitol.

Breakdown

Some tissues, especially the liver, also possess another enzyme, sorbitol dehydrogenase, which oxidizes sorbitol to fructose (see Fig. 2.43).

In the liver, this provides a way for dietary sorbitol to enter glycolysis or gluconeogenesis and be metabolized further (see Fig. 2.39).

This is also a useful pathway in sperm and in the seminal vesicles, where fructose is the preferred energy source.

Uses and complications of increased sorbitol

Sorbitol is used as a sweetener in many diabetic foods. It only has about one-half the sweetness of sucrose but, more importantly, it is safe because it is absorbed slowly from the intestine and also transported slowly across cell membranes. Therefore, at normal levels there is little chance of its accumulation.

Problems arise when the endogenous production of sorbitol increases. Since sorbitol does not cross cell membranes easily, it may remain trapped in the cells. Aldose reductase has a high K_m for glucose (about 60–70 mM). At normal blood glucose levels (3–5 mM) its activity is low, and the production of sorbitol is low. However, in poorly controlled diabetes, where blood glucose concentrations can reach sustained levels as high as 15–20 mM, there is an increased production of sorbitol, which may accumulate within cells. This causes the greatest problems in tissues that lack sorbitol dehydrogenase to break down the sorbitol. For example:

- In the lens and retina of the eye the increased sorbitol exerts a strong osmotic effect, causing water retention; the lens swells and becomes opaque, leading to cataract formation.
- In Schwann cells, the increased levels of sorbitol disrupt cell structure and function, and demyelination of nerves and peripheral neuropathy ensues.

- What are the main functions of glycolysis?
- How does the metabolism of pyruvate differ in anaerobic and aerobic glycolysis?
- Describe the main pathways of production and utilization of acetyl CoA.
- What is the significance of the irreversible, oxidative decarboxylation of pyruvate to carbohydrate metabolism?
- Name the main enzyme and coenzymes involved in the oxidative decarboxylation of pyruvate.
- What is the significance of the inhibition of pyruvate dehydrogenase?
- List four main functions of the TCA cycle.
- Name the two processes of ATP production and give an example of where each occurs.
- How does the electron transport chain produce ATP?
- Give a physiologic example of uncoupling of the electron transport chain.
- Describe the principle of respiratory control.
- What are the different roles of liver and muscle glycogen in the body?
- What is the basic outline of glycogen synthesis (name the site, the three main enzymes, and the three stages)?
- Explain the mechanism for the hormonal regulation of glycogen metabolism.
- What is the purpose of the Rapoport–Luebering shunt?
- In what physiologic states does the affinity of hemoglobin for 2,3-BPG differ from that in the normal adult?
- What is the significance of the sorbitol pathway in the development of complications of diabetes?
- What is the clinical significance of excessive ethanol ingestion?
- Which of the enzyme systems involved in ethanol catabolism cause a lower alcohol tolerance in some races?

3. Production of NADPH

Pentose phosphate pathway and pyruvate–malate cycle

Pentose phosphate pathway

The pentose phosphate pathway (PPP), otherwise known as the hexosemonophosphate shunt or the phosphogluconate pathway, provides an alternative route for the metabolism of glucose. Most of the pathways that have already been discussed are concerned with the generation of ATP. However, in the pentose phosphate pathway no ATP is directly consumed or produced; instead, the pathway is important for the production of reducing power in the form of NADPH and of ribose.

Like NADH, NADPH can be thought of as a high-energy molecule, but instead of transferring its electrons to the electron transport chain to make ATP, it is used for reductive synthetic reactions.

Location

Mainly the liver, lactating mammary glands, adipose tissue, adrenal cortex, and red blood cells (RBCs).

Site

Cell cytosol.

Main functions

The main functions of the pentose phosphate pathway are:

- Generation of NADPH necessary for reductive biosynthetic reactions; for example, fatty acid and cholesterol synthesis.
- Production of five-carbon, ribose sugar units for nucleotide and nucleic acid synthesis.
- In RBCs, NADPH is used to regenerate the reduced form of the antioxidant glutathione, which protects the cells against damage from reactive oxygen intermediates.

Pathway

The pathway has two stages:

- An irreversible oxidative phase (Fig. 3.1), which consists of three irreversible reactions, results in the formation of ribulose-5-phosphate, CO_2 and two molecules of NADPH per molecule of glucose-6-phosphate oxidized.
- A reversible non-oxidative phase (Fig. 3.2) that consists of a series of five, reversible sugar–phosphate interconversions, whereby ribulose-5-phosphate is converted either to ribose-5-phosphate for nucleotide synthesis or to intermediates of glycolysis such as glyceraldehyde-3-phosphate or fructose-6-phosphate. The pathway is therefore linked with the needs of glycolysis.

The sum of the reactions for the reversible phase is:

$$2 \text{xylulose-5-phosphate} + \text{ribose-5-phosphate} \leftrightarrow 2 \text{fructose-6-phosphate} + \text{glyceraldehyde-3-phosphate}.$$

It is not necessary to know the names of all the intermediates of the reversible phase; just be aware that it involves the interconversion of three, four, five, and seven carbon sugars, as shown in steps 1 to 5 in Fig. 3.2.

Fate of fructose-6-phosphate

The fate of fructose-6-phosphate formed in the pentose phosphate pathway depends on the specific needs of the tissue. For example, in liver, adipose tissue, and the adrenal cortex, fructose-6-phosphate promotes the synthesis of fatty acids.

How does this occur?

In the well-fed state, glucose is taken up by the liver and other tissues and phosphorylated to glucose-6-phosphate, which enters the pentose phosphate pathway to form fructose-6-phosphate. Accumulation of fructose-6-phosphate allosterically activates the rate-limiting enzyme of glycolysis, phosphofructokinase, which, in turn, allows the

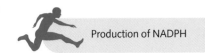

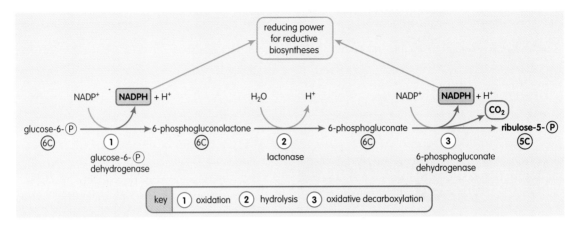

Fig. 3.1 The pentose phosphate pathway: phase I, the irreversible oxidative phase. Three irreversible reactions result in the production of two molecules of NADPH.

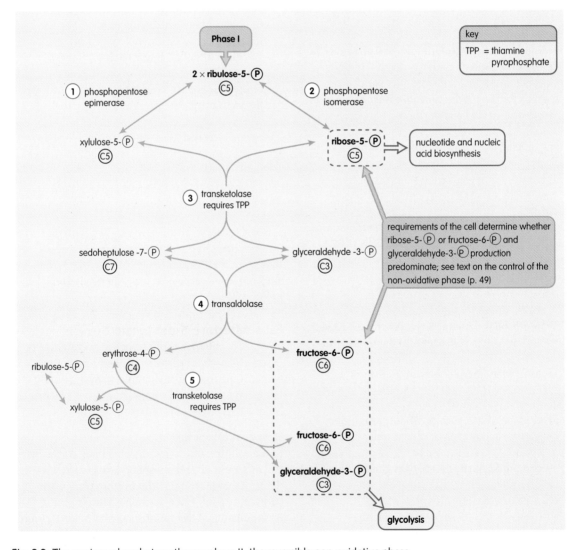

Fig. 3.2 The pentose phosphate pathway: phase II, the reversible non-oxidative phase.

formation of pyruvate. This is oxidatively decarboxylated to acetyl CoA, which can be used for fatty acid synthesis.

In RBCs, fructose-6-phosphate has a different fate. It is converted back to glucose-6-phosphate by the enzyme phosphoglucose isomerase to re-enter the pentose phosphate pathway, therefore creating a cycle and thus a continual supply of substrate for the pentose phosphate pathway. This allows the continued production of NADPH required for the regeneration of reduced glutathione, the antioxidant which protects RBCs (see Fig. 3.4).

Control of the pentose phosphate pathway

The main control of the pathway is exerted at the first step, that is, the glucose-6-phosphate dehydrogenase reaction.

Features are:
- This is an essentially irreversible reaction.
- The main controlling factor is the ratio of NADPH to $NADP^+$.
- As the cell uses up NADPH (e.g., during fatty acid synthesis) the concentration of $NADP^+$ increases. This activates the pathway, increasing NADPH formation to compensate.
- Therefore, the pentose phosphate pathway is activated by a low $NADPH:NADP^+$.

Control of the nonoxidative phase is by the requirement for products, namely ribose-5-phosphate and NADPH (see Fig. 3.2). The individual needs of the cell for either of these determine whether production of ribose-5-phosphate, or fructose-6-phosphate and glyceraldehyde-3-phosphate predominates. For example:
- If the NADPH requirement is greater than the ribose-5-phosphate requirement; for example, in cells that take part in a lot of reductive synthetic reactions, all of the ribose-5-phosphate formed is converted to fructose-6-phosphate and glyceraldehyde-3-phosphate. These are converted back to glucose-6-phosphate to re-enter the pentose phosphate pathway and therefore generate more NADPH.
- If the ribose-5-phosphate requirement is greater than the need for NADPH; for example, in cells with a high turnover and rate of nucleic acid formation, fructose-6-phosphate and glyceraldehyde-3-phosphate are converted to ribose-5-phosphate by further sugar interconversions.

Pyruvate–malate cycle

The pyruvate–malate cycle (Fig. 3.3) has two functions:
- The production of NADPH in the reaction catalyzed by the malic (malate dehydrogenase-decarboxylating) enzyme.
- The transport of acetyl CoA units from the mitochondria to the cytosol, the site of fatty acid synthesis by the citrate shuttle.

Glycolysis produces pyruvate, which enters the mitochondria, where it is oxidatively decarboxylated to acetyl CoA, from which fatty acids can be synthesized. However, fatty acid synthesis takes place in the cell cytosol, so that acetyl CoA requires a transport mechanism or "carrier" to enable it to leave the mitochondria, namely, the citrate shuttle (discussed further in Chapter 4).

Sources of NADPH for fatty acid synthesis

The pentose phosphate pathway is the main source of NADPH: two molecules of NADPH are produced for each molecule of glucose entering the pathway.

The pyruvate–malate cycle probably contributes between 25 and 40% of the total NADPH, depending on the source of the acetyl units (i.e., glucose, amino acids or lactate). For each acetyl CoA transferred from the mitochondria to the cytosol, one NADPH molecule is generated.

The pyruvate–malate cycle shows an interrelationship between glucose metabolism and fatty acid synthesis. When the need for ATP is low, the oxidation of acetyl CoA by the TCA cycle is minimal, thus providing acetyl CoA for fatty acid synthesis. Remember that these pathways are not all active at the same time.

The roles of NADPH

NADPH in lipid biosynthesis

NADPH, like NADH, is a high-energy molecule, but its electrons, instead of being transferred to oxygen via the electron transport chain, are used for reductive biosyntheses, particularly for lipid

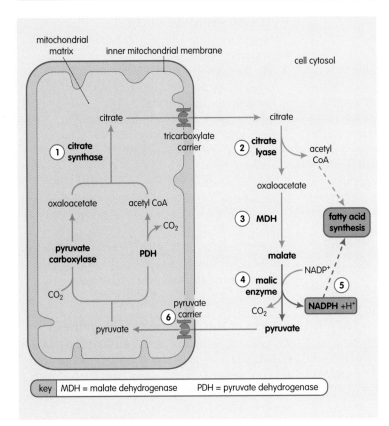

Fig. 3.3 The pyruvate–malate cycle operates between the cell cytosol and mitochondria. The reaction sequence is as follows:
1. Oxaloacetate and acetyl CoA condense to form citrate, which leaves the mitochondria via the tricarboxylate carrier.
2. Citrate is cleaved in the cytosol by citrate lyase back to oxaloacetate and acetyl CoA.
3. Acetyl CoA can be used for fatty acid synthesis whereas oxaloacetate is reduced to malate.
4. Malate is oxidatively decarboxylated by the malic enzyme, re-forming pyruvate.
5. The reaction produces a significant amount of NADPH, which is used mainly for fatty acid synthesis.
6. Pyruvate is transported back into the mitochondria via a pyruvate carrier, where some of it is carboxylated to oxaloacetate and some converted to acetyl CoA.

synthesis. Each cycle of lipid synthesis, in which the growing fatty acid chain is lengthened by two carbon atoms, employs two reductions, each requiring NADPH as cofactor. The pentose phosphate pathway and pyruvate–malate cycle both generate the NADPH necessary for fatty acid synthesis. Deficiency of NADPH leads to inhibition of fatty acid synthesis (see Chapter 4 for a more in-depth discussion of fatty acid synthesis).

NADPH in the production of glutathione

Glutathione is a tripeptide of three amino acids, glutamate, cysteine, and glycine, and is found in most cells. It can exist in two forms: an active, reduced form and an inactive, oxidized form (Fig. 3.4). Reduced glutathione contains a reactive thiol group (—SH) on the cysteine residue, which can reduce hydrogen peroxide (H_2O_2) and other reactive oxygen intermediates (free radicals), detoxifying them. That is, glutathione is an antioxidant and protects cells from damage.

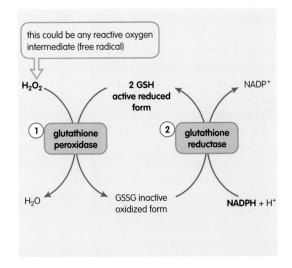

Fig. 3.4 The antioxidant action of glutathione. Glutathione (GSH) is an antioxidant. It reduces hydrogen peroxide and other reactive oxygen intermediates, inactivating them. In doing so it undergoes oxidation to its inactive, oxidized form (GSSG). NADPH is required for the regeneration of the active reduced form of glutathione by glutathione reductase, enabling it to continue its role as an antioxidant.

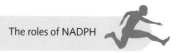

Role of NADPH in glutathione metabolism (numbers refer to Fig. 3.4)

1. Glutathione (GSH) reduces hydrogen peroxide, inactivating it. The reaction, catalyzed by glutathione peroxidase (an enzyme containing selenium), produces oxidized, inactive glutathione.
2. The active, reduced form of glutathione is regenerated by glutathione reductase, which requires NADPH as a reducing agent.

Therefore, NADPH indirectly provides the reducing power to inactivate hydrogen peroxide. This pathway is important in all cells of the body, but especially in RBCs.

Importance of NADPH in RBCs

RBCs do not contain mitochondria; therefore, they rely entirely on glycolysis and the pentose phosphate pathway. This means their only source of NADPH is the pentose phosphate pathway. Inhibition of the pathway would lead to a decrease in NADPH and therefore decreased activity of glutathione reductase. The amount of inactive, oxidized glutathione would increase, rendering the RBCs sensitive to oxidative damage by H_2O_2. This is seen in glucose-6-phosphate dehydrogenase deficiency, an X-linked condition in which oxidative damage leads to:

- The oxidation of hemoglobin to methemoglobin, which cannot transport oxygen effectively (see below).
- The oxidation of membrane proteins and lipids, destabilizing them, leading to an increased chance of cell lysis and thus hemolytic anemia (see below).

Action of free radicals

Reactive oxygen intermediates are formed from molecular oxygen in most cells, as either by-products of aerobic metabolism or from exogenous sources; for example, smoking, radiation, and the side effects of drugs and chemicals. They are highly reactive and attack cell components such as proteins, DNA, and polyunsaturated fatty acids in cell membranes, resulting in disruption of membrane structure and cell integrity. Free radicals are thought to be partly responsible for the cell damage associated with inflammation, ageing and certain cancers. They are detoxified by two main mechanisms, which are outlined below.

Enzyme inactivation

Several enzymes are responsible for the inactivation of free radicals:

- Glutathione peroxidase (a selenium-containing enzyme) removes hydrogen peroxide (see Fig. 3.4).
- Catalase (an iron-containing enzyme) removes hydrogen peroxide according to the reaction:

$$H_2O_2 \rightarrow H_2O + \tfrac{1}{2}O_2$$

- Superoxide dismutase detoxifies the superoxide radical ($O_2^{\bullet-}$) as shown below:

$$2O_2^{\bullet-} + 2H^+ \rightarrow H_2O_2\ O_2.$$

Superoxide dismutase exists in two forms: a copper- and zinc-containing cytoplasmic form and a manganese-containing mitochondrial form.

Deficiency of any of the trace elements contained in these enzymes can lead to their inhibition and thus an increase in cellular damage by free radicals (see Chapter 8).

Nonenzymatic inactivation: dietary antioxidants

Vitamins A, C, and E are antioxidants (see Chapter 8). There is no substantial evidence available to support the theory that increased dietary intake of these vitamins alone reduces the incidence of heart disease or cancer.

Prevention of oxidation of hemoglobin

The oxidation of the iron (Fe^{2+}; ferrous form) in hemoglobin by H_2O_2 or other free radicals yields methemoglobin (Fe^{3+}; ferric form), which cannot transport oxygen effectively. Methemoglobin is usually only present at low concentrations because RBCs possess an efficient enzyme system, NADH-dependent cytochrome b_5 reductase (methemoglobin reductase), which catalyzes the reduction of methemoglobin to hemoglobin (Fig. 3.5).

The generation of excessive amount of free radicals and the action of certain drugs or toxins can

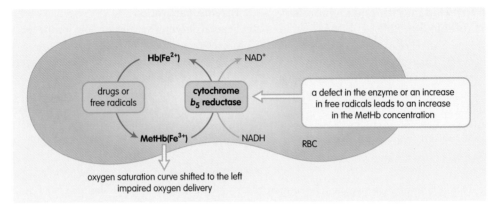

Fig. 3.5 The reduction of methemoglobin. A defect in the enzyme cytochrome b_5 reductase can lead to methemoglobinemia and cyanosis.

result in the increased formation of methemoglobin. In this scenario, the cytochrome b_5 reductase system cannot cope, and the concentration of methemoglobin in the blood rises, leading to methemoglobinemia. Because methemoglobin cannot carry oxygen, this results in poor perfusion of tissues and cyanosis (a dusky blue discoloration of skin). If adequate amounts of NADPH are present, the levels of glutathione in RBCs can cope with the excess free radicals and drugs and thus prevent oxidation of hemoglobin.

Newborn babies have only low concentrations of cytochrome b_5 reductase and are therefore susceptible to methemoglobinemia.

Drug metabolism

A continual supply of reduced glutathione is required in the liver for the conjugation and detoxification of certain drugs and steroid hormones. This increases their excretion, thus preventing accumulation and toxicity. NADPH is necessary to maintain a continuous supply of reduced glutathione, as already described.

The pentose phosphate pathway in RBCs provides the NADPH necessary to keep glutathione in a reduced state; glutathione protects RBCs from oxidative damage. A failure of these pathways leads to:

- Decreased membrane flexibility and leakiness of RBCs.
- The oxidation of hemoglobin and an increase in RBC breakdown, leading to hemolysis and a hemolytic anemia.

Glucose-6-phosphate dehydrogenase deficiency

Glucose-6-phosphate dehydrogenase (G6PDH) controls the rate-limiting step of the pentose phosphate pathway (see Fig. 3.1). Although G6PDH deficiency is an uncommon cause of anemia in the U.S., it affects 130 million people worldwide, particularly in Africa, the Mediterranean and South-East Asia. Remember, RBCs lack mitochondria and rely on glycolysis for ATP production. ATP is necessary for the maintenance of RBC membrane flexibility and shape, enabling their passage through small vessels. It also maintains osmotic equilibrium via ATP-dependent pumps in RBC membranes. The inheritance of G6PDH deficiency is sex-linked, affecting males and being carried by females. Carriers have about half the normal G6PDH activity, but have some degree of protection against *Plasmodium falciparum*, which causes malaria, giving carriers an evolutionary advantage. Over 400 different mutations have been identified in the gene coding for G6PDH, but only certain variants cause hemolytic anemia.

Pathogenesis

The mechanism is that a decrease in G6PDH activity leads to decreased NADPH formation and therefore decreased production of reduced glutathione (Fig. 3.6). RBCs are thus more susceptible to oxidative damage. Damage to the RBC membrane creates "bite" or "blister" cells. Damage to hemoglobin causes its oxidation to methemoglobin, and the

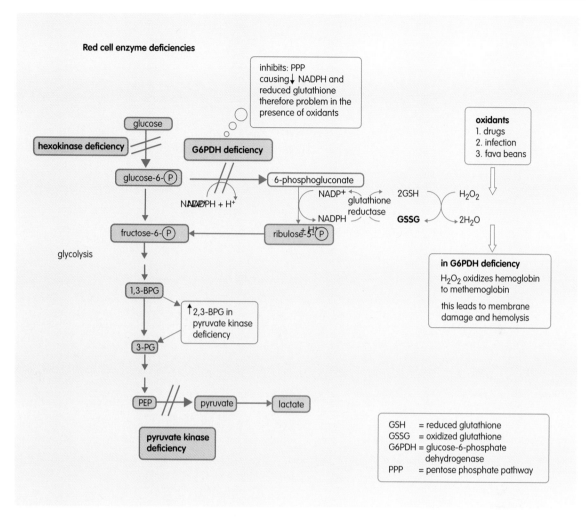

Fig. 3.6 Red blood cell enzyme deficiencies.

globin chains are precipitated as Heinz bodies. Both can be observed on the blood film during a hemolytic crisis.

There are two types of G6PDH deficiency: type A is commonly found in Afro-Caribbeans. The G6PDH activity falls with increasing cell age, that is, when the cells are first made they have a normal enzyme activity. Type A is self-limiting and mild. Type B is commonly found in people of Mediterranean descent and is more serious. The enzyme activity is reduced throughout the life span of the cell. Any factor that causes oxidative stress leads to a large intravascular hemolysis.

The precipitating factors that cause oxidative stress and hemolysis are:
• Drugs: antibiotics (sulfamethoxazole), antimalarials (quinine, primaquine,) and antipyretics (aspirin).
• Infection is the most common precipitating factor.
• Favism, only in type B. Consumption, or even the inhalation of the pollen, of fava beans (broad beans) leads to hemolysis.
• Neonatal jaundice.

Treatment is to avoid precipitants; in severe cases, consider a blood transfusion.

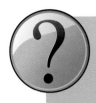

- What are the main functions of the pentose phosphate pathway?
- Describe the concept of reducing power and its importance to reductive biosynthetic reactions.
- How is NADPH involved in methemoglobinemia and drug metabolism?
- What are the positive and negative effects of glucose-6-phosphate dehydrogenase deficiency?
- Describe the origin of NADPH and its role in lipid synthesis.

4. Lipid Metabolism and Transport

Lipid biosynthesis

Overview of fatty acid biosynthesis
Fatty acids are an essential fuel and major energy source. The diet supplies a lot of the fat used by the body, but a number of tissues can also synthesize fatty acids *de novo* from acetyl CoA.

Working definition
Fatty acid synthesis (lipogenesis) consists of a cyclical series of reactions, in which a molecule of fatty acid is built up by the sequential addition of two carbon units derived from acetyl CoA into a growing fatty acid chain.

Fatty acid synthesis is not simply a reversal of the degradative pathway (i.e., β oxidation) but consists of its own set of reactions.

Location
Mainly in the liver, adipose tissue and lactating mammary glands; there is a small amount in the kidney.

Site
Cell cytosol.

Fig. 4.1 shows an overview of lipid biosynthesis and the main steps involved in the formation of palmitate. Construction of this 16-carbon saturated fatty acid begins with the formation of acetyl CoA in the mitochondria. It is transported into the cell cytosol, where it is carboxylated to malonyl CoA and then undergoes a characteristic sequence of reactions catalyzed by fatty acid synthase. It would be a good idea to have a look at this diagram now, before you embark on the rest of this chapter.

The pentose phosphate pathway and the pyruvate–malate cycle generate the NADPH necessary for fatty acid synthesis (about 60% from the pentose phosphate pathway and 40% via the malic enzyme; see Chapter 3). The steps of fatty acid synthesis are now considered in more detail.

Production of acetyl CoA
Pyruvate dehydrogenase (PDH) catalyzes the irreversible, oxidative decarboxylation of pyruvate to acetyl CoA in the mitochondrial matrix (Fig. 4.2). Details of this reaction are covered in Chapter 2. Acetyl CoA can also be produced by the degradation of fatty acids, ketone bodies or amino acids.

Transport of acetyl CoA from mitochondria to the cytosol
The same pathway, namely the pyruvate–malate cycle, that produces NADPH for fatty acid synthesis also transports acetyl CoA from the mitochondria to the cell cytosol (see Fig. 4.2). The part of the cycle that transports acetyl CoA is called the citrate shuttle. Acetyl CoA is produced in the mitochondria but fatty acid synthesis occurs in the cytosol. The CoA portion of the molecule cannot cross the mitochondrial membrane. However, by condensing with oxaloacetate to form citrate, the acetyl group can be carried across by the tricarboxylate carrier. In the cytosol, citrate is cleaved by citrate lyase to release oxaloacetate for recycling and acetyl CoA for fatty acid synthesis.

Fate of acetyl CoA: the TCA cycle vs fatty acid synthesis
Normally in mitochondria, any citrate formed enters the TCA cycle for oxidation and the generation of ATP. However, when the concentration of ATP is high, enzymes of the TCA cycle, especially isocitrate dehydrogenase, are inhibited because there is no need to generate further energy. The concentration of citrate rises, which activates the tricarboxylate transporter and so citrate is transported into the cytosol. As ATP is also needed for fatty acid synthesis, the high levels of both ATP and citrate favour lipogenesis.

Production of malonyl CoA from acetyl CoA
This is the irreversible, rate-limiting step of fatty acid synthesis (Fig. 4.3). The carboxylation of acetyl CoA

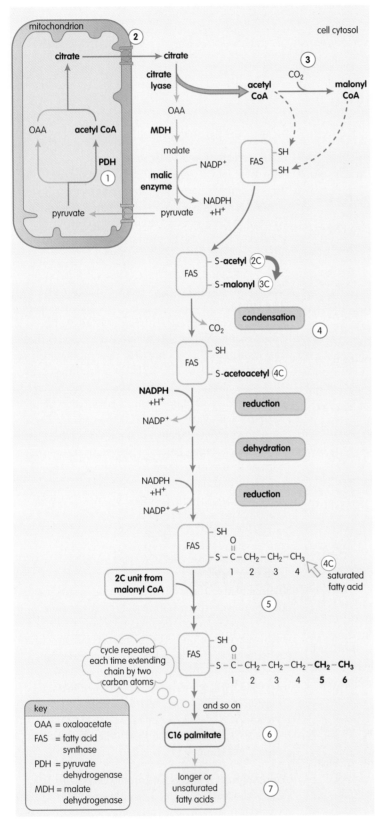

Fig. 4.1 An overview of fatty acid biosynthesis. The steps involved in the formation of palmitate:

1. Formation of the precursor acetyl CoA from pyruvate in mitochondria.
2. Transport of acetyl CoA into the cytosol. Acetyl CoA combines with oxaloacetate to form citrate (citrate shuttle).
3. The carboxylation of acetyl CoA to malonyl CoA by acetyl CoA carboxylase.
4. The initiation of the synthesis of a new fatty acid molecule requires both acetyl CoA and malonyl CoA. They attach to the enzyme, fatty acid synthase, and condense to form acetoacetyl-ACP. This then undergoes a characteristic sequence of reactions catalyzed by fatty acid synthase to make a four-carbon saturated fatty acid.
5. Fatty acid synthase also catalyzes the sequential addition of a further two carbon units from malonyl CoA to the growing fatty acid chain.
6. Elongation by fatty acid synthase stops on formation of palmitate (C16).
7. Further elongation and insertion of double bonds are carried out by other enzymes.

Fig. 4.2 Production of acetyl CoA and its transport by the citrate shuttle.

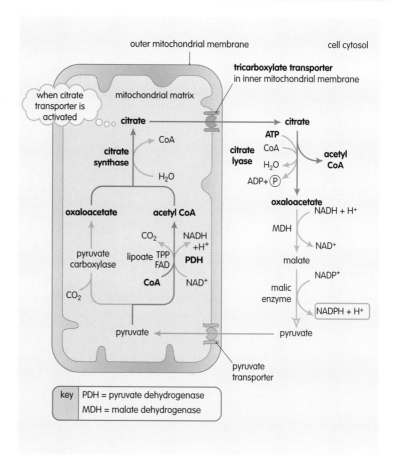

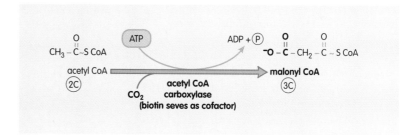

Fig. 4.3 Carboxylation of acetyl CoA to malonyl CoA by acetyl CoA carboxylase.

is catalyzed by acetyl CoA carboxylase, which requires the vitamin biotin as a cofactor. Biotin is covalently attached to a lysine residue of the enzyme and takes part in the reaction. The biotin group of the enzyme is first carboxylated, creating an active carboxyl group for further transfer to acetyl CoA.

Biotin is therefore a carrier of activated carboxyl group, and as such is the cofactor for other carboxylases, including pyruvate carboxylase (see Chapter 5).

Fatty acid synthase

Fatty acid synthesis requires several enzymes. In bacteria, these enzymes are all separate, but in eukaryotes they are joined together, forming a multi-enzyme complex called fatty acid synthase. Fatty acid synthase is a dimer of two identical subunits, each with seven different enzymatic activities that catalyze a different reaction of fatty acid synthesis. Each subunit also contains the acyl carrier protein. Subunits of fatty acid synthase are folded into three

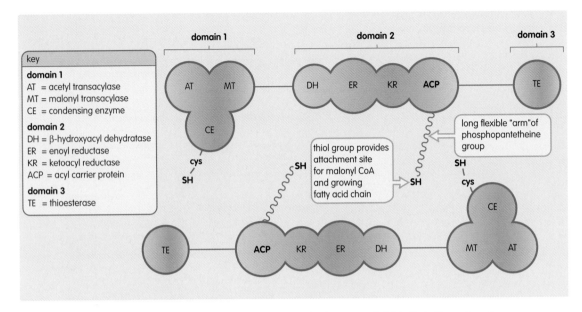

Fig. 4.4 Structure of fatty acid synthase: a dimer of two identical subunits, each folded into three domains.

domains joined by flexible regions (Fig. 4.4). Both the acyl carrier protein and one of the enzymes, the condensing enzyme (β-ketoacyl synthase), contain important thiol (sulphydryl) groups.

Function of the acyl carrier protein

The acyl carrier protein contains the vitamin pantothenic acid as a 4'-phosphopantetheine prosthetic group, which contains a terminal thiol group. This is similar to the pantothenic acid group of coenzyme A (see Chapter 2). All the intermediates of fatty acid synthesis are joined to the acyl carrier protein. The phosphopantetheinyl group forms a long flexible arm that carries the growing acyl chain from one active site to the next within the fatty acid synthase. This enhances the efficiency of the overall synthetic process.

Stages of fatty acid synthesis
Formation of saturated fatty acids

The stages of fatty acid synthesis are illustrated in Fig. 4.5.

1. Addition of acetyl and malonyl groups

Acetyl transacylase catalyzes the transfer of the acetyl group from acetyl CoA to the thiol group (SH) of the acyl carrier protein. It is then transferred to the thiol group of the β-ketoacyl synthase. Malonyl

transacylase then transfers the malonyl group from malonyl CoA to the acyl carrier protein.

2. Condensation

β-Ketoacyl synthase catalyzes the condensation of acetyl (2C) and malonyl (3C) groups to form acetoacetyl-ACP (4C). The reaction is driven by the loss of CO_2. The energy derived from ATP that was used to carboxylate acetyl CoA to malonyl CoA (see Fig. 4.3) had been stored in malonyl CoA; decarboxylation releases this energy and thus helps to drive elongation. The next three steps convert the acetoacetyl-ACP to a four-carbon, saturated acyl chain.

3. Reduction

The keto group at C3 (the β carbon) is reduced to an alcohol group by β-ketoacyl reductase. The reducing agent for this reaction is NADPH.

4. Dehydration

The removal of water by β-hydroxyacyl dehydratase introduces a double bond.

5. Reduction

Enoyl reductase catalyzes the second reduction producing a saturated four-carbon fatty acyl chain. This completes the first elongation cycle.

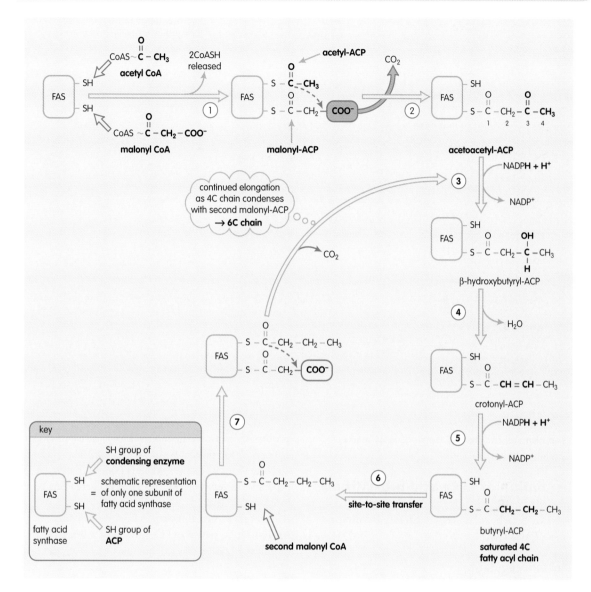

Fig. 4.5 Stages of fatty acid synthesis. Numbers 1 to 7 correspond to the text. The seven-stage synthesis of fatty acids has its cyclical part in steps 3–7, which add two carbons to the growing fatty acid chain for each cycle of the pathway.

6. Site-to-site transfer

The four-carbon chain is transferred to the thiol group of the cysteine residue of the β-ketoacyl synthase.

7. Addition of a second malonyl CoA to the acyl carrier protein

The four-carbon chain condenses with malonyl CoA and steps 2–6 are repeated to form a saturated six-carbon acyl chain.

The cycle is in fact repeated a further six times until a 16-carbon chain, palmitate, is made, i.e.,

seven cycles altogether (see Fig. 4.5). The enzyme thioesterase then catalyzes the release of palmitate. Therefore, the synthesis of one molecule of palmitate uses one molecule of acetyl CoA and seven of malonyl CoA. The overall reaction for the synthesis of palmitate is:

$$8\,\text{acetyl CoA} + 14\,\text{NADPH} + 14\,\text{H}^+ + 7\,\text{ATP} \rightarrow$$
$$\text{palmitate} + 14\,\text{NADP}^+ + 8\,\text{CoA} + 7\,\text{ADP} +$$
$$7\,\text{Pi} + 7\,\text{H}_2\text{O}$$

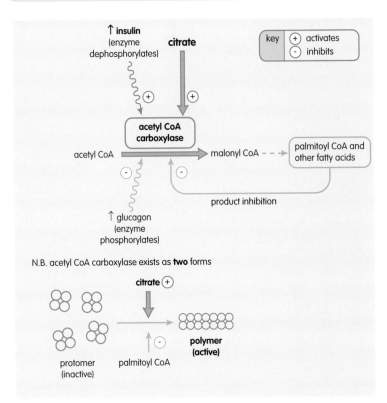

Fig. 4.6 Regulation of fatty acid biosynthesis. Insulin and glucagon control acetyl CoA carboxylase via reversible phosphorylation, whereas citrate and palmitoyl CoA allosterically regulate the enzyme.

Remember, all the carbon atoms of fatty acids originally come from acetyl CoA.

Regulation of fatty acid biosynthesis

The main control point is the reaction catalyzed by acetyl CoA carboxylase (Fig. 4.6). Control may be considered at two levels:

Allosteric regulation

Acetyl CoA carboxylase can exist in two forms: an inactive protomer or subunit form and an active polymer or filamentous form. Citrate activates acetyl CoA carboxylase by promoting the polymerization of

> It is worth remembering the characteristic set of reactions, namely the reduction, dehydration, reduction motif of fatty acid synthesis. The opposite of these reactions is the oxidation, hydration, and oxidation in the TCA cycle (Chapter 2) and fatty acid breakdown.

protomers to active filaments. How? A rise in citrate concentration indicates that acetyl CoA and ATP are available for fatty acid synthesis (since an increase in ATP inhibits enzymes of the TCA cycle leading to a build-up of citrate).

Acetyl CoA carboxylase is inhibited by the final product, palmitoyl CoA, which causes the depolymerization of its filaments.

Reversible phosphorylation

Acetyl CoA carboxylase is also controlled by hormone-dependent reversible phosphorylation in a way similar to glycogen synthase (see Chapter 2). Glucagon activates a cAMP-dependent protein kinase which phosphorylates acetyl CoA carboxylase, inactivating it. Insulin promotes dephosphorylation and activation of the enzyme and thus lipid synthesis.

Synthesis of triacylglycerol

Fatty acids are stored as triacylglycerol molecules in the cytosol of adipose cells. Please note: the term *triglyceride*, a synonym of triacylglycerol, is commonly used in clinical medicine. Triglycerides consist of a glycerol backbone esterified with three fatty acids. Triacylglycerol formation can be thought

Fig. 4.7 Triacylglycerol synthesis consists of three distinct stages, as described in the text.

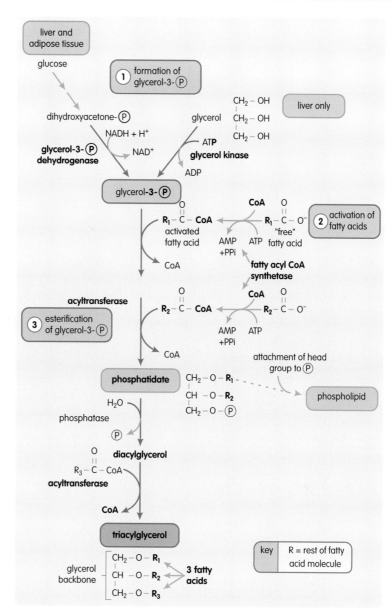

of in three main stages (the numbers correspond to Fig. 4.7).

1. Formation of glycerol-3-phosphate
This occurs either directly by the phosphorylation of glycerol by glycerol kinase or by the reduction of the glycolytic intermediate, dihydroxyacetone phosphate, by glycerol-3-phosphate dehydrogenase.

2. Activation of fatty acids
Fatty acyl CoA synthetase activates the fatty acids by attaching them to CoA. The reaction requires ATP.

3. Esterification of glycerol-3-phosphate
Acyl transferase adds the activated fatty acids to glycerol-3-phosphate in stages. During the synthesis of triacylglycerol, the intermediate phosphatidate formed can also be used for the synthesis of phospholipids, for example through the addition of choline to form phosphatidyl choline, which is used for membrane biosynthesis.

Nomenclature of fatty acids
Fatty acids vary in chain length and in the degree of unsaturation. The configuration of the double bonds

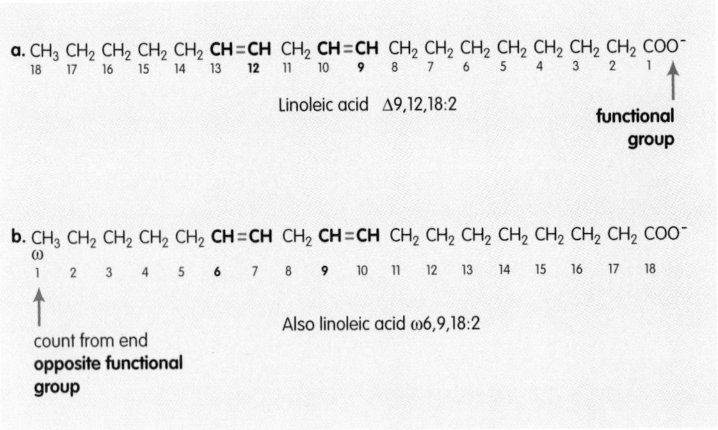

Fig. 4.8 The two ways of defining the position of a double bond:
a. By counting from the functional group.
b. By counting from the end opposite (ω) the functional group.

in most unsaturated fatty acids in animals is *cis* (*cis* refers to the orientation of the substituent groups, i.e., methyl groups to the double bond). *Cis* means that the methyl groups are on the same side of the double bond compared with *trans*, which indicates that they are on opposite sides.

There are two ways of defining the position of a double bond: by counting from the functional group and by counting from the end opposite to the functional group (Fig. 4.8).

Counting from the functional group (COOH)

Used by chemists; the position of the double bond is represented by the symbol Δ, followed by a number. For example, $\Delta 9,12, 18:2$ means an 18-carbon fatty acid containing two double bonds between the carbon atoms 9 and 10 and 12 and 13; that is, linoleic acid (see Fig. 4.8a).

Counting from the end opposite to the functional group

Used by biologists and more confusing! The symbol ω is used to depict the end opposite to the functional group (the methyl-terminal carbon). For example, $\omega 6,9, 18:2$ is an 18-carbon fatty acid containing two double bonds between the carbon atoms 6 and 7 and 9 and 10. From Fig. 4.8b, it can be seen, however, that this is also linoleic acid.

Modification of fatty acids

Elongation of fatty acids

Fatty acid synthase only produces palmitate (C16) and a small amount of stearate (C18). Other enzymes are required to make longer fatty acids.

These enzymes are found on the endoplasmic reticulum and in mitochondria.

Endoplasmic reticulum pathway

This pathway is similar to the normal pathway and steps of fatty acid synthesis. However, there are two main differences:

- The enzymes are all separate and are located on the cytosolic face of the smooth endoplasmic reticulum.
- The intermediates are bound to CoA rather than to an acyl carrier protein.

Mitochondrial pathway

This pathway is basically a reversal of fatty acid breakdown (β oxidation). It is important for the elongation of short-chain fatty acids, that is, those containing 14 carbon atoms or less, and it takes place in the mitochondrial matrix. Two carbon units are added directly from acetyl CoA, not malonyl CoA.

Desaturation of fatty acids

This pathway is located in the membrane of the smooth endoplasmic reticulum (Fig. 4.9). The system is in fact an electron transport chain consisting of three enzymes:

- NADH-cytochrome b_5 reductase.
- Cytochrome b_5.
- Fatty acyl CoA desaturase.

Two pairs of electrons are passed down the chain: one pair comes from the single bond of the fatty acid and one pair from NADH. Mammalian systems have four different desaturase enzymes capable of producing double bonds at positions $\Delta 4$, $\Delta 5$, $\Delta 6$, and $\Delta 9$.

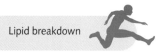

Fig. 4.9 The synthesis of unsaturated fatty acids. The desaturation pathway, located in the smooth endoplasmic reticulum, is responsible for the introduction of double bonds at positions $\Delta 4$, $\Delta 5$, $\Delta 6$, and $\Delta 9$.

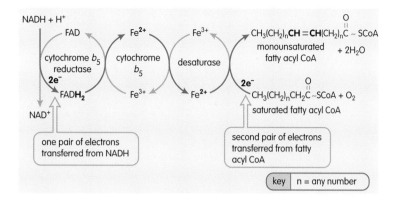

Unsaturated fatty acids are necessary for the synthesis of important membrane phospholipids and intracellular messengers such as prostaglandins.

Essential fatty acids

Mammals can only form double bonds at the positions $\Delta 4$, $\Delta 5$, $\Delta 6$, and $\Delta 9$ but lack the enzymes needed to create double bonds beyond the ninth carbon atom. Therefore, certain polyunsaturated fatty acids (PUFAs) that are vital for health cannot be synthesized endogenously and must be taken in from the diet. The principal essential fatty acids are linoleic (C18:2) and α-linolenic (C18:3) acids, of the $\omega 6$ and $\omega 3$ series, respectively (see Fig. 4.10). From these, other important unsaturated fatty acids can be made. For example, arachidonic acid (C20:4) is synthesized from linolenic acid and is the precursor molecule for prostaglandins, leukotriene and thromboxane molecules. Fish oils are a particularly good source of the $\omega 3$ series.

Essential fatty acids (EFAs)				
ω series	No. of C atoms	No. of double bonds	Position of double bonds	Name
$\omega 3$ series $\omega 3,6,9$	18	3	cis $\Delta 9,12,15$	α-linolenic acid
$\omega 6$ series $\omega 6,9$	18	2	cis $\Delta 9,12$	linoleic acid
$\omega 6,9,12$	18	3	cis $\Delta 6,9,12$	γ-linolenic acid (made from linolenic acid)
$\omega 6,9,12,15$	20	4	cis $\Delta 5,8,11,14$	arachidonic acid

Fig. 4.10 Essential fatty acids.

Lipid breakdown

Triacylglycerol stores in adipose tissue serve as the body's major fuel reserve. Fatty acids are easily mobilized to provide energy during prolonged exercise or starvation. The oxidation of fat yields about 9 kcal/g (38.6 kJ) of energy compared with only 4 kcal/g (16.8 kJ) for protein and carbohydrate.

An overview of fatty acid breakdown
Working definition
Fatty acid breakdown is the process by which a molecule of fatty acid is degraded by the sequential removal of two carbon units, producing acetyl CoA, which can then be oxidized to CO_2 and H_2O by the TCA cycle.

Location
Many tissues, especially liver and muscle. Certain tissues are unable to oxidize fatty acids, namely the brain, RBCs, and adrenal medulla, because they lack the necessary enzymes.

The four stages of lipid breakdown
Lipid breakdown can be conveniently divided into four main stages.

1. Hydrolysis of triacylglycerol by lipase: lipolysis

Lipolysis occurs in the cell cytosol of adipose cells. The hydrolysis of triacylglycerol produces glycerol and free fatty acids. Glycerol travels to the liver, where it is phosphorylated and oxidized to dihydroxyacetone phosphate, which in turn is isomerized to glyceraldehyde-3-phosphate. This intermediate is on both the glycolytic and gluconeogenic pathways. It can therefore be converted into pyruvate or glucose in the liver. The free fatty acids travel in the blood bound to albumin and are taken up by muscle or liver cells for oxidation.

2. Activation of fatty acids

Before they can be oxidized, fatty acids are activated by attachment to CoA to form acyl CoA molecules; this takes place in the cell cytosol.

3. Transport into mitochondria

β Oxidation occurs in the mitochondrial matrix. The acyl CoA molecules are transported into the mitochondria by the carnitine shuttle.

4. β Oxidation

Fatty acids are degraded by a cyclical sequence of four reactions: oxidation, hydration, oxidation, and thiolysis. This results in the shortening of the fatty acid chain by two carbon atoms per sequence. The two carbons are removed as acetyl CoA. For even-numbered saturated fatty acids this is straightforward, but other enzymes are necessary for the oxidation of unsaturated and odd-numbered fatty acids (see later).

These steps are now considered in more detail.

Lipolysis

The initial event in the breakdown of fat is the hydrolysis of triacylglycerol stores in adipose tissue. Triacylglycerol is converted into glycerol and three free-fatty acids in two steps (Fig. 4.11):

1. A hormone-sensitive lipase hydrolyzes triacylglycerol at the C1 and C3 positions to form monoacylglycerol.
2. A monoacylglycerol-specific lipase removes the remaining fatty acid.

The glycerol produced cannot be metabolized by adipose tissue because adipose tissue does not contain glycerol kinase. Glycerol is transported to the liver, where it is phosphorylated, either to be used again to make triacylglycerol or to be converted to dihydroxyacetone phosphate (DHAP), a glycolytic intermediate. The free fatty acids produced are either re-esterified to triacyglycerol in the adipose tissue or travel in the blood to be taken up by the cells for oxidation.

Activation of fatty acids to fatty acyl CoA

Fatty acyl CoA synthetase (thiokinase) activates fatty acids by attaching them to CoA. The reaction

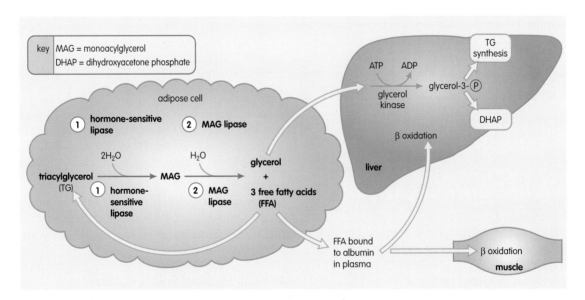

Fig. 4.11 Hydrolysis of triacylglycerol to glycerol and free fatty acids (numbers refer to the text).

occurs on the cytosolic face of the outer mitochondrial membrane and requires ATP, which is hydrolyzed to AMP and pyrophosphate (PPi), breaking a high-energy phosphate bond. The reaction is made irreversible by the rapid hydrolysis of the pyrophosphate to two free inorganic phosphates by pyrophosphatase, consuming a second high-energy phosphate bond (Fig. 4.12). Therefore, the activation of a fatty acid consumes 2ATP equivalents. Fatty acids are non-polar molecules and can easily diffuse out of cells, but the attachment to a polar molecule, such as CoA, "traps" the fatty acid inside.

Transport of fatty acyl CoA molecules into mitochondria

The activation of fatty acids occurs in the cytosol, but the enzymes for β oxidation are in the mitochondrial matrix. The inner mitochondrial membrane is relatively impermeable to long-chain acyl CoA molecules, so a special transporter system is required to carry the fatty acid across. The carnitine shuttle consists of three enzymes: a translocase and two carnitine acyl transferases, CAT I and II, as shown in Fig. 4.12.

β Oxidation

Acyl CoA molecules inside the mitochondrial matrix undergo β oxidation in a cyclical sequence of four reactions (numbers refer to Fig. 4.13).

1. Oxidation

The oxidation of acyl CoA introduces a double bond between the C2 and C3 atoms. The $FADH_2$ formed enters the electron transport chain to produce 1.5 ATP (see Chapter 2). In the mitochondria there are three types of acyl CoA dehydrogenase, which act on long-, medium- and short-chain fatty acids. A deficiency in medium-chain acyl CoA dehydrogenase has been recognized (this is discussed further below).

2. Hydration

Hydration is the addition of water across the double bond between C2 and C3 by Δ2 enoyl-CoA hydratase.

3. Oxidation by NAD^+

β-Hydroxyacyl CoA dehydrogenase converts the OH group at C3 (the β carbon) to a keto group. The NADH produced enters the electron transport chain to yield 2.5 ATP molecules. These three reactions of oxidation (dehydrogenation), hydration, and again oxidation resemble the last three reactions of the

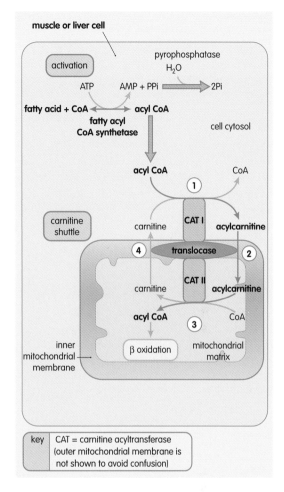

Fig. 4.12 Activation of fatty acids and their transport into mitochondria by the carnitine shuttle.
1. The acyl group is transferred from CoA to carnitine by carnitine acyl transferase I, an enzyme found on the cytosolic side of the inner mitochondrial membrane.
2. Acylcarnitine is transported across the membrane by the translocase to the mitochondrial matrix.
3. The acyl group is transferred back to CoA by carnitine acyl transferase II, located on the inner surface of the inner mitochondrial membrane.
4. Carnitine is returned to the cytosolic side in exchange for another molecule of acylcarnitine.

TCA cycle which convert succinate to oxaloacetate (see Chapter 2).

4. Thiolytic cleavage by CoA

Thiolase cleaves the molecule to release acetyl CoA, and acyl CoA is shortened by two carbon atoms. The shortened acyl CoA is ready to undergo another sequence of β oxidation. The four steps are repeated

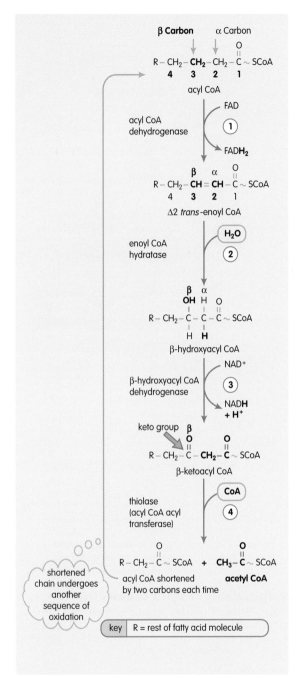

Fig. 4.13 β Oxidation pathway. The cyclical sequence of four reactions—oxidation, hydration, oxidation and thiolysis—shortens the fatty acid chain by two carbons each cycle. This continues until the fatty acid is completely oxidized to acetyl CoA.

until the fatty acid is oxidized completely to acetyl CoA. The last round of oxidation produces two molecules of acetyl CoA.

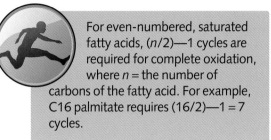

For even-numbered, saturated fatty acids, $(n/2)$—1 cycles are required for complete oxidation, where n = the number of carbons of the fatty acid. For example, C16 palmitate requires $(16/2)$—1 = 7 cycles.

ATP yield from the oxidation of the fatty acid palmitate

Each round of β oxidation produces one molecule each of $FADH_2$, NADH, and acetyl CoA. The β oxidation of palmitate requires seven cycles, producing 7 $FADH_2$, 7 NADH, and 8 acetyl CoA in total (see Fig. 2.21).

ATP yield

The activation of palmitate to palmitoyl CoA consumes 2 molecules of ATP. β oxidation generates:

- 7 $FADH_2$, which are oxidized by the electron transport chain to generate 10.5 ATP.
- 7 NADH, which are oxidized by the chain to generate 17.5 ATP.
- 8 acetyl CoA, which are oxidized by the TCA cycle to generate 80 ATP (remember, oxidation of each acetyl CoA by the TCA cycle yields 10 ATP).

Therefore, the total energy generated from the oxidation of a molecule of palmitate is 106 ATP.

Oxidation of odd-numbered fatty acids

The oxidation of odd-numbered fatty acids (Fig. 4.14) is essentially the same as for even-numbered fatty acids, except that the last round of β oxidation produces one molecule of acetyl CoA and one of propionyl CoA (3C) instead of two molecules of acetyl CoA. Propionyl CoA is metabolized to succinyl CoA, which can then enter the TCA cycle.

Oxidation of unsaturated fatty acids

In the oxidation of unsaturated fatty acids, most of the reactions are the same as for saturated fatty acids

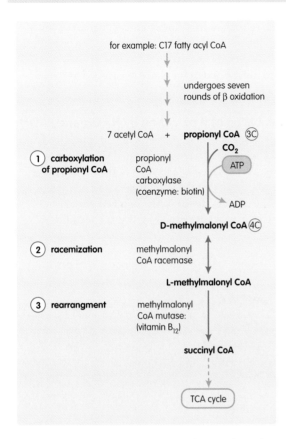

Fig. 4.14 Oxidation of odd-numbered fatty acids produces propionyl CoA, which is metabolized to succinyl CoA in three steps to enter the TCA cycle.

except two additional enzymes are involved, enoyl CoA isomerase and 2,4-dienoyl reductase. Naturally occurring unsaturated fatty acids contain *cis* double bonds. The enzymes of β oxidation, particularly enoyl CoA hydratase, which is specific for the *trans* configuration of double bonds, do not easily metabolize these. However, enoyl CoA isomerase converts a *cis* to a *trans* double bond, thus enabling β oxidation to proceed.

During the oxidation of some unsaturated fatty acids, for example, linoleic acid (*cis* Δ9,12, 18:2), the intermediate 2,4-dienoyl CoA is produced. This, again, is not a substrate for enoyl CoA hydratase; however, NADPH-dependent 2,4-dienoyl reductase reduces it to *trans* enoyl CoA, thus enabling β oxidation to continue. This 2,4-dienoyl CoA reductase enzyme has only recently been described. It was previously thought that an epimerase enzyme was required for oxidation of unsaturated fatty acids, but it is now known that this enzyme is only present in peroxisomes and not in mitochondria.

Peroxisomal β oxidation

Oxidation of fatty acids can also occur in peroxisomes, in the kidney and in the liver. Approximately 5–10% of the total oxidation of fatty acids occurs in peroxisomes, with the rest in mitochondria. The pathway of β oxidation in mitochondria and peroxisomes is identical; it is the enzymes that are different. The enzymes of peroxisomes are more versatile and can oxidize a wider range of substrates, including prostaglandins. The main function of peroxisomal oxidation is the shortening of long-chain fatty acids (e.g., those greater than 22–24 carbon atoms), preparing them for β oxidation by the mitochondrial system.

Different enzymes of peroxisomal and mitochondrial β oxidation
Oxidation
The FAD-containing enzyme acyl CoA dehydrogenase passes its electrons directly to oxygen, so no ATP is formed. Energy is dissipated as heat instead.

Hydration and oxidation
These are performed by the bifunctional enzyme which has both enoyl CoA hydratase and 3-hydroxyacyl CoA dehydrogenase activity.

Thiolysis
Thiolase cleaves acyl CoA, releasing acetyl CoA and a shortened acyl chain.

Oxidation continues until acyl CoA molecules are fewer than 22 carbons in length, at which point they diffuse out of the peroxisomes, via a pore-forming protein in the peroxisomal membrane, for further oxidation in mitochondria.

Regulation of lipid breakdown

The control of lipid breakdown is exerted at three levels (Fig. 4.15): lipolysis, carnitine shuttle and β oxidation.

Control of lipolysis
Hormone-sensitive lipase (see Fig. 4.11) is regulated by reversible phosphorylation. Adrenaline during exercise, and glucagon and adrenocorticotrophic hormone (ACTH) during starvation, activate adenylate cyclase, which increases the levels of cAMP. This activates a cAMP-dependent protein kinase, which phosphorylates lipase, activating it. The same cAMP-dependent protein kinase also phosphorylates acetyl CoA carboxylase, inhibiting

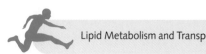
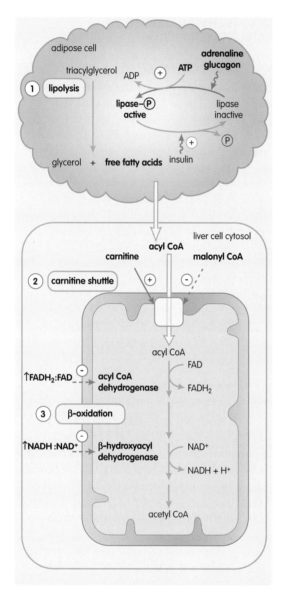

Fig. 4.15 Regulation of lipid breakdown. Control is exerted at three levels: **1.** lipolysis; **2.** the carnitine shuttle; **3.** β oxidation.

it (see Fig. 4.6); that is, it stimulates lipolysis but inhibits fatty acid synthesis. This is similar to the reciprocal mechanism of control of glycogen phosphorylase and synthase by reversible phosphorylation (see Fig. 2.34). Insulin brings about the dephosphorylation of lipase, inhibiting lipolysis.

Carnitine shuttle
Malonyl CoA inhibits carnitine acyl transferase I (CAT I), thus inhibiting the entry of acyl groups

into mitochondria. An increase in malonyl CoA is produced during fatty acid synthesis and ensures that newly synthesized fatty acids are not transported into mitochondria for oxidation as soon as they are made.

Inhibition of β oxidation by NADH and FADH$_2$
The oxidation reactions require a supply of FAD and NAD, which are regenerated via the electron transport chain. The enzymes of β oxidation have to compete with the dehydrogenase enzymes of the TCA cycle for NAD$^+$ and FAD because both pathways are usually active at the same time.

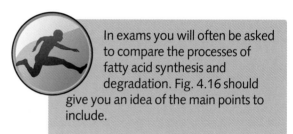

In exams you will often be asked to compare the processes of fatty acid synthesis and degradation. Fig. 4.16 should give you an idea of the main points to include.

Errors of fatty acid metabolism
Medium-chain fatty acyl CoA dehydrogenase deficiency
Medium-chain fatty acyl CoA dehydrogenase deficiency has an incidence of 1:10,000 births. It is thought that the deficiency of this enzyme leads to a decreased oxidation of fatty acids and therefore an increase in, and a greater reliance on, glucose oxidation. When glycogen reserves become exhausted, severe hypoglycemia occurs. It is believed that this is the cause of death in some cases of sudden infant death syndrome (crib death).

Jamaican vomiting sickness
This is thought to be caused by eating the unripe fruit of the ackee tree. The fruit contains a toxin, hypoglycin, which is in fact an unusual amino acid that inhibits both short- and medium-chain acyl CoA dehydrogenases. This results in the inhibition of β oxidation and therefore the oxidation of glucose takes place instead. Once glycogen reserves are depleted, hypoglycemia occurs.

Fig. 4.16 Comparison of fatty acid synthesis and degradation.

Comparison of fatty acid synthesis and degradation		
	Synthesis	**Degradation**
Active	after meals: fed state	fasting and prolonged exercise
Main tissues involved	liver and adipose tissue	muscle and liver
Site	cytosol	mitochondria
2C donor/product	acetyl CoA	acetyl CoA
Active fatty acid carrier	attached to ACP	attached to CoA
Enzymes	FAS: enzymes all part of multi-enzyme complex	probably not associated
Oxidant/reductant	NADPH	NAD^+ and FAD
Allosteric control	citrate activates acetyl CoA carboxylase; palmitoyl CoA inhibits it	malonyl CoA inhibits CAT I
Hormonal control	insulin activates acetyl CoA carboxylase; adrenaline and glucagon inhibit it	adrenaline and glucagon activate lipase; insulin inhibits it
Product	palmitate	acetyl CoA

Cholesterol metabolism

Role of cholesterol in the body

Cholesterol has many functions in the body, including being:

- An essential component of cell membranes.
- A precursor of the five major classes of steroid hormones: progestagens, estrogens, androgens, glucocorticoids, and mineralocorticoids.
- A precursor of bile acids and vitamin D.

The body therefore requires a continuous supply of cholesterol.

Sources of cholesterol

Cholesterol can either be obtained from the diet or be synthesized endogenously by the body. Regulatory mechanisms try to balance the amount of cholesterol made by the body daily with both the dietary intake and the amount excreted either in bile or as bile salts in order to enable control of the plasma cholesterol level. Failure of this control may lead to high plasma cholesterol levels and an increased risk of atherosclerosis and consequent coronary heart disease, stroke, and peripheral vascular disease.

Cholesterol synthesis

Cholesterol is a 27-carbon steroid molecule. All 27 carbon atoms of cholesterol come from acetyl CoA. It is one of a large group of compounds derived from the five-carbon isoprene group (others include ubiquinone and the vitamins A, E and K). The easiest way to view cholesterol synthesis is to divide it into two stages (Fig. 4.17):

- Stage I: The formation of the isoprene unit, isopentenyl pyrophosphate (IPP). This is formed by the condensation of three molecules of acetyl CoA to 3-hydroxy-3-methylglutaryl CoA (HMG-CoA), followed by the loss of CO_2.
- Stage II: The progressive condensation of isoprene units to form cholesterol. Six five-carbon isoprene units link up to form squalene (30C atoms) which cyclizes to lanosterol, from which cholesterol arises.

Location

Cholesterol is made by most tissues (except RBCs) but the main site of synthesis is the liver.

Site

Cell cytosol, although some of the enzymes are found in the endoplasmic reticulum. These stages are now considered in more detail and are clearly illustrated in Fig. 4.17.

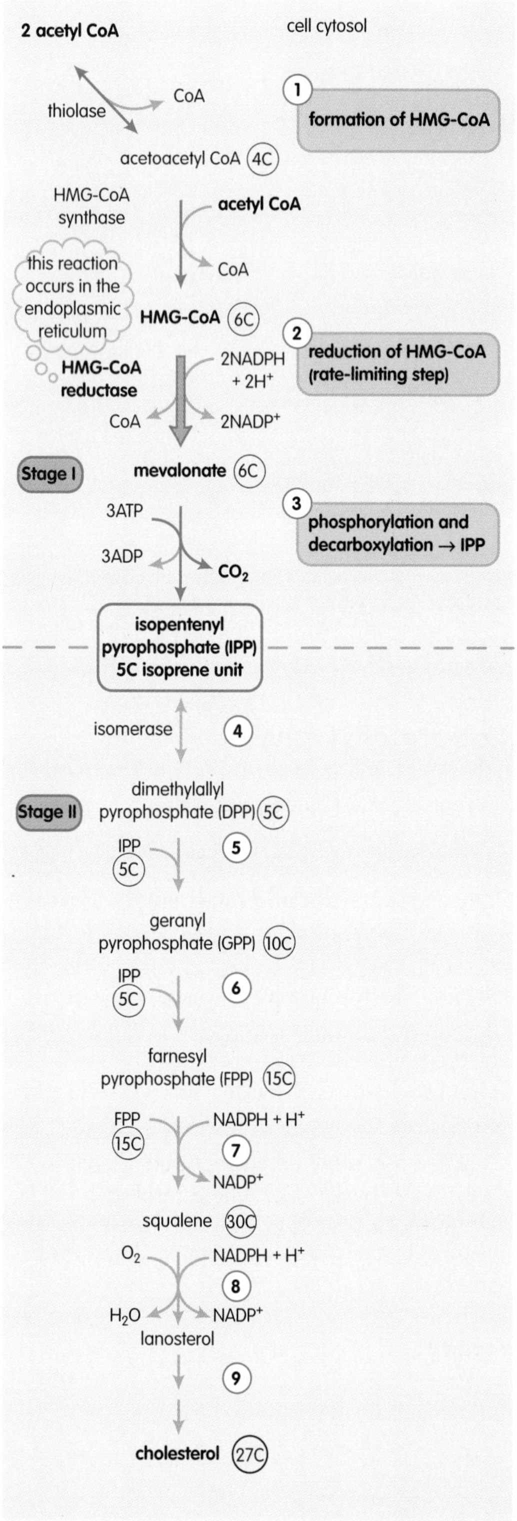

Fig. 4.17 Cholesterol synthesis. This multistep pathway is divided into two stages (numbers refer to the text).

Stage I: Formation of IPP

1. Formation of HMG-CoA from acetyl CoA

This occurs in two steps:

- Two molecules of acetyl CoA condense to form acetoacetyl CoA (4C).
- HMG-CoA synthase catalyzes the addition of a third molecule of acetyl CoA to form HMG-CoA (6C).

HMG-CoA is also an intermediate in the synthesis of ketone bodies. However, ketone body formation occurs in the mitochondria, whereas the reactions of cholesterol synthesis occur in the cell cytosol. The liver therefore contains two isoenzymes of HMG-CoA synthase: a cytosolic enzyme for cholesterol synthesis and a mitochondrial enzyme for ketone body formation.

2. Reduction of HMG-CoA to mevalonic acid (mevalonate)

This is the irreversible, rate-limiting step of cholesterol synthesis and thus the most important control site. The enzyme HMG-CoA reductase is found in the endoplasmic reticulum and requires NADPH as a reducing agent.

3. Phosphorylation and decarboxylation of mevalonate to IPP

Mevalonate is converted to IPP in three reactions requiring three molecules of ATP. The first two reactions are phosphorylations forming a pyrophosphome-valonate intermediate (not shown in Fig. 4.17), which is then decarboxylated to form isopentenyl pyrophosphate (IPP).

Stage II: Progressive condensation of isoprene units to cholesterol

4. Isomerization of IPP to dimethylallyl pyrophosphate

The five-carbon isoprene units then link up in a stepwise fashion as shown in Fig. 4.17.

5. IPP and dimethylallyl pyrophosphate condense to form the 10-carbon, geranyl pyrophosphate

6. Another IPP condenses with geranyl pyrophosphate to form the 15-carbon, farnesyl pyrophosphate

7. Squalene synthase catalyzes the reductive condensation of two molecules of farnesyl pyrophosphate, forming the 30-carbon molecule, squalene

All three condensation reactions (5, 6, and 7) release pyrophosphate (which "drives" the reactions), making them favorable.

8. Cyclization of squalene to lanosterol (30C) by squalene monoxygenase

9. Conversion of lanosterol to cholesterol

The exact pathway is not known, but it is thought to consist of about 20 steps! Basically, three methyl groups are removed to produce a 27-carbon molecule followed by the migration of the double bond to the $\Delta5$ position to produce cholesterol (Fig. 4.18).

Regulation of cholesterol synthesis

Regulation is necessary in order to prevent high plasma cholesterol levels, which may lead to cholesterol deposition in arterial walls and the formation of atherosclerotic plaques. Indeed, the primary control site is the rate-limiting enzyme HMG-CoA reductase (Fig. 4.19).

Product inhibition

HMG-CoA reductase is allosterically inhibited by cholesterol. HMG-CoA reductase inhibition is a mechanism of action of drugs inhibiting cholesterol synthesis (statins).

Short-term hormonal regulation

- HMG-CoA reductase is also regulated by hormone-dependent reversible phosphorylation by a similar mechanism to glycogen synthase (see Fig. 2.34) and acetyl CoA carboxylase.

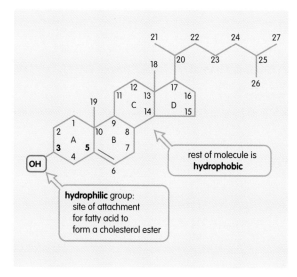

Fig. 4.18 Structure of cholesterol.

- Glucagon activates a cAMP-dependent protein kinase that reversibly phosphorylates HMG-CoA reductase, inhibiting it and therefore decreasing the rate of cholesterol synthesis.
- Insulin dephosphorylates the enzyme, leading to its activation and an increase in cholesterol synthesis.

Long-term regulation of HMG-CoA reductase

- This is the most important control mechanism.
- The amount of cholesterol, both dietary and endogenous, taken up by cells affects the amount of HMG-CoA reductase synthesized.
- A high cholesterol level in cells causes a decrease in the rate of transcription of the HMG-CoA reductase gene, inhibiting it and leading to a reduction in cholesterol synthesis.

High intracellular levels of cholesterol also suppress the synthesis of cholesterol receptors, resulting in a decrease in the uptake of cholesterol by the cell. A low intracellular cholesterol concentration stimulates receptor synthesis. This is the most important mechanism of the regulation of cholesterol level in plasma.

Packaging of cholesterol

Most of the cholesterol in the blood is in the form of cholesterol esters, formed by the addition of a fatty acid to the C3-OH group (see Fig. 4.18). Esterification makes the cholesterol more hydrophobic, enabling it to be packaged, stored, and transported more easily. Two enzyme systems are responsible for the esterification of cholesterol (numbers refer to Fig. 4.20):

1. In cells:
   - If the cholesterol taken up or synthesized by cells is not immediately required, then it is esterified by acyl CoA:cholesterol acyl transferase (ACAT).
   - ACAT transfers a fatty acid from a fatty acyl CoA to cholesterol, forming a cholesterol ester that can be stored in the cell.
2. In the high-density lipoproteins:
   - A similar enzyme, known as lecithin:cholesterol acyl transferase (LCAT), is found associated with high-density lipoproteins (HDLs).
   - HDL is responsible for picking up free cholesterol from peripheral tissues and transporting it to the liver; that is, it acts as a cholesterol scavenger.

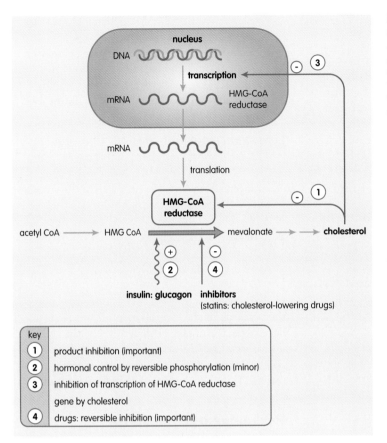

Fig. 4.19 Control of HMG-CoA reductase. This enzyme is not only affected by cholesterol as its product in an allosteric fashion but also because cholesterol actually downregulates the transcription of HMG-CoA reductase, which catalyzes the rate-limiting step of cholesterol synthesis.

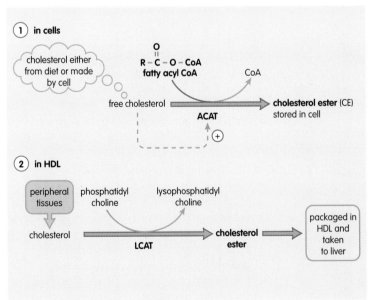

Fig. 4.20 Two enzyme systems are responsible for the esterification of cholesterol—acyl CoA:cholesterol acyl transferase in cells, and lecithin:cholesterol acyl transferase in HDL.

- LCAT catalyzes the transfer of a fatty acid from the phospholipid, phosphatidylcholine, to cholesterol.
- HDL then carries cholesterol esters to the liver, either to be reused or excreted.

For patients with a high plasma cholesterol (hypercholesterolemia), treatment includes drugs that reversibly inhibit HMG-CoA reductase. Therefore, these drugs, known as statins, decrease the rate of cholesterol synthesis by cells. Cells compensate for lower cholesterol levels by increasing the synthesis (and thus the number) of cholesterol receptors on the cell surface. This increases cholesterol uptake by the cells and therefore reduces plasma cholesterol.

Transport of lipids

Lipoproteins

Lipids are insoluble in aqueous solution and therefore are transported in the plasma in association with proteins in the form of lipoproteins (Fig. 4.21). Lipoproteins function both to solubilize the lipids and to provide an efficient transport system for them. If the system fails, the plasma lipid concentration will increase. Long term, a high plasma cholesterol level is associated with an increased risk of atherosclerosis.

Some apolipoproteins are only weakly associated with lipoprotein complexes and can be transferred easily between them. They have a number of functions, including acting:

- As recognition sites or ligands for receptors.
- As structural components.
- As activators or coenzymes for enzymes involved in lipid metabolism.

The functions of the major apolipoproteins are summarized in Fig. 4.22.

Classes of lipoprotein

There are five main classes of lipoproteins: chylomicrons (CMs), very-low-density lipoproteins (VLDLs), intermediate-density lipoproteins (IDLs), low-density lipoproteins (LDLs), and high-density lipoproteins (HDLs). They are classified according to increasing density, with CMs having the lowest density and HDLs the highest. Remember, protein is more dense than lipid and so HDLs, with the highest density, must contain the most protein. Lipoproteins differ in composition, size, function, and the apolipoproteins present on their surface. These properties are summarized in Fig. 4.23.

Pathways of lipid transport

Lipids can either be obtained from the diet (exogenous lipids) or synthesized by the body (endogenous lipids). There are two different pathways for lipid transport in the body:

- Exogenous pathway: CMs transport dietary lipid absorbed from the intestine to the tissues (Fig. 4.24).
- Endogenous pathway: VLDLs, IDLs and LDLs form a continuous cascade. The VLDLs transport endogenously synthesized triacylglycerol from the liver to the tissues (Fig. 4.25).

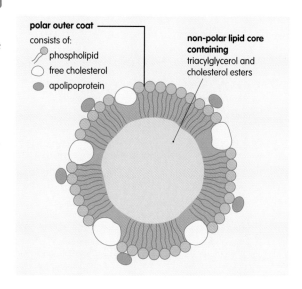

Fig. 4.21 The basic structure of a lipoprotein particle consists of a nonpolar lipid core containing triacylglycerol (TG) and cholesterol esters surrounded by a polar outer coat of phospholipids and free cholesterol, which also contains proteins known as apolipoproteins.

73

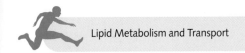

Functions of the major apolipoproteins	
Apolipoprotein	**Function**
A-I	activates lecithin:cholesterol acyl transferase
A-II	activates hepatic lipase
B-48	structural chylomicrons (CM)
B-100	structural; binds to the apoB/E (LDL) receptor increases cholesterol uptake
C-I	cofactor for lecithin:cholesterol acyl transferase
C-II	activates lipoprotein lipase
C-III	inhibits lipoprotein lipase?
E	binds to apo. B/E (LDL) receptor and increases uptake of LDL and remnant particles including CM remnants

Fig. 4.22 Functions of major apolipoproteins.

These pathways can now be considered in more detail.

Exogenous pathway (numbers refer to Fig. 4.24)

1. CM formation

CMs are assembled in intestinal mucosal cells from dietary fat. They contain mainly triacylglycerol with some cholesterol and apolipoprotein B-48. These newly formed chylomicrons are referred to as nascent CMs.

2. Circulation of CMs

Nascent CMs travel in the lymphatic system to enter the blood via the thoracic duct. When they reach the blood they acquire apolipoprotein C-II and E from HDL.

Classification and properties of lipoproteins				
Class	**Main composition**	**Diameter (nm)**	**Source and function**	**Major apolipoproteins**
CM	90% triacylglycerol	500	transport of **dietary** triacylglycerol	A-I, II, B-48, C-I, II, III, E
VLDL	65% triacylglycerol	43	transport of **endogenously** synthesized triacylglycerol from the liver to peripheral tissues	B-100, C-I, II, III, E
IDL	35% phospholipid 25% cholesterol	27	formed by partial breakdown of VLDL, precursor of LDL	B-100, C-III, E
LDL	50% cholesterol 25% protein	22	formed by breakdown of IDL; carries cholesterol to peripheral tissues	B-100
HDL	55% protein 25% phospholipid	8	formed in the liver and intestine; 2 main functions: • reverse cholesterol transport removes cholesterol from tissues and takes it to liver; "cholesterol scavenge" • exchanges apolipoproteins and cholesterol esters with chylomicrons and VLDL	A-I, II, C-I, II, III, D, E

Fig. 4.23 Classification and properties of lipoproteins.

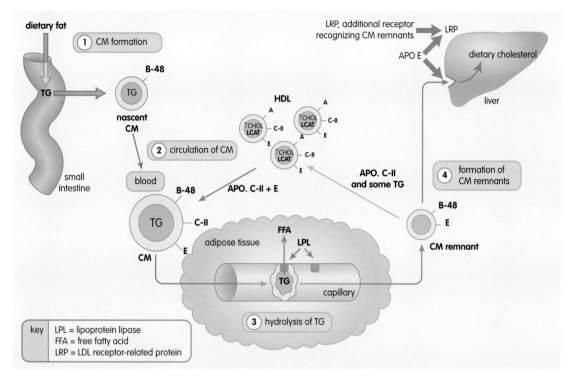

Fig. 4.24 Exogenous pathway of lipid transport (numbers refer to the text below).

3. Hydrolysis of triacylglycerol

CMs are carried in the blood to tissues; for example, adipose tissue and muscle. As they pass through the capillaries of tissues, the enzyme lipoprotein lipase, found on the luminal surface of the capillary endothelium, is activated by apolipoprotein C-II on the surface of the CMs. Lipoprotein lipase hydrolyzes a large part of the CMs' triacylglycerol to glycerol and free fatty acids. The fatty acids are taken up by cells, either for oxidation or resynthesis to triacylglycerol.

4. Formation of CM remnants

The removal of triacylglycerol leaves behind a much smaller CM remnant particle. Apolipoprotein C-II is returned to HDL. Apolipoproteins B-48 and E are recognized by remnant receptors on liver cells and the CM remnants are taken up by the liver and degraded (see Fig. 4.19).

Endogenous pathway (numbers refer to Fig. 4.25)

The liver is the main site of lipid synthesis.

1. Assembly of VLDLs

VLDLs are synthesized in the liver, mostly from triacylglycerol, and are released as nascent VLDL particles containing surface apolipoprotein B-100. Like CMs, VLDLs acquire apolipoprotein C-II and E from HDL. VLDL transports endogenous triacylglycerol to peripheral tissues.

2. Hydrolysis by lipoprotein lipase (LPL) in tissues

Lipoprotein lipase removes triacylglycerol in the same way as for CMs. VLDLs become smaller in size and more dense (VLDL remnants). Cholesterol released from the remnants contributes to the inhibition of HMG-CoA reductase and thus to the decrease in endogenous synthesis of cholesterol by the liver.

3. Formation of IDL and LDL

Some triacylglycerol, phospholipids and apolipoprotein C-II are transferred to HDL, converting VLDL to the denser lipoprotein, IDL. Cholesterol esters are transferred from HDL to IDL in exchange for triacylglycerol and phospholipid by cholesterol ester transfer protein (CETP). Some of the IDLs are taken up by the liver via receptors

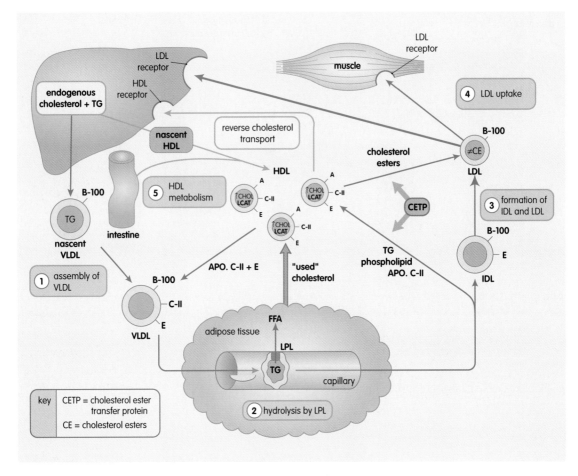

Fig. 4.25 Endogenous pathway of lipid transport (numbers refer to the text below).

that recognize both apolipoprotein B and apolipoprotein E on the surface of IDL (not shown in Fig. 4.25); but the rest forms LDL (note that the well-known LDL-receptor is in fact an apoB/E receptor).

4. LDL provides cholesterol for peripheral tissues
LDL binds to LDL receptors on cell membranes and is internalized by receptor-mediated endocytosis. The LDL receptor recognizes apolipoprotein B-100 on the LDL. Lysosomal enzymes hydrolyze LDL, releasing free cholesterol into the cell.

5. HDL metabolism
HDL is made in the liver and has two main functions:
• It accepts the free cholesterol from peripheral tissues and lipoproteins and esterifies it by the action of LCAT (see Fig. 4.20). The cholesterol esters formed are either transferred to VLDL or IDL to form LDL, or are carried back to the liver by "reverse cholesterol transport."

• HDL also exchanges apolipoproteins with other lipoproteins (CMs and VLDL) as already described.

Effects of cholesterol inside cells
Cholesterol inhibits HMG-CoA reductase activity and therefore cholesterol synthesis. It does this by both product inhibition and by the inhibition of the transcription of the HMG-CoA reductase gene (see Fig. 4.19). Cholesterol also inhibits LDL receptor synthesis. An increased cholesterol concentration in the cell down-regulates the synthesis of LDL receptors by decreasing the rate of transcription of the LDL receptor gene. This limits the uptake of cholesterol.

If cholesterol is not immediately required by the cell, the enzyme ACAT esterifies cholesterol for storage in cells (see Fig. 4.20).

Whereas an increase in LDL-cholesterol is harmful, an increase in HDL-cholesterol has a protective effect because it removes cholesterol from tissues and takes it to the liver for degradation and excretion. It is known that one or two glasses of red wine each day increase the levels of HDL. Unfortunately, this is seen only with one or two glasses, so most people will not notice this beneficial effect!

Disorders of lipid metabolism and transport

The dyslipidemias are a group of disorders caused by a defect at a stage in the course of either lipoprotein formation, transport or degradation (Fig. 4.26). They result in the accumulation of lipids in the blood and, in most cases, an increased risk of atherosclerosis (coronary disease, stroke and peripheral vascular disease). Thus dyslipidemias occur as a result of a deficiency in either:

- An enzyme; for example, LPL deficiency.
- An apolipoprotein; for example, apolipoprotein C-II deficiency.
- A receptor; for example, LDL receptor defect.

Disorders of lipid metabolism: dyslipidemias			
Type	Name	Cause	Effect on lipoproteins
I	**familial LPL deficiency or apo C-II deficiency** autosomal recessive	decreased or absent LPL activity	increased CMs cause a milky serum increased triacylglycerol may cause acute pancreatitis
IIa	**familial hypercholesterolemia** autosomal dominant (1:5000)	defect or total absence of LDL receptors (occasionally caused by a defect in apolipoprotein B-100)	decreased uptake of LDL by tissues and increased plasma cholesterol concentration homozygotes have no receptors and die of coronary heart disease in childhood
IIb	**familial combined hyperlipidemia** autosomal dominant	overproduction of apo B by liver	increased VLDL secretion leads to increased LDL [increased plasma cholesterol and triacylglycerol]
III	**familial dysbetalipoproteinemia**	abnormal apolipoprotein E decrease in remnant clearance by liver	increased remnant particles (IDL); increased risk of peripheral vascular disease and coronary heart disease
IV	**familial hypertriglyceridemia**: mild form	overproduction of VLDL by the liver	increased VLDL
V	**familial hypertriglyceridemia**: severe form	overproduction of VLDL by the liver	increased VLDL and increased CMs

Fig. 4.26 Disorders of lipid metabolism: dyslipidemias (hyperlipidemias).

The dyslipidemias

This is a group of inherited disorders of lipid metabolism. They are also called hyperlipidemias; dyslipidemia is a better term because some disorders of lipoprotein metabolism actually involve a decrease in lipoprotein (e.g., HDL) concentration. Fig. 4.26 shows the classification of these disorders based on the Fredrickson classification. In practice his classification is now rarely used. The correct clinical classification divides dyslipidemias into hypercholesterolemia, hypertriglyceridemia, and mixed disorders.

Here, the main clinical features of the more important dyslipidemias are considered. There are two complementary approaches to the treatment of dyslipidemias: diet and/or drugs. The main drugs used to control lipid metabolism are listed in Fig. 4.27.

Familial lipoprotein lipase or apolipoprotein C-II deficiency (Type I)

This is a rare, autosomal recessive disorder, due to either a deficiency of the enzyme lipoprotein lipase (LPL) or apolipoprotein C-II required for the activation of LPL. It results in a failure of the clearance of chylomicrons from the bloodstream; therefore, it is also called familial chylomicronemia. Its main clinical features, diagnosis and management are discussed in Fig. 4.28.

Familial hypercholesterolemia (FH) (Type IIa)

Familial hypercholesterolemia is the most common and the most important inherited lipid disorder. It is an autosomal dominant disease with a prevalence of 1:500 (0.2%) for heterozygotes and $1:10^6$ for homozygotes. The cause in the majority of patients (95%) is a defect in the LDL receptor: either a decrease in the actual number of receptors or malfunctioning receptors (for example, a mutation in the apoB-100 binding site). A smaller number of patients (5%) have a defective apoB-100 molecule. For all patients, there is a defect in the uptake of LDL, leading to an increase in plasma LDL concentration. In homozygotes, no LDL receptors are present, leading to grossly elevated plasma cholesterol levels, as high as 20 mmol/L. This causes a massive deposition of cholesterol in the arterial walls and skin. These patients usually develop coronary heart disease in childhood and, if untreated, rarely survive to adult life.

Main drugs used to control lipid metabolism	
Drug	**Mechanism of action**
statins: simvastatin, lovastatin	inhibit **HMG-CoA reductase**, decreasing cholesterol synthesis; cell compensates for lower intracellular cholesterol by increasing LDL receptor synthesis, resulting in increased cholesterol uptake, thus leading to decreased plasma cholesterol
fibrates: bezafibrate, gemfibrozil	activate LPL (main effect), thus lowering plasma TG; slightly suppress HMG-CoA reductase, decrease the synthesis of apo B and increase apo A
anion exchange resins: cholestyramine, colestipol	bind bile acids in gastrointestinal tract preventing their reabsorption and therefore decrease plasma LDL levels
nicotinic acid	decreases VLDL production by liver and thus LDL; increases LPL activity, leading to decreased triacylglycerol
fish oils	reduce triacylglycerol synthesis in the liver

Fig. 4.27 Main drugs used to control lipid metabolism.

Clinical features and diagnosis of type I hyperlipidemia		
Clinical features	**Diagnosis**	**Management**
presents in childhood with: • eruptive xanthomas • lipemia retinalis and retinal vein thrombosis • recurrent abdominal pain • risk of pancreatitis • hepatosplenomegaly	based on the presence of high levels of chylomicrons in fasting sample of plasma stored overnight in fasting sample, white layer at top due to chylomicrons which float like cream	depends on serum triacylglycerol concentration: <2.0 mmol/L = normal 2.0–4.0 mmol/L = minor problem; check other risk factors >4.0 mmol/L = treatment required [diet or diet and drugs]

Fig. 4.28 The clinical features and diagnosis of type I hyperlipidemia, familial LPL deficiency (this is very rare).

Clinical features of FH	
Clinical Features	**Diagnosis and Management**
homozygotes: tendon xanthomata: thickening of Achilles tendon and xanthomata over extensor tendons of fingers xanthelasma: white yellow fatty deposits in skin of eyelid (non-diagnostic) premature arcus senilis: thin white rim around iris of eye	**diagnosis:** • fasting cholesterol usually > 16 mmol/L **management:** • diet: very low in cholesterol and saturated fat • drugs: statins, cholesterol binding resins, nicotinic acid (see Fig. 4.27) • low-density lipoprotein removal by plasmapheresis • liver transplant • gene therapy: trials are under way
heterozygotes: • as above but not as severe • may have no physical signs	**diagnosis:** fasting cholesterol >8 mmol/L **management:** • diet • cholesterol-lowering drugs

Fig. 4.29 The clinical features of familial hypercholesterolemia.

The clinical features, diagnosis, and management of familial hypercholesterolemia are discussed in Fig. 4.29. The prognosis for homozygotes is poor. Plasmapheresis, if used regularly, is successful in the short term. Liver transplantation offers the possibility of a cure. For heterozygotes, the prognosis is reasonable; still these patients tend to develop coronary heart disease earlier than the normal population and therefore require lipid-lowering treatment.

Do not confuse familial hypercholesterolemia with the polygenic form, common hypercholesterolemia.

Familial combined hyperlipidemia (Type IIb)

Familial combined hyperlipidemia is relatively common, with a prevalence of 1:300. The genetic basis is unclear, but it is probably autosomal dominant. The abnormality is an overproduction of apolipoprotein B, leading to an increased VLDL secretion from the liver, which results in an increased plasma LDL. Usually, both plasma cholesterol and triacylglycerol are elevated (Fig. 4.30).

Clinical features and diagnosis of familial combined *hyperlipidemia*	
Clinical features	**Diagnosis and management**
signs are usually present: • xanthelasma • arcus senilis	**diagnosis:** ↑ low-density lipoprotein and ↑ triacylglycerol (triglycerides; TG) with a positive family history of early coronary disease treatment is aimed at reducing cholesterol to <5.0 mmol/L and TG to <2.0 mmol/L **management:** • diet • fibrates reduce both cholesterol and TG, and high-density lipoprotein

Fig. 4.30 The clinical features and diagnosis of familial combined hyperlipidemia.

Remnant hyperlipidemia (familial dysbetalipoproteinemia) (Type III)

Remnant hyperlipidemia (familial dysbetalipoproteinemia) is rare, with a prevalence of 1:10,000. It occurs due to inheritance of an abnormal apolipoprotein E molecule. It results in the increased accumulation of IDL (remnants) in the blood. Patients have an increased risk of coronary heart disease.

The clinical features are palmar xanthomas (which are actually reasonably diagnostic) and tuberous xanthomas over the knees and elbows.

The diagnosis is made by measurement of a raised total cholesterol and triacylglycerol, and electrophoresis of the serum, showing a "broad β-band" due to excess of remnants (see Fig. 11.13).

Familial hypertriglyceridemia (Types IV and V)
Type IV

This is the mild form of hypertriglyceridemia. The prevalence is 1:600. It is an autosomal dominant disorder caused by an increased synthesis of VLDL by the liver, leading to a raised plasma VLDL.

Type V

This is the severe form of hypertriglyceridemia. Other risk factors such as obesity and alcohol are also implicated in its etiology, leading to an increase in plasma VLDL and chylomicrons.

Clinical features Physical signs are seen only with the severe form; for example, eruptive xanthomas and lipemia retinalis. Plasma triacylglycerol is very high, and consequently there is usually high plasma cholesterol. The increased triacylglycerol concentration is associated with an increased risk of pancreatitis.

Treatment The treatment is diet, aiming to reduce body weight and to modify any coexisting factors, such as alcohol, diabetes, or obesity. Drugs used include fibrates, nicotinic acid derivatives (which decrease VLDL synthesis), and fish oils.

Common hypercholesterolemia

This includes patients who have a raised serum cholesterol but do not have familial hypercholesterolemia. It has a polygenic inheritance; that is, it is influenced by several genes. The plasma cholesterol is not as high as in familial hypercholesterolemia and is influenced by the environment (e.g., diet). Dietary treatment alone is often successful.

Metabolic adaptation to starvation, exercise and diabetes are very common topics for exam questions. The use of ketone bodies as fuel is just one of the adaptation mechanisms. You must know which fuels are used and why.

Ketone bodies and ketogenesis

The roles of the ketone bodies

Ketone bodies, namely acetoacetic acid, 3-hydroxybutyric acid, and acetone, provide an alternative fuel for cells and are produced at low levels all the time. However, they are produced in significant quantities only during adverse states such as starvation, prolonged severe exercise, or uncontrolled diabetes. A severe increase in ketone bodies decreases blood pH (acidemia).

Starvation

In the fed state, the brain uses only glucose as its energy source, since fatty acids cannot cross the blood–brain barrier. During starvation, the brain adapts to using ketone bodies as its major fuel because they are soluble and can therefore cross the blood–brain barrier. This reduces the need for glucose when glycogen reserves are depleted. In this starved state, glucose would have to come from the breakdown of muscle protein into amino acids, which are then oxidized to glucose by gluconeogenesis. Therefore, the use of ketone bodies as a fuel spares glucose and preserves muscle protein. In starvation the production of ketone bodies is usually controlled, so that their rate of formation is equal to their rate of use. This prevents the accumulation of acidic ketone bodies, so the pH of the blood remains within normal limits.

Diabetes

In well-controlled diabetes, tissues receive an adequate glucose supply and ketone body production is minimal. Poorly controlled diabetes leads to the massive production of acidic ketone bodies, to the point where the rate of formation is far greater than the rate of use. This can lead to life-threatening, severe ketoacidosis, as the accumulation of hydrogen ions exceeds the buffering capacity of the blood.

Synthesis of ketone bodies

Ketone bodies are formed from acetyl CoA arising mainly from the β oxidation of fatty acids (Fig. 4.31).

Location

Liver mitochondria.

Pathway

The synthesis of ketone bodies (ketogenesis) is a five-step pathway (illustrated in Fig. 4.31). Three molecules of acetyl CoA condense to form HMG-CoA, which is then cleaved to acetoacetate. The first two reactions are the same as for cholesterol synthesis, but ketone bodies are formed in the mitochondria, whereas cholesterol is synthesized in the cytosol (see Fig. 4.17).

3-Hydroxybutyrate is formed by the reduction of acetoacetate. The ratio of 3-hydroxybutyrate to acetoacetate formed depends on the availability of NADH.

The spontaneous decarboxylation of acetoacetate forms acetone, but usually only a small amount is made. Acetone can be smelt on the breath when the concentration of ketone bodies is high, especially in people with poorly controlled diabetes.

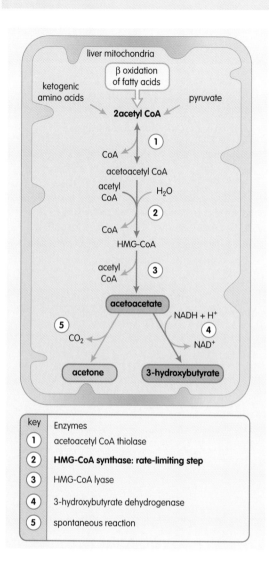

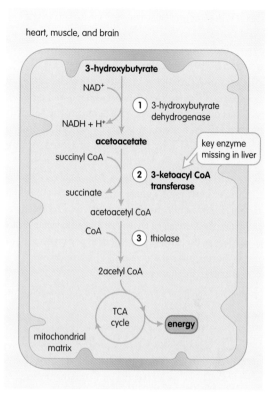

Fig. 4.32 Oxidation and utilization of ketone bodies. The pathway includes three reactions:
1. The oxidation of 3-hydroxybutyrate back to acetoacetate.
2. The activation of acetoacetate, which involves the transfer of CoA from succinyl CoA, catalyzed by 3-ketoacyl CoA transferase. Therefore, only tissues with this enzyme can oxidize ketone bodies (it cannot take place in the liver).
3. Thiolase cleaves acetoacetyl CoA to produce two molecules of acetyl CoA, which enter the TCA cycle for oxidation and ATP production.

Fig. 4.31 Synthesis of ketone bodies. The five-step pathway to synthesize ketone bodies takes place in liver mitochondria; the first two steps are the same as for cholesterol synthesis.

Control of the pathway

Acetyl CoA formed by β oxidation of fatty acids usually enters the TCA cycle. During starvation or diabetes, the oxaloacetate necessary for acetyl CoA to combine with, to form citrate, is directed to gluconeogenesis to help maintain the blood glucose. Therefore, acetyl CoA is used to form ketone bodies instead.

Use of ketone bodies

Ketone bodies are carried in the blood to various tissues, mainly the heart, muscle and the brain, where they are oxidized in mitochondria to acetyl CoA, which can enter the TCA cycle (Fig. 4.32). Ketone bodies are important sources of energy for these tissues. In fact, the heart uses ketone bodies as a fuel in preference to glucose. The liver cannot use ketone bodies despite being the site of their synthesis. This is because it lacks 3-ketoacyl CoA transferase. RBCs cannot metabolize ketone bodies because they have no mitochondria.

ATP yield from the oxidation of ketone bodies

The oxidation of 3-hydroxybutyrate produces two molecules of acetyl CoA. The oxidation of each acetyl CoA by the TCA cycle yields 10 molecules

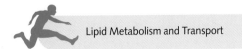

of ATP. There is no net formation of NADH (the NADH formed in the breakdown of 3-hydroxybutyrate is used in its synthesis). So, the oxidation of 3-hydroxybutyrate produces 20 molecules of ATP. However, in order to calculate the true, total ATP yield from the oxidation of a ketone body, it is necessary to take into account the origin of the acetyl CoA. For example, if the acetyl CoA used in the synthesis of 3-hydroxybutyrate arose from the oxidation of a fatty acid, a total of 26 molecules of ATP would be generated (Fig. 4.33). The ATP yield from the oxidation of a glucose molecule is 32 ATP (see Fig. 2.20). Therefore, the ATP yield from the oxidation of a ketone body is comparable with that of glucose, showing that ketone bodies are an excellent energy source and substitute for glucose during adverse states such as starvation.

ATP yield if acetyl CoA arose from a fatty acid	
	ATP yield
two ATP required to activate fatty acid → acyl CoA	−2
to form two acetyl CoA, fatty acid undergoes two rounds of β oxidation	
releases two NADH → electron transport chain	5
releases two FADH$_2$ → electron transport chain	3
oxidation of two molecules acetyl CoA by TCA cycle	20
total	26 ATP

Fig. 4.33 ATP yield from the oxidation of 3-hydroxybutyrate if the acetyl CoA from which it was synthesized was derived from a fatty acid.

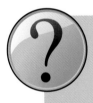

- How is fatty acid synthesis controlled?
- What is the importance of the class of acids to which linoleic acid belongs?
- How does insulin influence lipid breakdown?
- Describe the three main control sites of lipid breakdown.
- Describe the main functions of cholesterol.
- What are the risk factors for coronary heart disease?
- List the clinical features of familial hypercholesterolemia.
- What are the biochemical and clinical consequences of poor control of plasma cholesterol?
- What is the mechanism of action of statins?
- How are fatty acids implicated in sudden infant death syndrome?
- Describe the regulatory mechanisms for HMG-CoA reductase.
- What are the metabolic differences between the endogenous and exogenous transport of lipids?
- Outline the two pathways for lipid transport in the body.
- What is the role of ketone bodies in exercise?
- Name the tissues that can use ketone bodies.

5. Protein Metabolism

Biosynthesis of nonessential amino acids

Essential amino acids
In the body there are 20 amino acids, nine of which are essential; the other 11 are nonessential. The essential amino acids are those which cannot be synthesized by the body and therefore have to be obtained from the diet.

These nine essential amino acids are:
- Histidine (His) (infants only).
- Valine (Val).
- Leucine (Leu).
- Isoleucine (Ile).
- Lysine (Lys).
- Methionine (Met).
- Threonine (Thr).
- Phenylalanine (Phe).
- Tryptophan (Trp).

Histidine and arginine are regarded as essential only during periods of rapid cell growth such as infancy, childhood, or illness. At other times arginine is synthesized in sufficient quantities by the body.

Nonessential amino acids
These 11 amino acids can be synthesized by the body from intermediates of the TCA cycle and other metabolic pathways. They are:
- Tyrosine (Tyr).
- Glycine (Gly).
- Alanine (Ala).
- Cysteine (Cys).
- Serine (Ser).
- Aspartate (Asp).
- Asparagine (Asn).
- Glutamate (Glu).
- Glutamine (Gln).
- Arginine (Arg).
- Proline (Pro).

The pathways for the synthesis of these nonessential amino acids will be considered in this chapter.

Key reactions of amino acid metabolism
There are two main reactions essential to amino acid metabolism: transamination and oxidative deamination. You must know about them.

Transamination converts one amino acid into another
Working definition
Aminotransferases (or transaminases) catalyze the transfer of the α-amino group (NH_3^+) from an amino acid to an α-ketoacid (either pyruvate, oxaloacetate or, most often, α-ketoglutarate) (Fig. 5.1). A new amino acid and a new keto-acid are formed. If the acceptor is α-ketoglutarate, then glutamate is produced. All transamination reactions are fully reversible. Remember, the amino group is not released.

Site
Aminotransferases are found in both the cytosol and the mitochondria.

Mechanism
Aminotransferases all require pyridoxal phosphate (PLP), a vitamin B_6 derivative, as a cofactor. The pyridoxal phosphate is covalently linked to a lysine residue in the active site of the enzyme and therefore takes part in the reaction. The two most important aminotransferases are alanine aminotransferase (ALT) and aspartate aminotransferase (AST).

Aminotransferases are central to amino acid metabolism. They are used both for the synthesis of amino acids and for their breakdown. During breakdown, all amino groups are ultimately transferred to α-ketoglutarate because only glutamate can undergo rapid oxidative deamination.

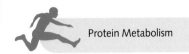

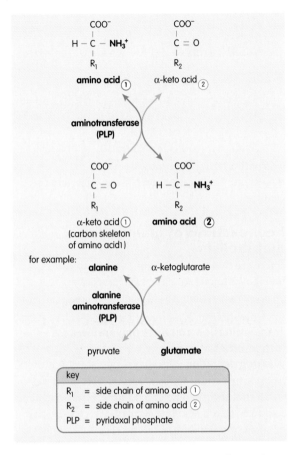

Fig. 5.1 Transamination reaction. Aminotransferases (or transaminases) catalyze the transfer of the α-amino group (NH$_3^+$) from an amino acid to an α-ketoacid (pyruvate, oxaloacetate, or, most often, α-ketoglutarate).

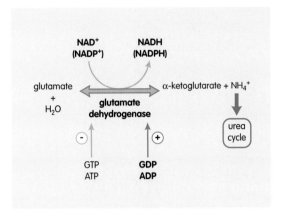

Fig. 5.2 Oxidative deamination of glutamate. Glutamate dehydrogenase removes the amino group from glutamate, leaving behind the carbon skeleton, α-ketoglutarate.

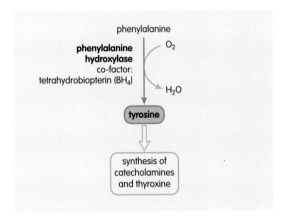

Fig. 5.3 Tyrosine synthesis. Tyrosine is formed by the hydroxylation of the essential amino acid phenylalanine by phenylalanine hydroxylase.

Oxidative deamination removes the amino group

Glutamate dehydrogenase removes the amino group from glutamate, leaving behind the carbon skeleton (Fig. 5.2). The ammonia formed enters the urea cycle (discussed later in this chapter) and the carbon skeletons (α-ketoacids) are all glycolytic and TCA cycle intermediates. Glutamate dehydrogenase is specific for glutamate and is unusual because it can use either NAD$^+$ or NADP$^+$ as a cofactor.

Site

Mitochondria.

Control

The reaction is reversible. ATP and GTP allosterically inhibit the enzyme; GDP and ADP activate it. Therefore, when energy levels are low,

amino acids are deaminated to provide α-ketoglutarate for the TCA cycle to generate energy. Deamination can also be achieved by other minor enzymes (see p. 92).

Biosynthetic pathways of nonessential amino acids

Tyrosine

Tyrosine is formed by the hydroxylation of the essential amino acid phenylalanine by phenylalanine hydroxylase (Fig. 5.3). This is an irreversible reaction; therefore, phenylalanine cannot be made from tyrosine. The enzyme requires the cofactor tetrahydrobiopterin, which takes part in the hydroxylation. The genetic deficiency of phenylalanine hydroxylase leads to phenylketonuria, a disease characterized by an accumulation of phenylalanine (this is discussed fully below). Tyrosine is the precursor of the catecholamines, namely dopamine, epinephrine, and norepinephrine as well as melanin and the hormone thyroxine. Its synthesis is regulated by the demand for these molecules.

Serine, glycine, and cysteine

These three amino acids are all formed from glycolytic intermediates. Both glycine and cysteine can be formed from serine.

Serine synthesis

There are a number of possible pathways available for the synthesis of serine (letters refer to Fig. 5.4).

a. The main pathway takes place in the cell cytosol. Serine is formed from the glycolytic intermediate 3-phosphoglycerate in three steps: oxidation, transamination to 3-phosphoserine, and hydrolysis to serine.

b. Serine can also be synthesized from glycine in mitochondria. Serine hydroxymethyl transferase transfers a hydroxymethyl group to glycine. The reaction is reversible; glycine and serine are thus interconvertible. The enzyme requires pyridoxal phosphate as a cofactor.

Glycine synthesis

c. Glycine synthesis takes place via two main pathways, both of which occur in mitochondria (see Fig. 5.4):

- Glycine can also be formed from CO_2, NH_4^+, and N^5N^{10}-methylene tetrahydrofolate (THF) (a donor of one-carbon units; see Chapter 6) in a reaction catalyzed by glycine synthase (glycine cleavage enzyme). This is probably the main pathway.
- From serine, by way of serine hydroxymethyl transferase (this is merely a reversal of serine synthesis).

Glycine has many functions in the body; for example:

- It is a component of proteins, especially collagen, and it is also used in glutathione, creatine, porphyrin and purine synthesis.
- It participates in the metabolism and excretion of drugs.
- It acts as an inhibitory neurotransmitter in the brain.

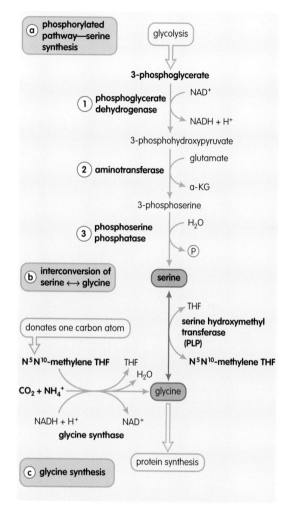

Fig. 5.4 Serine and glycine synthesis. A number of pathways are available to synthesize serine:
a. The main pathway occurs in the cell cytosol.
b. Serine is also synthesized from glycine in mitochondria by serine hydroxymethyl transferase. This is a reversible reaction and therefore is also a pathway for glycine synthesis.
c. Glycine can also be formed from CO_2, NH_4^+, and N^5N^{10}-methylene-THF in mitochondria.

Cysteine synthesis

Cysteine is formed from serine and the essential amino acid methionine in the cell cytosol (Fig. 5.5). Cysteine synthesis is dependent on an adequate supply of methionine in the diet. A large number of steps are involved and only the main ones are shown (numbers refer to Fig. 5.5):

1. Activation of methionine and the formation of homocysteine (details of this reaction are in Fig. 6.2).

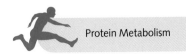
2. Condensation of serine with homocysteine to form cystathionine.
3. Hydrolysis by cystathionase to form cysteine and homoserine.

Alanine

Alanine is formed by a simple one-step transamination of pyruvate (Fig. 5.6). The formation

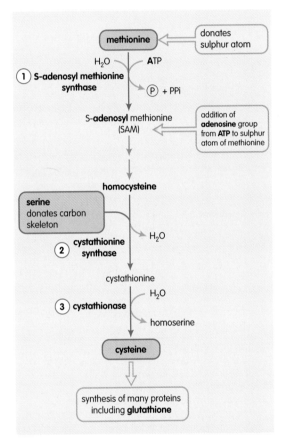

Fig. 5.5 Synthesis of cysteine. Cysteine is formed from serine and the essential amino acid methionine in the cell cytosol. Some of the steps have been omitted (numbers refer to text).

depends on the energy status of the cell and thus the demand for glycolysis.

Aspartate and asparagine

Asparagine is a derivative of the amino acid aspartate (Fig. 5.7).

1. Aspartate is formed by the transamination of oxaloacetate (a TCA cycle intermediate). Aspartate is an important amino acid in metabolism because of its role as an amino group donor in the urea cycle and in purine and pyrimidine synthesis.
2. Asparagine is formed by the transfer of an amide group from glutamine to aspartate. The reaction requires ATP and the equilibrium is in favor of asparagine synthesis.

Glutamate, glutamine, proline, and arginine

These amino acids are grouped together because glutamate is the precursor of the others. They are all formed from α-ketoglutarate (numbers refer to Fig. 5.8).

1. Glutamate is formed by the reductive amination of α-ketoglutarate by glutamate dehydrogenase. Glutamate has a key role in amino acid metabolism, since it is the only amino acid that can undergo rapid oxidative deamination (see Fig. 5.2). Glutamate is also formed by transamination of most other amino acids.
2. Glutamine is formed by the amination of glutamate by glutamine synthetase (like asparagine). Glutamine is used for purine and pyrimidine synthesis. As well as producing glutamine for protein synthesis, the reaction serves as a pathway for the removal of ammonia in the liver and the kidney.
3. Proline is synthesized from glutamate in three steps: reduction of glutamate to glutamate γ-semialdehyde, a spontaneous cyclization, and then reduction to proline.

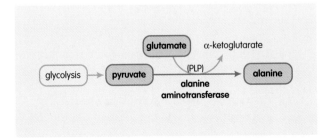

Fig. 5.6 Transamination of pyruvate to form alanine. Alanine is formed by a simple one-step transamination of pyruvate. The formation depends on the demand for glycolysis and thus the energy status of the cell.

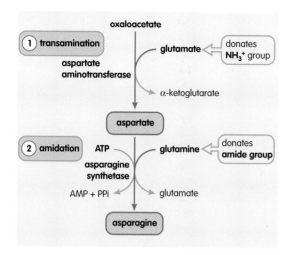

Fig. 5.7 Synthesis of aspartate and asparagine. Aspartate is formed by the transamination of oxaloacetate (1). Asparagine is formed by transfer of an amide group from glutamine to aspartate (2) (refer to text).

4. Arginine is formed by the reduction of glutamate to glutamate γ-semialdehyde, which is transaminated to ornithine. Ornithine is metabolized in the urea cycle to form arginine (discussed later in this chapter).

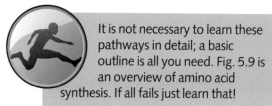

It is not necessary to learn these pathways in detail; a basic outline is all you need. Fig. 5.9 is an overview of amino acid synthesis. If all fails just learn that!

Protein breakdown and the disposal of nitrogen

Protein turnover
Most proteins in the body are constantly being synthesized from amino acids and degraded back to them. Therefore, there is a continual turnover of protein.

Amino acid pool
This is a "pool" of amino acids present in the body in dynamic equilibrium with tissue protein (Fig. 5.10). Amino acids are continually taken from the pool for protein synthesis and replaced by the hydrolysis of

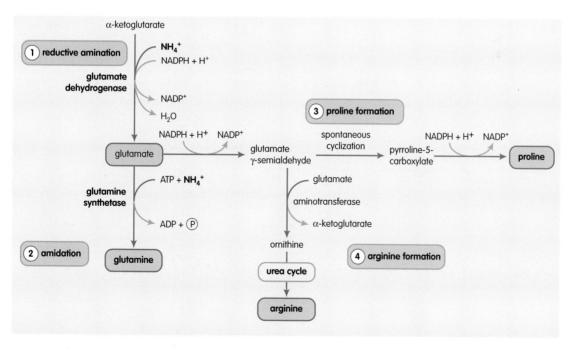

Fig. 5.8 Synthesis of glutamate, glutamine, proline and arginine. Glutamate is the precursor of the other amino acids in this group. They are all formed from α-ketoglutarate (numbers refer to text).

87

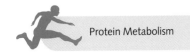

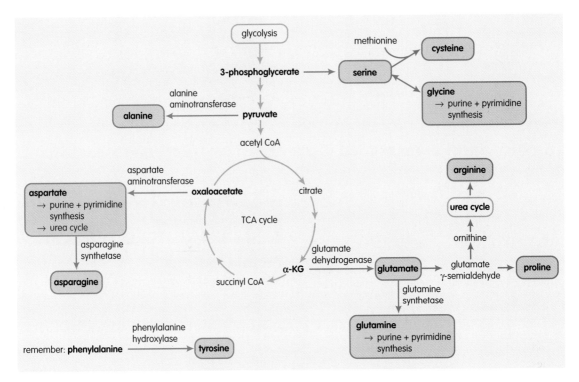

Fig. 5.9 Overview of the biosynthesis of nonessential amino acids. If all else fails, just learn this!

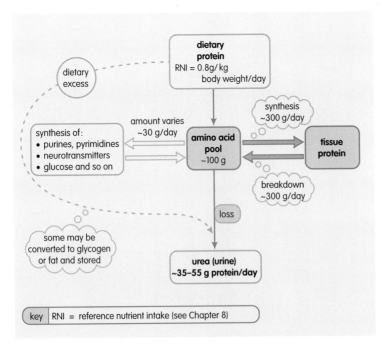

Fig. 5.10 Amino acid pool in the body is in dynamic equilibrium with tissue proteins.

Fig. 5.11 Daily turnover of tissue proteins. In an average 70-kg person the daily turnover of protein is about 300 g/day.

Daily turnover of tissue protein	
Amount	**Use**
70 g	turnover of digestive enzymes and gut cells
20 g	synthesis of plasma proteins
8 g	synthesis of hemoglobin
20 g	white blood cell turnover
75–100 g	turnover of muscle cells
80–100 g	various synthetic pathways
	N.B. under certain conditions (e.g. stress, infection or pregnancy) the synthesis of certain proteins may increase

dietary and tissue protein. Any amino acids not immediately used are lost, since protein cannot be stored.

In a healthy adult, the total amount of protein in the body is constant, so that the rate of protein synthesis is equal to the rate of protein breakdown. In an average 70 kg person, about 300 g of protein is synthesized each day and 300 g is degraded. Fig. 5.11 shows how this protein is used.

The amino acid pool can be thought of in terms of a sink without a plug. Therefore, it requires a continual daily filling because protein is not stored.

Nitrogen balance

The breakdown of protein leads to a net daily loss of nitrogen (as urea) from the body, which corresponds usually to about 35–55 g protein lost each day. Therefore, a normal diet must provide at least 35–55 g of protein every day. Under these conditions the body is said to be in nitrogen balance because the dietary intake is equal to the loss from the body.

Positive nitrogen balance

This occurs when nitrogen intake is greater than nitrogen loss from the body. Three conditions are associated with this:

- Growth.
- Pregnancy.
- Convalescence.

Negative nitrogen balance

This occurs when nitrogen intake is less than nitrogen loss from the body. Conditions associated with this are:

- Malnutrition.
- Starvation.
- Cachexia (seen in advanced stages of cancer).
- Posttraumatic state (surgery, severe burns or sepsis).
- Lack of an essential amino acid (remember, all 20 are needed for protein synthesis).

This is discussed further in Chapter 8.

Rate of protein turnover

Between 1 and 2% of the total body protein is turned over daily. The rate of protein turnover varies for individual proteins and with the function of the protein:

- Regulatory proteins; for example, digestive enzymes, lactate dehydrogenase, or RNA polymerase, have short half-lives (minutes to hours).
- Structural proteins; for example, collagen, have long half-lives and last for years.
- Hemoglobin has an intermediate half-life of about 120 days.

Protein degradation

There are two possible pathways for protein degradation; the end result of each is the breakdown

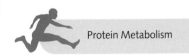
of proteins to their constituent amino acids by proteases.

Ubiquitin pathway

The ubiquitin pathway degrades abnormal proteins and short-lived cytosolic proteins; it is ATP-dependent and is located in the cell cytosol (Fig. 5.12).

Structure of ubiquitin

Ubiquitin is a small, basic protein that attaches to proteins to be destroyed. The attachment of ubiquitin targets the protein for degradation—it is a "tagging" system. At the carboxyl terminal of ubiquitin there is a glycine residue that attaches to lysine residues on target proteins to form ubiquitin-C-glycine–lysine-target protein.

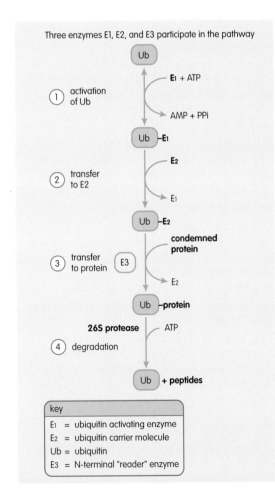

Fig. 5.12 Ubiquitin pathway degrades abnormal proteins and short-lived cytosolic proteins; it is ATP-dependent and is located in the cytosol (numbers refer to text).

The sequence of events

The ubiquitin pathway consists of four stages (steps below refer to Fig. 5.12): the enzymes E1, E2 and E3 participate in the pathway.

1. The activation of ubiquitin by attachment to E1, the ubiquitin activating enzyme. The reaction is driven by the hydrolysis of ATP.
2. The transfer of activated ubiquitin to E2, the ubiquitin carrier molecule.
3. E3 catalyzes the transfer of ubiquitin to the target protein. The E3 enzyme actually "reads" the N-terminal amino acid on proteins to determine whether a protein may be easily tagged with ubiquitin (see below).
4. The degradation of the labeled protein by 26S protease complex (also called megapain or endopeptidase) to peptides.

Lysosomal pathway

The lysosomal pathway degrades long-lived membrane or extracellular proteins and organelles; for example mitochondria. It is ATP-independent and is located in lysosomes (Fig. 5.13). Initially, the proteins must enter lysosomes, and there are two possible processes by which proteins can do this:

- Endocytosis, by which extracellular proteins enter cells for degradation in lysosomes.
- Autophagy for intracellular proteins or organelles; these are engulfed by the plasma membrane or endoplasmic reticulum to form autophagosomes.

The end result of both is the degradation of proteins by lysosomal proteases (cathepsins). Lysosomal activity, and therefore protein degradation, is increased in starvation (an increase in protein breakdown provides substrates for gluconeogenesis) and many disease states, including diabetes, hyperthyroidism and chronic inflammatory diseases.

Signals for degradation

Protein degradation (ubiquitinylation) is not random but is affected by some structural aspect of the protein.

N-end rule

This divides proteins into short- and long-lived by the nature of their N (amino)-terminal amino acid:

- Examples of stabilizing N-terminal residues are methionine, glycine, alanine and serine. These are not easily tagged by ubiquitin, and proteins containing these stabilizing residues have long half-lives.

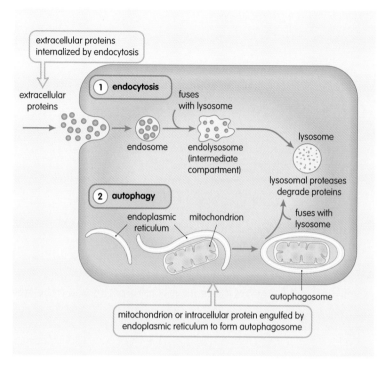

Fig. 5.13 Lysosomal pathway degrades long-lived, membrane or extracellular proteins and organelles; for example, mitochondria. Extracellular proteins enter cells by endocytosis where, as intracellular proteins, they are engulfed by the endoplasmic reticulum to form autophagosomes.

• Examples of destabilizing N-terminal residues are phenylalanine, tryptophan, aspartate, arginine and lysine. These are signals for rapid ubiquitin tagging.

It is the E3 enzyme that actually reads the N-terminal residues.

PEST region
Proteins containing PEST regions [–Pro–Glu–Ser–Thr] (named according to the one-letter nomenclature for amino acids) are rapidly degraded and have short half-lives. An example is cAMP-dependent protein kinase.

Conformational changes
The binding of ligands to receptors often causes a conformational change that may expose a PEST region or a region susceptible to the action of proteases.

Disposal of protein nitrogen and the urea cycle
An overview
Any amino acids surplus to the body's requirements are degraded. The amino group is removed, forming ammonia: however, ammonia is extremely toxic. Ammonia is therefore converted to a non-toxic compound, namely urea, by the urea cycle for excretion in the urine. A small amount of ammonia can also be incorporated into glutamine (see Fig. 5.8). The removal of the amino group from amino acids leaves behind the carbon skeletons (α-keto acids). Their metabolism is discussed later in this chapter.

The major site of amino acid degradation is the liver. Nitrogen disposal can be divided into two main stages:
• The removal of the amino group from amino acids.
• The formation of urea via the ornithine cycle.

These two stages are now considered in more detail.

Removal of amino group
There are two possible routes for the removal of the amino group.

Transdeamination
Transdeamination is transamination linked to oxidative deamination (see Figs 5.1 and 5.2):

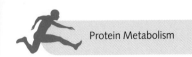
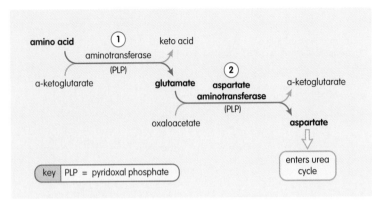

Fig. 5.14 Transamination route involves two transamination reactions (for details, see text below).

- In this case, transamination is the transfer of amino groups from amino acids to form glutamate in the cytosol.
- Oxidative deamination, catalyzed by glutamate dehydrogenase, removes the amino group from glutamate. The reaction occurs in mitochondria and the amino group released then enters the urea cycle.

Transamination
This involves two transamination reactions (numbers refer to Fig. 5.14):
1. The first transfers the amino group to α-ketoglutarate, forming glutamate.
2. In the second, aspartate aminotransferase transfers the amino group from glutamate to oxaloacetate, forming aspartate.

(Transamination involving essential amino acids is normally unidirectional since the body cannot synthesize the equivalent α-keto acid.)
   Aspartate then enters the urea cycle by condensing with citrulline. In this way, a second amino group enters the urea cycle, providing a second nitrogen atom to form urea. Deamination can also be achieved by other enzymes, but these are only minor pathways. For example, there is a non-specific L-amino acid oxidase, but it is not very important physiologically. There are also specific enzymes such as serine and threonine dehydratases, which deaminate serine and threonine, respectively, by removal of H_2O and NH_4, and cysteine desulphydrase, which deaminates cysteine and produces hydrogen sulphide as a byproduct.

Formation of urea by the ornithine cycle
The urea cycle consists of five reactions (described below) that synthesize the organic compound urea

from two inorganic compounds, CO_2 and NH_4 (Fig. 5.15). Urea, NH_2—CO—NH_2, contains two nitrogen atoms: one nitrogen is supplied by ammonia formed by the transdeamination of amino acids; the other derives from aspartate. The cycle uses a carrier molecule, ornithine, which is regenerated (this is similar to the way the TCA cycle uses oxaloacetate).

Location
Liver hepatocytes, mainly in the periportal cells.

Site
The first two reactions occur in mitochondria, the last three in the cytosol.

Urea cycle
Numbers refer to Fig. 5.15.

1. Formation of carbamoyl phosphate
This is the irreversible, rate-limiting step of the pathway, catalyzed by carbamoyl phosphate synthase I (CPS I). The reaction consumes two molecules of ATP. (There is also a carbamoyl phosphate synthase II enzyme in the cytosol but this is only involved in pyrimidine synthesis [see Chapter 6].)

2. Formation of citrulline
The carbamoyl group is transferred to ornithine by ornithine transcarbamoylase. Specific transporters for citrulline and ornithine are present in the inner mitochondrial membrane.

3. Synthesis of argininosuccinate
Argininosuccinate synthase catalyzes the condensation of citrulline with aspartate. The reaction is driven by the cleavage of ATP to AMP and pyrophosphate, which is rapidly hydrolyzed to two inorganic phosphates. Therefore the reaction consumes two ATP equivalents.

Fig. 5.15 The urea cycle consists of five reactions that synthesize the organic compound urea from two inorganic compounds: CO_2 and NH_4^+ (numbers refer to text).

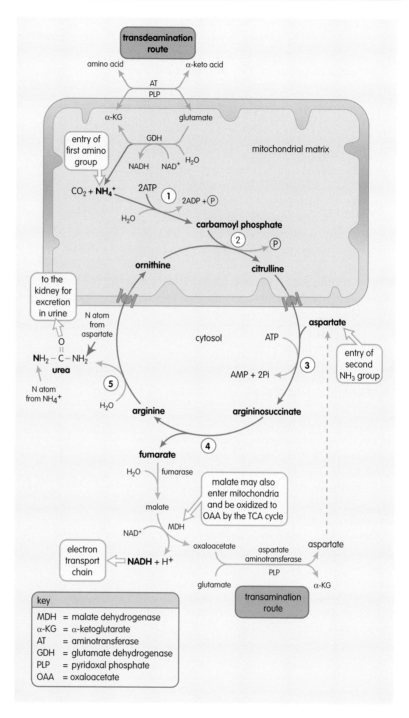

4. **Cleavage of argininosuccinate to fumarate and arginine by argininosuccinate lyase**
5. **Cleavage of arginine to ornithine and urea by arginase**

Arginase is specific to the liver, meaning that only the liver can produce urea. The urea formed is transported in the blood to the kidneys for excretion in urine.

Fate of fumarate

The fumarate formed is converted to malate by fumarase. Malate either can be converted to oxaloacetate and then aspartate in the cytosol, as shown in Fig. 5.15, or it can be transported into mitochondria and enter the TCA cycle first. There is evidence to suggest that both are possible and it is a matter of debate what actually happens. Either way, the NADH formed can be oxidized by the electron transport chain to produce 2.5 molecules of ATP.

The ATP yield

The overall reaction can be written as:
- Four ATP equivalents are consumed for every molecule of urea formed (reactions 1 and 3).
- The conversion of fumarate to oxaloacetate produces NADH, which is oxidized by the electron transport chain to generate 2.5 ATP.

Therefore, overall 1.5 ATP are consumed for every molecule of urea formed by the cycle (i.e., energy is required, not generated).

Control of the urea cycle

Control can be considered at two levels:

Short-term allosteric control

The main control of the urea cycle is by N-acetyl glutamate (formed from acetyl CoA and glutamate), which allosterically activates carbamoyl phosphate synthase I (CPS I), the enzyme which catalyzes the rate-limiting step of the urea cycle. How does this work? Following a protein-rich meal, the excess amino acids are deaminated, resulting in an increased concentration of glutamate and thus N-acetyl glutamate. N-acetyl glutamate activates CPS I, and thus the urea cycle, to cope with the extra nitrogen load.

Long-term regulation

Changes in the diet are thought to induce or repress transcription of the urea cycle enzymes. For example, in starvation, the increased breakdown of tissue protein induces the synthesis of enzymes to cope with the extra load of ammonia.

Why is it beneficial to form urea?

Ammonia is extremely toxic. By converting ammonia to urea (a nontoxic, organic compound), it can be excreted easily by the kidneys. Urea possesses a number of properties which favor its formation:
- It is a small, uncharged and water-soluble molecule. It can therefore diffuse across membranes easily and be excreted in the urine.

- Nearly 50% of its weight is nitrogen, making it a very efficient nitrogen carrier and excretory product.
- Little energy is used up in its synthesis—only about 1.5 ATP are required for every mole of urea formed.

A normal diet produces 35–55 g of urea each day. In birds, ammonia is converted to uric acid for excretion, which is quite insoluble.

Ammonia toxicity

Ammonia is one of the most toxic compounds produced by the body. Elevated levels (hyperammonemia) can cause symptoms of ammonia intoxication: tremors, slurred speech, and blurred vision. At very high concentrations, ammonia causes irreversible brain damage, coma, and death. It is therefore essential that ammonia is detoxified rapidly to urea by the liver.

Proposed mechanisms of ammonia toxicity

Ammonia toxicity affects the brain and central nervous system. Whereas the effects of ammonia toxicity are well-known, its mechanism of action is still unclear. An increase in the concentration of ammonia causes a shift in the equilibrium of the glutamate dehydrogenase reaction toward glutamate formation (Fig. 5.16). This leads to a depletion of α-ketoglutarate, which results in a decrease in TCA cycle activity and therefore ATP production. Shifting the equilibrium of the reaction also leads to an increase in the ratio of NAD+ to NADH, which also results in a decrease in ATP levels. The brain and nervous system require large amounts of energy and

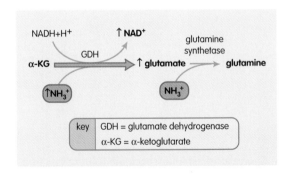

Fig. 5.16 Mechanisms of ammonia toxicity. An increase in the concentration of ammonia causes a shift in the equilibrium of the glutamate dehydrogenase reaction toward glutamate formation, which leads to the depletion of α-ketoglutarate, a substrate of the TCA cycle.

are therefore particularly susceptible to ammonia toxicity.

High levels of ammonia may also react with glutamate, forming glutamine, which may damage the brain directly. Decreasing the level of glutamate (a neurotransmitter) in the brain may also cause problems. Remember, these are only proposed mechanisms.

A genetic deficiency in each of the urea cycle enzymes has been identified; all are rare, the most common being ornithine transcarbamoylase deficiency. These deficiencies each result in a failure to synthesize urea, leading to hyperammonemia and irreversible mental retardation from ammonia toxicity. Ammonia toxicity is also seen in patients with liver damage due to cirrhosis.

Formation of glucose from non-carbohydrate sources

Role of protein as an energy source
Fed state
In the fed state, proteins undergo digestion in the stomach and small intestine to release amino acids, which are taken up by cells and used for the synthesis of proteins and other molecules. However, if amino acids are present in excess of the body's requirements, they can either be used directly as a fuel to produce ATP, or converted to glycogen or fat and stored for later use. Thus, that is they provide an "indirect" energy store: amino acids are never stored as protein.

Starvation
Following prolonged exercise or during starvation, the body has to rely on its energy stores for fuel. Glycogen reserves last only between 12 and 24 hours and are quickly depleted. The main concern is how to maintain the blood glucose concentration and provide fuel for the brain and RBCs. Fat, as has already been shown, cannot be converted to glucose

(see Fig. 2.15). In prolonged starvation the brain adapts to using ketone bodies as its main fuel, although it still requires some glucose, but RBCs cannot metabolize ketone bodies at all because they have no mitochondria (see Chapter 4). Therefore, alternative substrates for glucose production are required. These are provided via gluconeogenesis. Lactate and glycerol can provide some glucose, but the majority is obtained by the breakdown of muscle protein to release amino acids. Many of these amino acids produced from muscle protein are transaminated to alanine and glutamine, which are then released into the blood. Alanine is taken up by the liver for gluconeogenesis. Glutamine is taken up by the small intestine to be used as a fuel and by the kidney to form glucose, also via gluconeogenesis.

Gluconeogenesis
Gluconeogenesis is defined as the production of glucose from noncarbohydrate sources. For a period of starvation of longer than about 12 hours, or during prolonged exercise, glucose has to be formed from alternative substrates to maintain the blood glucose concentration. Gluconeogenesis is the process in which glucose is produced from:
- Glycerol (released by triacylglycerol hydrolysis) (see Fig. 4.11).
- Lactate (from anaerobic glycolysis in RBCs and active skeletal muscle).
- Amino acids (from the breakdown of muscle protein).

Location
Liver (however, in prolonged starvation it can also occur in the cortex of the kidney).

Site
Cell cytosol—except for the first step, the carboxylation of pyruvate, which occurs in mitochondria.

Pathway
Gluconeogenesis is not simply a reversal of glycolysis. Some of the reactions of glycolysis are reversible and are common to both glycolytic and gluconeogenic pathways. However, the three essentially irreversible reactions of glycolysis, namely those catalyzed by hexokinase, phosphofructokinase-1 (PFK-1) and pyruvate kinase, have to be bypassed. How this is achieved is shown in Fig. 5.17, and explained in stages 1–3 below.

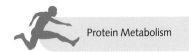

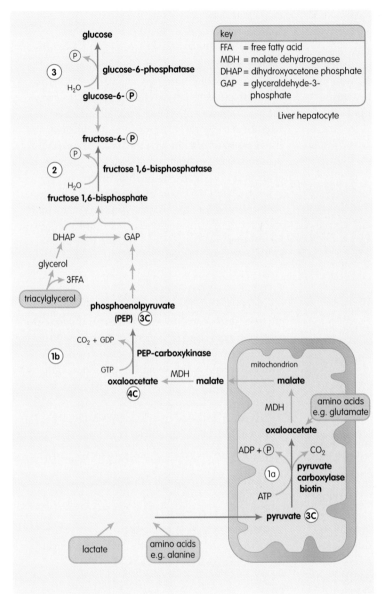

Fig. 5.17 Gluconeogenesis is not simply a reversal of glycolysis. The three essentially irreversible reactions of glycolysis have to be bypassed. The first reaction, the carboxylation of pyruvate to oxaloacetate, occurs in the mitochondrial matrix. The rest of the reactions occur in the cell cytosol. Details of the individual reactions 1 to 3 are found in the text.

1. Conversion of pyruvate to phosphoenolpyruvate (PEP)

The conversion of pyruvate to PEP occurs via two reactions:

a. The carboxylation of pyruvate to oxaloacetate. Pyruvate carboxylase is found in the mitochondria but PEP-carboxykinase and the other enzymes involved are in the cytosol. The oxaloacetate formed is unable to cross the inner mitochondrial membrane; therefore it is reduced to malate, which is transported into the cytosol where it is re-oxidized. Pyruvate carboxylase requires the vitamin biotin as a cofactor and has a similar mechanism to acetyl CoA carboxylase (see Chapter 4).

b. The decarboxylation and phosphorylation of oxaloacetate by PEP-carboxykinase.

2. Hydrolysis of fructose 1,6-bisphosphate

The hydrolysis of fructose 1,6-bisphosphate by fructose 1,6-bisphosphatase bypasses the PFK reaction (rate-limiting step of glycolysis).

3. Hydrolysis of glucose-6-phosphate

The hydrolysis of glucose-6-phosphate by glucose-6-phosphatase bypasses the irreversible hexokinase reaction to form free glucose. This enzyme is unique to the liver.

Amino acid breakdown

Amino acid breakdown involves two stages:
- The removal of amino groups by transamination and oxidative deamination (see Figs 5.1 and 5.2).
- The catabolism of the carbon skeletons.

The carbon skeletons of amino acids can be metabolized to intermediates of the TCA cycle and glycolytic pathway. In fact, the breakdown of all 20 amino acids converges to produce seven products: pyruvate, acetyl CoA, acetoacetyl CoA, α-ketoglutarate, succinyl CoA, fumarate, and oxaloacetate (Fig. 5.18). Depending on the energy status of the cell, these products can either be oxidized to generate energy or used to synthesize glycogen or fat.

Concepts of amino acid catabolism

Metabolically, amino acids can be classified into two types: ketogenic and glucogenic.

Ketogenic amino acids

These are amino acids that are broken down to either acetyl CoA or acetoacetyl CoA and are therefore able to form ketone bodies, hence ketogenic, meaning "ketone-forming." Only leucine and lysine are purely ketogenic (see Fig. 5.18). Isoleucine, phenylalanine, tryptophan and tyrosine are both ketogenic and glucogenic; that is, their breakdown yields some acetyl CoA and acetoacetyl CoA and some precursors of glucose.

Glucogenic amino acids

These are amino acids that can be broken down to either pyruvate or one of the intermediates of the TCA cycle. They can be channeled into gluconeogenesis for glucose synthesis, hence the term glucogenic ("glucose-forming").

Pathways of amino acid catabolism

Amino acids can be divided into seven groups, based on their breakdown product. Several breakdown pathways are possible for each amino acid, but only the main ones are discussed here:

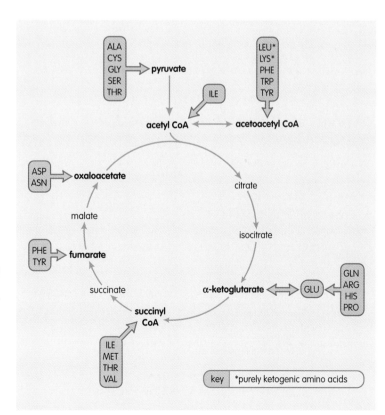

Fig. 5.18 Entry points of amino acid carbon skeletons into the TCA cycle and glycolytic pathways. The breakdown of all 20 amino acids converges to produce only seven products: pyruvate, acetyl CoA, acetoacetyl CoA, α-ketoglutarate, succinyl CoA, fumarate, and oxaloacetate. These products, depending on the energy status of the cell, can either be oxidized to generate energy or used to synthesize glycogen or fat.

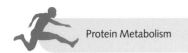

Protein Metabolism

- Five amino acids form pyruvate; that is alanine, serine, glycine, cysteine, and threonine (Fig. 5.19). Note that hydroxyproline can also be converted to pyruvate.
- Two amino acids form oxaloacetate: aspartate (transamination of aspartate by aspartate aminotransferase) and asparagine (hydrolysis of asparagine by asparaginase releases ammonia and forms aspartate, which can undergo transamination to oxaloacetate).
- Four amino acids form glutamate and α-ketoglutarate (Fig. 5.20).
- Four amino acids form succinyl CoA (Fig. 5.21).
- Phenylalanine and tyrosine form fumarate. The hydroxylation of phenylalanine by phenylalanine hydroxylase produces tyrosine (pathway for its synthesis [see Fig. 5.3]). Tyrosine is then transaminated and undergoes a series of reactions to form fumarate. Some acetoacetyl CoA is also

Breakdown of amino acids to pyruvate			
Amino acid	**Important reactions**	**Enzymes involved**	**Product**
alanine	transamination	alanine aminotransferase	pyruvate
serine	deamination and dehydration	serine dehydratase	pyruvate
glycine	methylation to serine followed by dehydration	serine hydroxymethyl transferase serine dehydratase	pyruvate
cysteine	two main steps: • oxidation to cysteine sulphinate • transamination	cysteine dioxygenase cysteine aminotransferase	pyruvate
threonine	aminoacetone pathway	threonine dehydrogenase	pyruvate

Fig. 5.19 Breakdown of amino acids to pyruvate. Six amino acids form pyruvate.

Breakdown of amino acids to glutamate and α-ketoglutarate			
Amino acid	**Important reactions**	**Enzymes involved**	**Product**
glutamine	hydrolysis	glutaminase	glutamate
glutamate	oxidative deamination	glutamate dehydrogenase	α-ketoglutarate
proline	two main steps: • oxidation → pyrroline-5-carboxylate • oxidation → glutamate	proline oxygenase dehydrogenase	glutamate
arginine	two steps: • cleaved to ornithine (part of urea cycle) • transamination	arginase aminotransferase	glutamate
histidine	two main steps: • deamination and hydrolysis to N-formiminoglutamate (FIGlu) • transfer of formimino group to THF	histidase glutamate formiminotransferase	glutamate

Fig. 5.20 Breakdown of amino acids to glutamate and α-ketoglutarate. Five amino acids form glutamate and α-ketoglutarate.

Fig. 5.21 Breakdown of amino acids to succinyl CoA. Four amino acids form succinyl CoA (only the important reactions are shown). (SAM, S-adenosylmethionine; BCAA, branched-chain amino acids.)

Breakdown of amino acids to succinyl CoA			
Amino acid	**Key reactions**	**Enzymes involved**	**Product**
isoleucine (BCAA)	three reactions: • transamination • oxidative decarboxylation • dehydrogenation	BCAA aminotransferase BCAA α-ketoacid dehydrogenase	succinyl CoA and acetyl CoA
valine (BCAA)	all BCAAs have a similar breakdown pathway	as above	succinyl CoA
methionine	condensation with ATP to form SAM; hydrolysis to homocysteine	SAM synthase	succinyl CoA
threonine	dehydration to α-ketobutyrate	threonine dehydratase	succinyl CoA

produced; therefore, it is both a ketogenic and glucogenic amino acid.

- Isoleucine forms acetyl CoA: its breakdown actually produces both acetyl CoA and succinyl CoA (see Fig. 5.21).
- Leucine, lysine, and tryptophan form acetoacetyl CoA (phenylalanine and tyrosine can also produce some acetoacetyl CoA). Leucine is a branched-chain amino acid and its breakdown is discussed below.

Lysine undergoes a number of reactions: a reduction to saccharopine, two oxidations to form aminoadipate, transamination to α-ketoadipate, and then further reactions to eventually form acetoacetyl CoA (it is not necessary to know this in detail). The breakdown of tryptophan is even more complicated!

Branched-chain amino acids (BCAA)

The BCAAs are isoleucine, leucine, and valine, all of which are degraded by a common pathway of three reactions:

- Transamination: a single enzyme, branched-chain amino acid aminotransferase, transaminates all three amino acids.
- Oxidative decarboxylation: again by one enzyme, the branched-chain α-ketoacid dehydrogenase, which requires thiamine pyrophosphate as a cofactor. A deficiency of this enzyme causes an accumulation of the ketoacids derived from BCAAs in the urine; this is called maple syrup urine disease (see below).
- Dehydrogenation.

Not all tissues can oxidize BCAAs: the liver has limited ability because it lacks the branched-chain amino acid aminotransferase. BCAAs are mainly oxidized by peripheral tissues, in particular, muscle.

You are not going to be asked to discuss the different degradation pathways of the amino acids. Know about transamination and deamination reactions and where the amino acid carbon skeletons feed into the TCA cycle; learn Fig. 5.18.

Regulation of amino acid catabolism

Gluconeogenesis is active during fasting and starvation (Fig. 5.22).

Hormonal control

In starvation, the levels of glucagon, cortisol, and adrenocorticotrophic hormone (ACTH) are high, which activates gluconeogenesis and inhibits glycolysis. The actions of glucagon are:

- It activates a cAMP-dependent protein kinase, which causes phosphorylation and inactivation of pyruvate kinase in the glycolytic pathway (see Fig. 2.10).

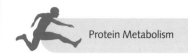
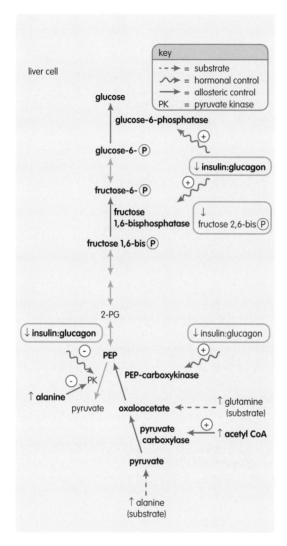

Fig. 5.22 Regulation of gluconeogenesis: fasting and starved state. Control is at two levels. Hormonal control: glucagon activates gluconeogenesis. Allosteric control: acetyl CoA activates pyruvate carboxylase. An increased supply of amino acids, alanine and glutamine activate gluconeogenesis.

- Through phosphorylation of a bifunctional enzyme, 6-phosphofructokinase-2/fructose 2,6-bisphosphatase, it decreases the concentration of fructose 2,6-bisphosphate, the allosteric activator of phosphofructokinase-1 (glycolytic enzyme) but inhibitor of fructose 1,6-bisphosphatase (gluconeogenic enzyme, see Fig. 2.8).

- It increases the rate of transcription and thus the rate of synthesis of PEP-carboxykinase.
- It inhibits the rate of transcription of pyruvate kinase.

Allosteric activation by acetyl CoA

During starvation, the rate of lipolysis and β oxidation is high, leading to a large increase in the amount of acetyl CoA. Acetyl CoA allosterically activates pyruvate carboxylase, stimulating gluconeogenesis. It has an opposite inhibitory effect on pyruvate dehydrogenase. Therefore, the pyruvate formed will be channelled into gluconeogenesis rather than into the TCA cycle. An increased supply of substrates, particularly of the amino acids alanine and glutamine, favors gluconeogenesis. A high concentration of cortisol favours mobilization of amino acids from muscle.

Disorders of amino acid metabolism

Disorders of amino acid metabolism are very rare inborn errors of metabolism that result in severe developmental abnormalities if left untreated. They include phenylketonuria, albinism, alkaptonuria, maple syrup urine disease, and histidinemia. You may see some of them when you do pediatrics. Phenylketonuria is the most important of these.

Phenylketonuria

Phenylketonuria (PKU) is an autosomal recessive disorder that is caused by the deficiency of the enzyme phenylalanine hydroxylase. In a small number of patients it may be due to a deficiency in the enzymes that synthesize its cofactor tetrahydrobiopterin (see Fig. 5.3). The disease is characterized by an increased plasma phenylalanine level. It has a prevalence of 1:10,000–20,000 live births.

Mechanism

Normally, phenylalanine hydroxylase catalyzes the hydroxylation of phenylalanine to tyrosine. Tyrosine is an extremely important amino acid: it is the precursor of dopamine, catecholamines, and melanin. In PKU, phenylalanine accumulates in the plasma and tissues and is converted into the phenylketones: phenylpyruvate, phenyllactate, and

Clinical features and diagnosis of PKU	
Clinical features	**Diagnosis and management**
central nervous system involvement: untreated, presents at 6–12 months with development delay, failure to thrive and seizures	all neonates are screened for raised phenylalanine levels at 5–7 days, when milk feeding is established (so the phenylalanine levels are adequate); part of Guthrie test
hypopigmentation: many affected infants are fair-haired, blue eyed and pale, since phenylalanine inhibits tyrosinase which converts tyrosine to melanin	**management:** • restriction of dietary phenylalanine • blood phenylalanine levels are monitored regularly and maintained in the normal range to allow normal growth and development

Fig. 5.23 Clinical features and diagnosis of phenylketonuria.

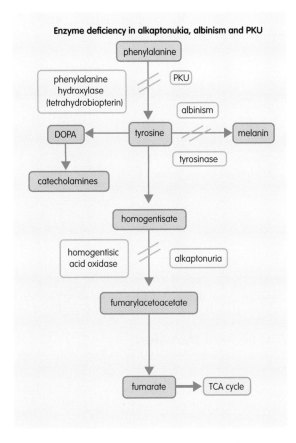

Fig. 5.24 Enzyme deficiencies in alkaptonuria, albinism and phenylketonuria (PKU).

phenylacetate. These are not normally produced in significant amounts. High levels of phenylalanine may impair development and in the long-term can cause mental retardation (Fig. 5.23).

Treatment
Treatment of phenylketonuria is by restriction of dietary phenylalanine. However, phenylalanine is an essential amino acid; therefore, too much dietary restriction can also cause poor growth and neurologic symptoms. Tyrosine cannot be made in patients with PKU and becomes an essential amino acid.

Pregnancy
In PKU patients, the restriction of dietary phenylalanine should be for life. It is particularly important during pregnancy when hyperphenylalaninemia in the mother may damage the fetus, causing microcephaly, mental retardation, and heart defects.

Alkaptonuria
Alkaptonuria is a rare, autosomal recessive disorder with a prevalence of 1:100,000. It is caused by a deficiency of the enzyme homogentisic acid oxidase, normally involved in the breakdown of tyrosine to fumarate (Fig. 5.24). Unlike other amino acid disorders, it does not produce serious effects until adult life.

Mechanism
The enzyme deficiency leads to an accumulation of homogentisate, which polymerizes to produce a black–brown pigment that is deposited in cartilage and other connective tissue. This process is called ochronosis.

Clinical features
Joint damage and arthritis. Homogentisate is excreted in the urine; on standing, the urine turns black because of the formation of alkapton. Sweat may also be black. There is no specific treatment.

Albinism
Albinism is a deficiency of the enzyme tyrosinase which converts tyrosine into melanin. The incidence is 1:13,000. The clinical features and management of albinism are discussed in Fig. 5.25.

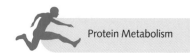

Histidinemia, homocystinuria, and maple syrup urine disease

These three diseases are described in Fig. 5.26.

> Disorders of amino acid metabolism are all rare autosomal recessive disorders, which mostly present in neonates with failure to thrive and developmental delay. The treatment is a restricted diet.

Amino acid metabolism in individual tissues

Amino acid transport

Several transporters exist for "carrying" amino acids across the cell membrane. The concentration of free amino acids outside the cell is much lower than the concentration of free amino acids inside. Therefore, most amino acid transporters function as active transport systems in which the movement of amino acids into cells, against their concentration gradient, is driven by the hydrolysis of ATP.

Five main transport systems exist, based on the specificity of the transporter for the side chain of the amino acid (Fig. 5.27). Thus there is one for basic amino acids, another for acidic amino acids, and so on.

The γ-glutamyl cycle

Unlike the specific transport systems described in Fig. 5.27, the γ-glutamyl cycle transports a wide

Clinical features and management of albinism	
Clinical features	**Management**
amelanosis: • whitish hair, pale skin, and grey-blue eyes • low pigment in iris and retina leads to failure to develop fixation reflex; resulting in nystagmus, photophobia and constant frowning • pale skin leads to sunburn and skin cancer	tinted contact lenses from early infancy may allow development of normal fixation in some patients high sun protection in the long term, results in severe visual impairment

Fig. 5.25 Clinical features and management of albinism.

Other amino acid disorders			
Disorder	**Enzyme defect**	**Biochemical feature**	**Clinical features**
histidinemia 1:10,000	histidase	↑ histidine in blood and urine	mental retardation
homocystinuria (rare)	cystathionine synthase (see Fig. 5.5)	↑ homocysteine in urine ↑ methionine in blood	failure to thrive, progressive mental retardation, and dislocation of lens in eye
maple syrup urine disease 1:200,000 (very rare)	branched-chain α-ketoacid dehydrogenase	↑ excretion of branched-chain amino acids, valine, leucine and isoleucine and their α-ketoacids in plasma and urine; compounds smell like maple syrup	neonates present with metabolic acidosis, hypoglycemia, and seizures delay in diagnosis leads to neurologic problems

Fig. 5.26 Genetically determined amino acid disorders.

range of amino acids into cells, being particularly active for neutral amino acids.

Function

The γ-glutamyl cycle is responsible for the active transport of amino acids into cells via the synthesis and breakdown of a glutathione carrier (Fig. 5.28). Three molecules of ATP are required for the transport of each amino acid molecule into the cell and the regeneration of glutathione.

Location/site

Kidney renal tubular cells and the endoplasmic reticulum of hepatocytes and brain cells.

Amino acid metabolism

Amino acids are taken up into tissues by active transport and are used for protein synthesis. Excess amino acids are not stored by the body; those not immediately required are degraded. The role of protein as an energy source has already been outlined; here we consider amino acid metabolism in individual tissues during the absorptive (fed) state and postabsorptive state.

Absorptive (fed) state

A summary of amino acid metabolism in tissues during the fed (absorptive) state is given in Fig. 5.29.

Small intestine

After a protein-rich meal, protein digestion takes place in the small intestine. The amino acids released

Specific transport systems for amino acids		
Amino acid specificity	Amino acids transported	Diseases resulting from a defect of the carrier system
small, neutral amino acids	alanine, serine, threonine	nonspecific
large, neutral and aromatic amino acids	isoleucine, leucine, valine, tyrosine, tryptophan, phenylalanine	Hartnup's disease: a defect in the intestinal and renal transporter for neutral amino acids
basic amino acids	arginine, lysine, cysteine, ornithine	cystinuria: a defect in kidney tubular reabsorption of all four basic amino acids
proline and glycine	proline, glycine	glycinuria
acidic amino acids	glutamate, aspartate	nonspecific

Fig. 5.27 Specific transport systems for amino acids.

Fig. 5.28 γ-Glutamyl cycle for amino acid transport.
1. Glutathione is formed in the cell and transported to the external surface of the plasma membrane.
2. The enzyme, γ-glutamyl transpeptidase, catalyzes the transfer of a γ-glutamyl group from glutathione to the amino acid. This enables uptake of the γ-glutamyl amino acid by the cell (or the cells of other organs if it travels in the blood first).
3. γ-Glutamyl cyclotransferase releases the amino acid for use by the cell.
4. The glutathione is reformed by the action of oxoprolinase, γ-glutamyl-cysteinyl synthetase, and glutathione synthetase in three ATP-dependent reactions.

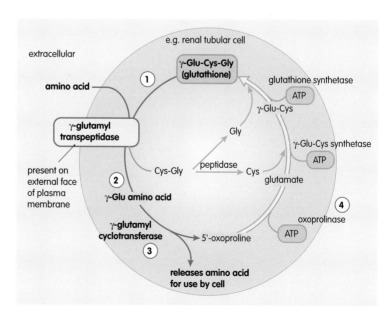

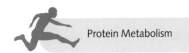

are absorbed by intestinal epithelial cells. A large proportion of amino acids are transaminated to alanine, which is released into the portal vein and taken to the liver. Therefore, alanine is the major amino acid secreted by the gut and the principal carrier of nitrogen in the plasma.

Liver

Alanine and other diet-derived amino acids received from the small intestine have a number of possible fates:

- Protein synthesis.
- Transamination to glutamate, which may be oxidatively deaminated to produce NH_4^+, which in turn enters the urea cycle (some NH_4^+ comes from the hydrolysis of glutamine in the small

intestine). The urea formed is taken to the kidneys for excretion. Some of the glutamate formed may also be used for protein synthesis.

Postabsorptive state

The postabsorptive state is the period four to eight hours after a meal when there is no dietary supply of amino acids. A summary of amino acid metabolism in tissues in the postabsorptive state is given in Fig. 5.30.

Muscle

The breakdown of muscle protein releases amino acids, which are transaminated to alanine and glutamine. Glutamine is formed in two steps: transamination to glutamate and amidation to glutamine. Nucleic acid turnover provides the

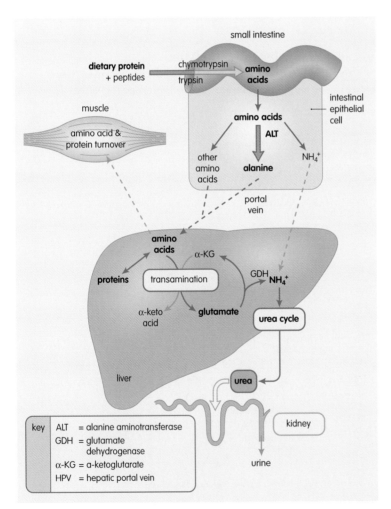

Fig. 5.29 Summary of amino acid metabolism in tissues during the absorptive state.

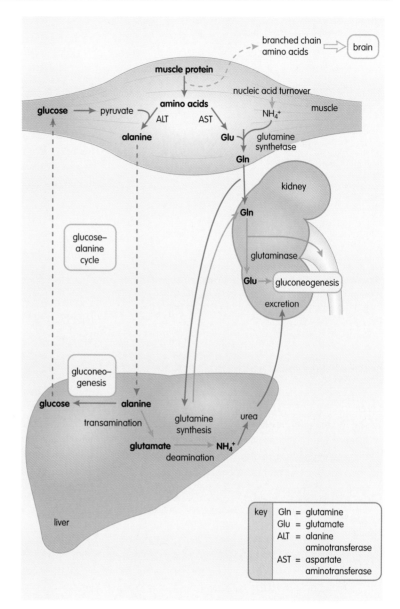

Fig. 5.30 Summary of amino acid metabolism in tissues in the postabsorptive state (refer to text for explanation).

NH$_4^+$ for this reaction. The released glutamine is taken up by the intestine and the kidney. The formed alanine goes to the liver. The breakdown of muscle protein also releases branched-chain amino acids, which are taken up primarily by the brain (especially valine).

Intestine

Glutamine has two main fates; respective degrees depend on the energy status of the cell:

- Firstly, it can be used for nucleotide synthesis to compensate for the very high turnover rate of intestinal cells (see Chapter 6).
- Secondly, it undergoes hydrolysis to glutamate to release NH$_4^+$, which travels to the liver to enter the urea cycle.

The glutamate formed is transaminated either to alanine or citrulline (a urea cycle

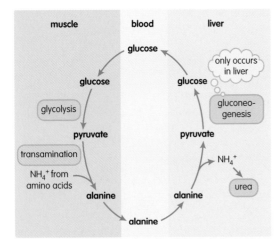

Fig. 5.31 The glucose–alanine cycle shows how carbon skeletons alternate between protein and glucose. Alanine released by muscle is converted back to glucose in the liver by gluconeogenesis. The glucose formed is taken back to the muscle for use.

intermediate), both of which are taken to the liver.

Liver

In the liver alanine is either:

- Converted to pyruvate and then to glucose by gluconeogenesis, providing an energy source for the muscle. The reactions constitute the glucose–alanine cycle (Fig. 5.31).

or

- Transaminated to glutamate. The balance between these two processes depends on the energy state of the cell.

Glutamate can be deaminated to form NH_4^+, which enters the urea cycle. During starvation or acidosis, glutaminase activity is reduced, resulting in a decrease in glutamine hydrolysis and NH_4^+ production. This leads to a decrease in the urea cycle and amino acid breakdown. A reciprocal increase is seen in the activity of glutamine synthetase and amino acid synthesis.

Kidney

Glutamine released from muscle is taken up by kidney cells. It is hydrolyzed by glutaminase to release ammonia for excretion. In starvation, glutamate serves as a substrate for gluconeogenesis (see Fig. 5.17).

The glucose–alanine cycle

The glucose–alanine cycle (see Fig. 5.31) makes carbon skeletons alternate between protein and glucose. Alanine from muscle is converted back to glucose in the liver—glucose is, in turn, used by muscle. This is very similar to the Cori cycle, in which lactate formed by active skeletal muscle is taken to the liver to be converted back to pyruvate and then to glucose by gluconeogenesis. The glucose formed is then taken back to muscle (see Chapter 7).

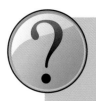

- Define essential and nonessential amino acids, and list the essential ones.
- What is the significance of transamination reactions in amino acid metabolism?
- Contrast the two main pathways of protein degradation.
- Why is the ornithine cycle alone insufficient for amino acid degradation?
- Positive nitrogen balance is a good thing in healthy individuals. Discuss.
- What metabolic reactions inform the body when proteins need to be broken down?
- Describe the control of gluconeogenesis.
- How does the role of protein as an energy source vary in the fed and the fasted state?
- Give examples of glucogenic and ketogenic amino acids.
- Gluconeogenesis is glycolysis in reverse. Discuss.
- How is amino acid catabolism controled?
- Explain the benefits and potential problems associated with treatment of phenylketonuria.
- Explain the biochemical mechanism of the Guthrie test for phenylketonuria.
- Compare and contrast amino acid metabolism in the absorptive and post-absorptive states.

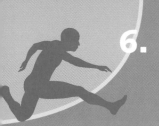

6. Purines, Pyrimidines and Heme

One-carbon pool

Concepts

Single carbon units can exist in a number of oxidation states; for example, methane, formaldehyde and methanol. They are used in the synthesis and elongation of many organic compounds. In order to do this, carbon units require a carrier to "activate" them and to enable their transfer to the molecule being synthesized. The main carriers used are folate and S-adenosyl methionine. The one-carbon pool refers to single carbon units attached to these carriers.

S-adenosyl methionine

S-adenosyl methionine (SAM) is a high-energy compound formed by the condensation of the amino acid methionine with ATP. It contains an activated methyl group, which can be transferred easily to a variety of molecules. SAM is the main methyl group donor used in biosynthetic reactions; for example, the methylation of noradrenaline to adrenaline.

Folate

The active form of folate is 5,6,7,8-tetrahydrofolate (THF). THF is a carrier of a number of one-carbon units which bind to its nitrogen atoms at positions N^5, N^{10} or both, to form the compounds shown in Fig. 6.1. THF receives these one-carbon fragments from donors such as serine, glycine or histidine, and transfers them to intermediates in the synthesis of other amino acids, purines, and thymidine.

Students always tend to find the concept of the one-carbon pool confusing. All you need to realize is that THF and SAM are just carriers of one-carbon groups, which are used in the synthesis of a range of molecules, mainly amino acids, purines, and pyrimidines. These THF compounds are all interconvertible except the N^5-methyl group; along with SAM they comprise the one-carbon pool.

Folate metabolism
Formation of THF

THF is formed by the two-step reduction of folate by dihydrofolate reductase (Fig. 6.2). Dihydrofolate reductase is competitively inhibited by methotrexate, a folic acid analog used in the treatment of certain cancers. By inhibiting folate synthesis, methotrexate can decrease the amount of THF available for purine and pyrimidine formation, thus decreasing DNA and RNA synthesis in cells.

Methyl-folate trap

Reactions involving the transfer of methyl groups result in the formation of N^5-methyl THF (Fig. 6.3). Unlike the other THF compounds, this is not interconvertible; therefore, the THF cannot be released and is trapped. Normally, however, the methionine salvage pathway is present. Methionine is formed by methylation of homocysteine using N^5-methyl THF as the methyl group donor, releasing the THF. Homocysteine methyltransferase catalyzes the reaction and requires vitamin B_{12} as an essential cofactor (methylcobalamin). In vitamin B_{12} deficiency this pathway is inhibited and THF remains as N^5-methyl THF. Eventually, all of the body's folate can become trapped, resulting in folate

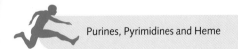

One-carbon units and corresponding THF compounds	
One-carbon unit	Compound
—CH=NH	N^5-formimino THF
—CHO	N^5-formyl THF
—CHO	N^{10}-formyl THF
=CH—	N^5,N^{10}-methenyl THF
—CH$_2$—	N^5,N^{10}-methylene THF
—CH$_3$	N^5-methyl THF

Fig. 6.1 Compounds formed by the binding of THF to various one-carbon compounds.

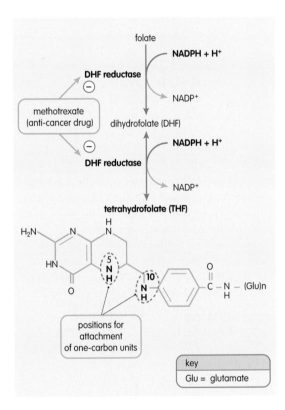

Fig. 6.2 Formation of tetrahydrofolate (THF). THF is formed by the two-step reduction of folate by dihydrofolate reductase.

deficiency secondary to B_{12} deficiency (see also Chapter 8). This results in decreased nucleotide synthesis and DNA and RNA formation. As blood cells require high levels of nucleotides for their turnover, they are particularly sensitive to folate deficiency, which can lead to megaloblastic anemia.

Amino acids and the one-carbon pool

The synthesis and breakdown of certain amino acids produces THF carriers that can then be used in the synthesis of other amino acids and nucleotides. The following reactions demonstrate the use of the one-carbon pool.

Formation of SAM from methionine (numbers refer to Fig. 6.3)

1. Condensation of ATP and methionine to form SAM.
2. SAM contains an activated methyl group that can be donated to a number of acceptor molecules, forming S-adenosyl homocysteine.
3. The hydrolysis of S-adenosyl homocysteine releases adenosine to form homocysteine.
4. Homocysteine can be used either for the synthesis of the amino acid cysteine (see Chapter 5), or for
5. The regeneration of methionine in the methionine salvage pathway.

Serine to glycine conversion

The reaction sequence for the conversion of serine to glycine is shown in Fig. 6.4.

Purine metabolism

Structure and function of purines

The purines are the nitrogenous bases adenine, guanine and hypoxanthine. Purines have a double-ring structure, consisting of a six-carbon ring and a five-carbon ring. They are nearly always found with a pentose sugar (5C) attached to the nitrogen atom at N9 to form a nucleoside; for example, adenosine. The sugar is usually ribose or deoxyribose. Phosphorylation of the sugar at the C5 position leads to the formation of mono-, di- and tri-nucleotides as shown in Fig. 6.5. The phosphate groups cause these molecules to be negatively charged. The main functions of purines are listed in Fig. 6.6.

An overview of purine metabolism

The diet provides negligible amounts of purines because they are broken down in the gut to form uric

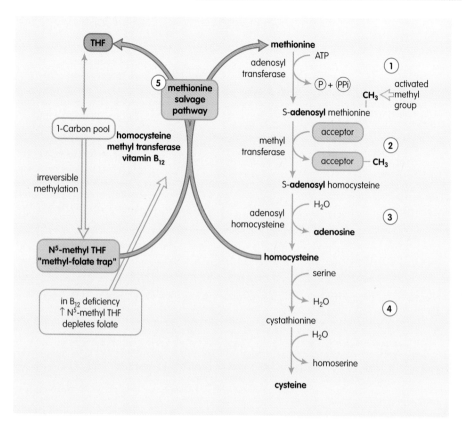

Fig. 6.3 Formation of S-adenosyl methionine (SAM) and the methionine salvage pathway. SAM is formed by condensation of ATP and methionine. It contains an activated CH3 group that can be transferred to a number of acceptor molecules. Homocysteine released from hydrolysis of S-adenosyl homocysteine can either be used for synthesis of the amino acid cysteine or for the methionine salvage pathway. The methionine salvage pathway reverses the methyl-folate trap (numbers refer to the text).

Fig. 6.4 Serine to glycine conversion.
1. Serine hydroxymethyl transferase transfers a methyl group from serine to tetrahydrofolate (THF) forming N^5,N^{10}-methylene THF and glycine.
2. This methyl group can then be used for the synthesis of thymidine (discussed later in this chapter).
3. The glycine cleavage enzyme (glycine synthase) oxidatively decarboxylates glycine, generating N^5,N^{10}-methylene THF and CO_2.

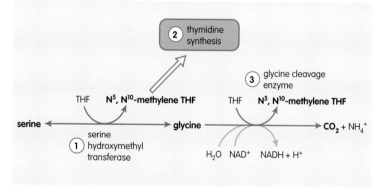

acid. Two pathways are concerned with the formation of purine nucleotides (Fig. 6.7).

I. De novo synthesis of purines

The purine ring is assembled on a molecule of ribose-5-phosphate; therefore, the purines are synthesized as mononucleotides as opposed to free bases. The location of this pathway is in the cytosol of liver cells (hepatocytes) and there are two stages:

- The formation of inosine monophosphate. Eleven reactions are necessary to form inosine monophosphate (IMP), the nucleotide of hypoxanthine. The first reaction forms 5-phosphoribosyl-1-pyrophosphate (PRPP). The

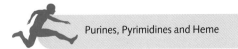

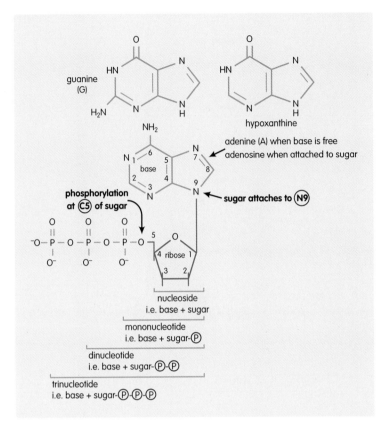

Fig. 6.5 Structure of purines, nucleosides and nucleotides. Purines are the nitrogenous bases adenine, guanine and hypoxanthine. They can either exist as free bases or with a pentose sugar, usually ribose or deoxyribose attached at the N9 position to form a nucleoside. For example, adenine is the free base, adenosine is the nucleoside; or guanine is the free base, guanosine is the nucleoside. The nucleoside of hypoxanthine is called inosine. Phosphorylation of the sugar at the C5 position leads to the formation of mono-, di- and tri-nucleotides as shown.

Main functions of purines	
Functions	**Examples**
building blocks of DNA and RNA	adenine and guanine
components of cofactors, particularly adenine	NAD^+, FAD, CoA
components of high-energy compounds in cell	ATP, GTP, AMP, etc.
components of regulatory compounds	ATP, ADP, NAD^+, etc.
components of signaling molecules	cAMP, cGMP, GTP, G-proteins
components of neurotransmitters	cGMP

Fig. 6.6 Main functions of purines.

rest of the reactions are concerned with the construction of the purine ring by the addition of five carbon and four nitrogen atoms from amino acids (aspartate, glycine, and glutamine), CO_2 and THF derivatives to PRPP.

- The conversion of IMP to AMP and guanosine monophosphate (GMP).

II. Salvage pathways
The turnover of nucleic acids leads to the release of free purines. These free bases are recycled by the salvage pathway, which re-attaches a sugar and a phosphate group to reform the nucleotide.

Breakdown of purines
AMP and GMP are broken down to the free bases hypoxanthine and xanthine, respectively (see Fig. 6.7). These are converted into uric acid, which is excreted by the kidneys. Uric acid is insoluble. When present at high levels in the blood it may precipitate out forming crystals which may cause gout. These pathways will now be considered in more detail.

Purine formation
De novo synthesis of purines
The sources of the carbon and nitrogen atoms for the synthesis of the purine ring are shown in Fig. 6.8.

Fig. 6.7 Overview of purine metabolism. Two pathways are concerned with the formation of purine nucleotides:

I. *De novo* synthesis of purines, where the purine ring is assembled on a molecule of ribose-5-phosphate. The pathway consists of two stages:

   a. Formation of IMP, which occurs in 11 reactions. The purine ring is constructed by addition of C and N atoms from a number of sources: amino acids, CO_2 and THF derivatives.

   b. IMP is then converted to either GMP or AMP.

II. Salvage pathways "recycle" free purines released during nucleic acid turnover by re-attaching a sugar phosphate unit to them.

There is only one pathway for purine breakdown, which converts the purines to the free bases hypoxanthine and xanthine; these are then oxidized to uric acid for excretion by the kidney.

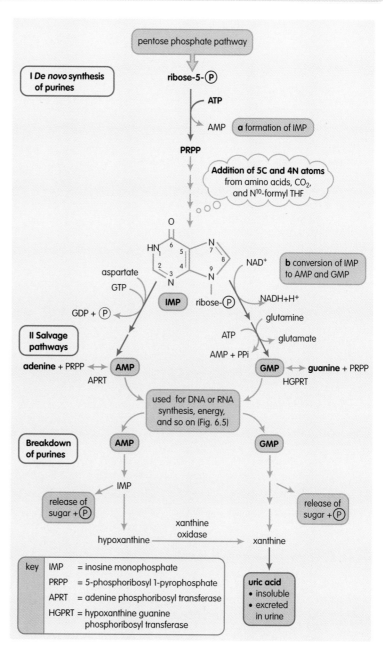

key

IMP	=	inosine monophosphate
PRPP	=	5-phosphoribosyl 1-pyrophosphate
APRT	=	adenine phosphoribosyl transferase
HGPRT	=	hypoxanthine guanine phosphoribosyl transferase

Formation of IMP

This first stage of purine synthesis has 11 reactions (numbers refer to Fig. 6.9):

1. 5-Phosphoribosyl-1-pyrophosphate (PRPP) synthesis: PRPP synthetase catalyzes the phosphorylation of ribose-5-phosphate at the C1 position, forming 5-phosphoribosyl-1-pyrophosphate. This irreversible reaction requires two molecules of ATP (as ATP is hydrolyzed to AMP) and serves to "activate" ribose-5-phosphate.

2. The synthesis of 5-phosphoribosylamine. PRPP glutamyl amidotransferase catalyzes the addition of an amide group from glutamine to the C1 position, displacing the pyrophosphate. This starts the formation of the purine ring at N9, and is the irreversible rate-limiting step of the pathway.

3. The addition of glycine requires ATP.

4. The addition of the formyl group from N^5N^{10}-methenyl THF produces C8 of the five-carbon ring.

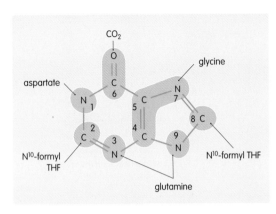

Fig. 6.8 Sources of the carbon and nitrogen atoms of the purine ring (THF, tetrahydrofolate.)

5. The addition of the second amide group from glutamine requires ATP.
6. Closure of the five-carbon ring requires ATP.
7. Carboxylation at the C6 position.
8. The addition of aspartate. The whole molecule attaches at position C6, requiring ATP.
9. The removal of the carbon skeleton of aspartate as fumarate, leaving behind the amino group to form N1 of the six-carbon ring.
10. The addition of a second formyl group from N^{10}-formyl THF.
11. Closure of the six-carbon ring.

The formation of IMP requires six molecules of ATP in total.

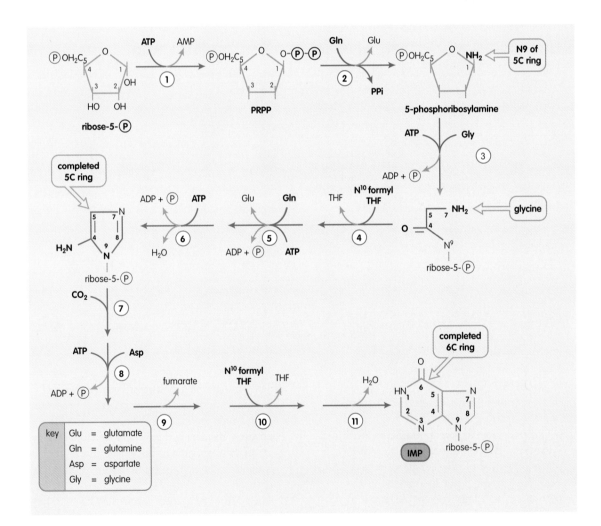

Fig. 6.9 Formation of inosine monophosphate (IMP). This first stage of purine synthesis has 11 reactions (numbers refer to text).

In purine formation, the five-carbon ring is synthesized first. The order of assembly is very useful to know:
1. N9 from glutamine
2. C4, C5, N7 from glycine
3. C8 from N^{10}-formyl THF
4. N3 from glutamine
5. C6 from CO_2
6. N1 from aspartate
7. C2 from N^{10}-formyl THF

Conversion of IMP to AMP and GMP

IMP is converted to GMP by the addition of an amino group at the C2 position; two steps are involved (Fig. 6.10):
1. Oxidation at C2 by IMP dehydrogenase, forming xanthosine monophosphate (XMP).
2. Insertion of the amino group from glutamine by GMP synthase to form GMP.

The synthesis of GMP requires ATP; that is, the reciprocal nucleotide is required.

AMP is formed from IMP by converting the keto group at the C6 position to an amino group; again two steps are involved (see Fig. 6.10):

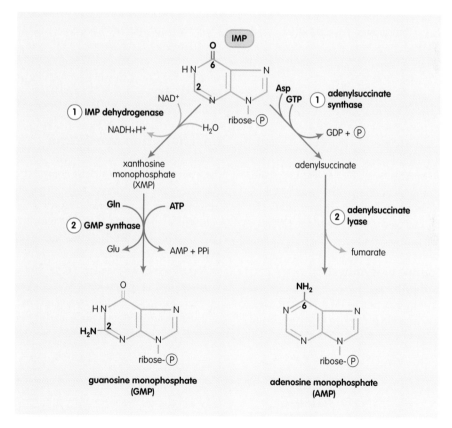

Fig. 6.10 Conversion of inosine monophosphate (IMP) to AMP and GMP. Both conversions involve two steps. Conversion of IMP to GMP involves:

1. Oxidation at the C2 position by IMP dehydrogenase, forming xanthosine monophosphate.
2. The amino group of glutamine is then inserted at the C2 position by GMP synthase to form GMP. This reaction requires the reciprocal nucleotide, ATP.

Conversion of IMP to AMP involves:
1. Addition of aspartate at the C6 position to form adenylsuccinate. This reaction requires the reciprocal nucleotide, GTP.
2. Adenylsuccinate lyase then eliminates the C-skeleton of aspartate as fumarate, leaving behind the amino group at C6 to form AMP.

1. The addition of aspartate at the C6 position by adenylsuccinate synthase. This reaction requires GTP (again the reciprocal nucleotide).
2. The elimination of the carbon skeleton of aspartate as fumarate, leaving behind the amino group.

Regulation of purine biosynthesis

Purine synthesis is controlled allosterically by feedback inhibition at four major control sites:

- PRPP synthetase. This is inhibited by the end products GMP and AMP. Since PRPP is also an intermediate in both the salvage pathway and pyrimidine synthesis (discussed later in this chapter), this is not the major control site.
- PRPP amidotransferase. This irreversible, rate-limiting reaction is unique to purine synthesis. It is allosterically inhibited by the end products IMP, AMP, and GMP.
- Adenylsuccinate synthase. This is inhibited by the end product AMP.
- IMP dehydrogenase. This is inhibited by the end product GMP.

If regulation is lost because of a defect in one of these four regulatory enzymes, this may lead to the overproduction of AMP and GMP, in excess of the requirements for nucleic acid synthesis and other functions. The excess purines are broken down to uric acid, which may become deposited in tissues, leading to symptoms of gout.

ATP yield of purine biosynthesis

The formation of IMP requires six molecules of ATP (see Fig. 6.9); the conversion of IMP to AMP uses one GTP; the conversion of IMP to GMP uses two molecules of ATP (see Fig. 6.10). Therefore, seven molecules of ATP are required to form one molecule of AMP and eight ATP are required to form a molecule of GMP.

Thus, in terms of energy, the *de novo* pathway is an expensive process. The salvage pathway, however, provides an alternative way of forming purine nucleotides without using much ATP.

Salvage pathways

When nucleic acids and nucleotides are broken down, the free bases are released. The salvage pathway recycles these free bases by re-attaching ribose-5-phosphate to them (Fig. 6.11). It is a one-step pathway and the ribose-5-phosphate is transferred to the free bases from PRPP. The release of pyrophosphate makes the reactions irreversible. Only two enzymes are necessary: adenine phosphoribosyl transferase (APRT) and hypoxanthine guanine phosphoribosyl transferase (HGPRT). The pathway is simple and requires much less ATP than *de novo* synthesis because the bases do not have to be made first.

Lesch–Nyhan syndrome

Lesch–Nyhan syndrome is a very rare, X-linked disorder caused by an almost complete absence of the salvage enzyme hypoxanthine guanine phosphoribosyl transferase (HGPRT). HGPRT catalyzes the addition of 5-phosphoribosyl-1-pyrophosphate (PRPP) to the purine bases, guanine, and hypoxanthine in the salvage pathway; that is, it recycles free bases (see Fig. 6.11). In Lesch–Nyhan syndrome a decreased level of HGPRT results in:

- Increased guanine and hypoxanthine in excess of their requirements, which are broken down to

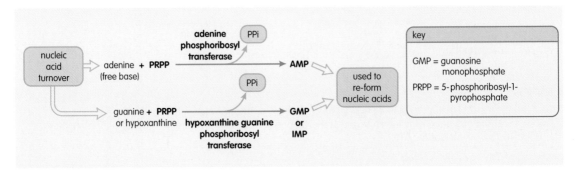

Fig. 6.11 Salvage pathways. When nucleic acids and nucleotides are broken down, free bases are released. The salvage pathway recycles these free bases by re-attaching ribose-5-phosphate to them by transfer from PRPP.

form large amounts of uric acid, leading to severe hyperuricemia and gout.

- Increased levels of PRPP, which is therefore used for the *de novo* synthesis of purines, leading to purine overproduction and severe neurological disturbances.

The salvage pathway for adenine is normal. It is thought that the level of HGPRT activity is related to the severity of symptoms. For example:

- If HGPRT activity is less than 2%, moderate mental retardation is present.
- If HGPRT activity is less than 0.2%, severe mental retardation and self-mutilation occur.

The prognosis is very poor; sufferers usually die by the age of 5 years. The clinical features and diagnosis of Lesch–Nyhan syndrome are discussed in Fig. 6.12.

Breakdown of purines

The breakdown of purines occurs in two stages: the breakdown of the nucleotide to a free base hypoxanthine or xanthine, and the formation of uric acid (Fig. 6.13).

I. Breakdown of the nucleotide to a free base: hypoxanthine or xanthine

Three reactions are necessary (numbers refer to Fig. 6.13):

1. The removal of the phosphate group by a nucleotidase.

Clinical features and treatment of Lesch–Nyhan syndrome	
Clinical features	**Diagnosis and treatment**
hyperuricemia causing: • kidney stones • arthritis • gout severe neurological disturbances: • spasticity and mental retardation • self-mutilation (bite fingers and lips to the bone) symptoms begin at about 3 months	**diagnosis:** • orange nappy (urine) • hypoxanthine guanine phosphoribosyl transferase activity • symptoms **treatment:** • allopurinol lowers uric acid levels and helps to control gout and arthritis • with time, high purine levels result in worsening of neurological symptoms because no treatment is possible • boys usually die from kidney failure because of high sodium urate deposits causing kidney stones

Fig. 6.12 Clinical features and treatment of Lesch–Nyhan syndrome.

Fig. 6.13 Breakdown of purines. Breakdown of purines occurs in two stages:
I. The breakdown of the nucleotide to a free base, hypoxanthine or xanthine. For both AMP and GMP, three reactions are necessary, although the order differs:
1. removal of the phosphate group.
2. removal of ribose as ribose-1-phosphate.
3. release of amino group.
II. Formation of uric acid by the oxidation of hypoxanthine and xanthine by xanthine oxidase.

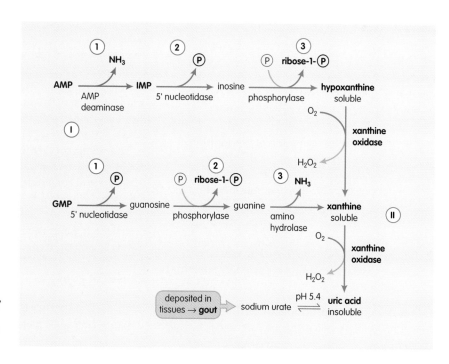

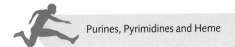

2. The removal of ribose as ribose-1-phosphate by nucleoside phosphorylase.
3. The release of the amino group.

Both AMP and GMP are degraded by the same three reactions; only the order differs (shown in Fig. 6.13). AMP and IMP form hypoxanthine and GMP forms xanthine.

II. Formation of uric acid
Only two steps are necessary, and are catalyzed by the same enzyme (see Fig. 6.13):
1. The oxidation of hypoxanthine to xanthine by xanthine oxidase.
2. The oxidation of xanthine to uric acid by the same enzyme.

Xanthine oxidase is the key enzyme involved in purine degradation. It is unusual because it is a molybdenum- and iron-containing flavoprotein that uses molecular oxygen as an oxidizing agent.

In humans, the uric acid formed is excreted in the urine. Uric acid is insoluble. The acidic pH of urine allows it to precipitate out at high concentrations as sodium urate. Hyperuricemia, that is high serum levels of uric acid, may lead to gout (see below).

Xanthine oxidase inhibitors
Xanthine oxidase is the key enzyme involved in controlling the amount of uric acid produced. Treatment with xanthine oxidase inhibitors decreases the amount of uric acid formed and increases the amounts of the soluble precursors hypoxanthine and xanthine, which are easily excreted in the urine. Allopurinol, an analog of hypoxanthine, is the most commonly used xanthine oxidase inhibitor. It has a number of actions:
- It is a competitive inhibitor of xanthine oxidase.
- The salvage enzyme can catalyze the addition of ribose-5-phosphate to allopurinol, forming allopurinol ribonucleotide. This can inhibit the rate-limiting enzyme of *de novo* purine synthesis, namely by PRPP amidotransferase, leading to a decrease in the level of purines and also of the PRPP pool.
- Allopurinol can be metabolized by xanthine oxidase to oxypurinol, an even stronger inhibitor of xanthine oxidase.

Other breakdown products of purines
In mammals other than primates, uric acid is further degraded by splitting of the purine ring to form

Clinical features and diagnosis of gout	
Clinical features	**Diagnosis**
hyperuricemia recurrent attacks of acute arthritis caused by deposition of sodium urate crystals in joints; usually only one joint affected (big toe > 90%) kidney stones and ↑ chance of renal disease tophi under skin and around joints	synoval fluid examination: affected joint is aspirated and fluid examined under microscope for long, needle-shaped, negatively birefringent crystals hyperuricemia does not necessarily cause gout

Fig. 6.14 Clinical features and diagnosis of gout.

allantoin, which is highly soluble. The reason why humans and monkeys have lost the ability to break down uric acid may be because it has some evolutionary advantage. It is possible that, when we lost the ability to synthesize vitamin C, we also lost the enzyme uricase, which degrades uric acid to a soluble product. However, uric acid does have a beneficial effect: it is an effective scavenger of free oxygen radicals and can take over the role of vitamin C as an antioxidant. Remember, only humans and monkeys can get gout!

Gout
The prevalence of gout varies from about 0.1–0.2% in Europe to as high as 10% in the Maori population of New Zealand. It is caused by an abnormality of uric acid metabolism, resulting in hyperuricemia and the deposition of sodium urate crystals in joints, soft tissues and the kidney (Fig. 6.14).

The risk factors are that:
- Gout predominantly affects men in middle life. It does not occur before puberty (unless it is part of Lesch–Nyhan syndrome).
- In women, it occurs only after the menopause (the male to female ratio is 8:1).
- It is an inherited condition in some families.

Causes of gout
Genetic
- Decreased HGPRT levels; to 2–5% of normal. Similar to Lesch–Nyhan syndrome but not as severe.

- Overactive PRPP synthetase, involved in the regulation of purine biosynthesis (see above). Overactivity causes release from normal control, leading to increased rates of *de novo* synthesis of purines.
- Insensitive PRPP amidotransferase, the rate-controlling enzyme of purine synthesis. A mutant form has full activity but no regulatory sites, therefore feedback control is lost, causing overproduction of purines.
- The excess purines produced in these conditions are broken down to uric acid, leading to hyperuricemia and gout.

Secondary causes
- Increased purine turnover; for example, in leukemia, myeloproliferative disorders, and due to the use of cytotoxic drugs in control of cancers.
- Decreased excretion of uric acid; for example, drug therapy (thiazides, aspirin), lead toxicity, excess alcohol.

Management of gout
Acute attacks are treated with anti-inflammatory drugs: colchicine or nonsteroidal anti-inflammatory drugs (e.g., indomethacin) provide relief within 24–48 hours.

Long-term prophylaxis is aimed at decreasing uric acid levels.
- Simple measures are weight reduction, decreased alcohol intake and withdrawal of drugs such as salicylates and thiazides.

Aspirin is absolutely contraindicated in gout because it impairs the excretion of uric acid by the renal tubules, aggravating hyperuricemia.

- Allopurinol is a xanthine oxidase inhibitor. It is the main drug used for the prophylaxis of gout (see above).
- Probenecid, a uricosuric drug, is an alternative to allopurinol. It has a direct action on the renal tubule, preventing the reabsorption of uric acid in the kidney, causing it to be excreted.

Pyrimidine metabolism

Structure and function of pyrimidines
Structure
There are three main pyrimidines: thymine, cytosine, and uracil. Like purines, the pyrimidines are mostly found associated with a five-carbon sugar attached at N1 to form the nucleosides thymidine, cytidine and uridine (Fig. 6.15). The sugar may be mono-, di-, or tri-phosphorylated to form the corresponding nucleotides.

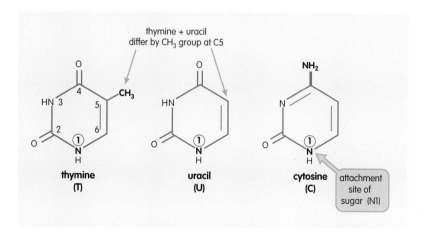

Fig. 6.15 Structure of pyrimidines. Like purines, the pyrimidines are mostly found associated with a five-carbon sugar attached at N1 to form nucleosides.

Functions

Pyrimidines are the building blocks of DNA and RNA: thymine and cytosine are present in DNA and cytosine and uracil are present in RNA.

Nucleotide derivatives are activated intermediates in a number of synthetic reactions; for example, UDP-glucose, the precursor of glycogen (see Chapter 2).

Biosynthesis of pyrimidines

There are three main stages in the biosynthesis of pyrimidines (Figs. 6.16, 6.17, and 6.18):

a. The construction of the pyrimidine ring to form uridine monophosphate (UMP).

b. The conversion of UMP to uridine triphosphate (UTP) and cytidine triphosphate (CTP), the ribonucleotides found in RNA.

c. The formation of the deoxyribonucleotides dCTP and dTTP found in DNA see (Fig. 6.18).

All of the three stages take place in the cell cytosol and will now be considered in more detail.

Construction of the pyrimidine ring

Unlike purine synthesis, the pyrimidine ring is synthesized before attachment to ribose-5-phosphate, that is, it is formed as a free base. The ring is derived from glutamine, aspartate and CO_2 (see Fig. 6.17). There are six steps in the reaction sequence (numbers refer to Fig. 6.16).

1. The synthesis of carbamoyl phosphate by carbamoyl phosphate synthase II (CPSII). This is the rate-limiting step. Carbamoyl phosphate is also the precursor of urea; however, urea is formed by the mitochondrial enzyme, carbamoyl phosphate synthase I (see Chapter 5).

2. The addition of aspartate.

3. Closure of the ring by dihydroorotase. The first three enzymes are actually present as a single

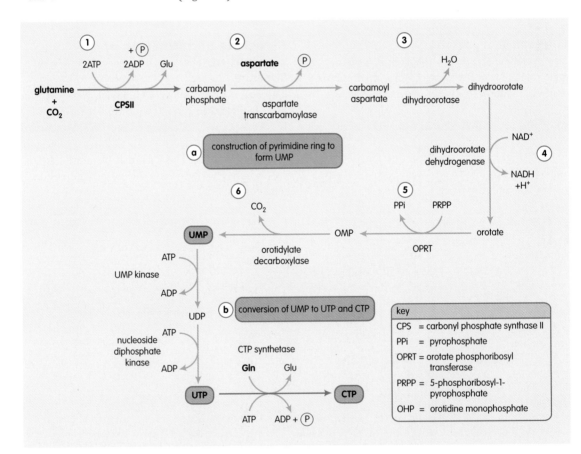

Fig. 6.16 Pyrimidine synthesis: there are three main stages in the biosynthesis of pyrimidines. Construction of the pyrimidine ring from glutamine, aspartate and CO_2 to form uridine monophosphate. UMP can then be converted to UDP, UTP and CTP, the ribonucleotides of RNA (numbers refer to text). The third stage of pyrimidine synthesis is shown in Fig. 6.17.

polypeptide chain, forming a multi-functional enzyme, CAD of carbamoyl phosphate synthase II, aspartate trans-carbamoylase and dihydroorotase. In a similar way to fatty acid synthase, the enzymes are linked together to minimize side reactions and loss of substrate.

4. The oxidation of dihydroorotate to orotate using NAD^+.

5. Conversion of the free pyrimidine to a nucleotide by the addition of ribose-5-phosphate from PRPP. This is catalyzed by orotate phosphoribosyl transferase (OPRT) and is driven by the hydrolysis of pyrophosphate to two free molecules of inorganic phosphate. PRPP is thus required for the synthesis of both purines and pyrimidines.

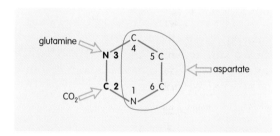

Fig. 6.17 The pyrimidine ring. The ring is derived from glutamine, aspartate and CO_2.

6. The decarboxylation of orotidine monophosphate (OMP) to UMP by orotidylate decarboxylase. Both OPRT and orotidylate decarboxylase are also found together as a single polypeptide.

Conversion of UMP to UDP, UTP and CTP— the ribonucleotides of RNA

UMP is phosphorylated to UDP and UTP, as shown in Fig. 6.16. CTP is formed from UTP by amination, that is, the addition of an NH_2 group from glutamine to position 4 of the pyrimidine ring. Both UTP and CTP are used for RNA synthesis.

Formation of the deoxyribonucleotides dCTP and dTTP (see Fig. 6.18)

1. Formation of dCTP. Ribonucleotide reductase reduces CDP to dCDP by removing the C2 hydroxyl group on ribose, converting it to deoxyribose. The enzyme requires thioredoxin as a cofactor. The actual mechanism is quite complicated but can be divided into three steps (not shown in Fig. 6.18):

   • Ribonucleotide reductase contains two thiol (SH) groups and it is these that actually reduce the ribose.

   • Thioredoxin also contains two thiol groups that are oxidized to enable the thiol groups on the enzyme to be re-formed.

   • NADPH then reduces the cofactor to regenerate the reduced form.

Fig. 6.18 Pyrimidine synthesis: the formation of deoxyribonucleotides.
1. Ribonucleotide reductase reduces CDP to deoxyCDP by removal of the C2 hydroxyl group on ribose, converting it to deoxyribose. The dCDP formed is phosphorylated to dCTP.
2. dTTP is formed by the methylation of dUMP. Thymidylate synthetase transfers a methyl group from N^5,N^{10}-methylene THF to position 5 of the pyrimidine ring, forming dTMP, which can be phosphorylated to dTTP (numbers refer to text below). DHF, dihydrofolate; THF, tetrahydrofolate.

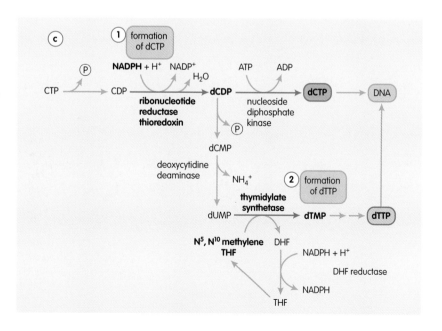

The dCDP formed is phosphorylated by nucleoside diphosphate kinase to dCTP.

2. Formation of dTTP. dTTP is formed by the methylation of dUMP. Dephosphorylation and deamination convert dCDP to dUMP, the precursor of dTMP. Thymidylate synthetase catalyzes the transfer of a methyl group from N^5,N^{10}-methylene THF to position 5 of the pyrimidine ring, forming dTMP. The reaction is unusual because N^5,N^{10}-methylene THF undergoes oxidation itself to dihydrofolate, that is, it transfers the methyl group and a hydrogen atom. Dihydrofolate reductase regenerates the THF. dTMP can be phosphorylated by dTMP kinase and nucleoside diphosphate kinase to dTTP.

Regulation of pyrimidine synthesis

The rate-limiting step in humans is the formation of carbamoyl phosphate by carbamoyl phosphate synthase II. CPSII is inhibited by the end products of pyrimidine synthesis, namely UDP and UTP. The reaction is activated by ATP and PRPP.

Regulation of deoxyribonucleotide synthesis

Ribonucleotide reductase actually catalyzes the irreversible reduction of all four nucleoside diphosphates (ADP, GDP, CDP, and UDP) to their corresponding deoxy forms and is therefore subject to regulation. The enzyme has four subunits (two B1 and two B2). Each B1 subunit has two allosteric sites distinct from the active site: an activity site and a substrate specificity site. The binding of the product dATP to the activity site inhibits the enzyme. The binding of the substrate, a ribonucleotide (e.g. ATP),

to the substrate specificity site activates the enzyme.

Salvage pathways

The salvage pathways for pyrimidines are similar to those for purines (Fig. 6.19). The breakdown of nucleotides releases free pyrimidines that are salvaged by the enzyme uracil/thymine phosphoribosyl transferase (UTPRT), which re-attaches a ribose-5-phosphate to them, reforming the mononucleotides. PRPP donates the ribose-5-phosphate. The enzyme UTPRT cannot salvage cytosine. Therefore cytidine (nucleoside) is deaminated to uridine; this can then be converted to uracil, which can be salvaged.

Breakdown of pyrimidines

Purines are excreted with their ring still intact as uric acid. The pyrimidine ring, however, can be split and broken down to soluble structures (Fig. 6.20). Uracil and cytosine are broken down to β-alanine, which forms acetyl CoA. Thymine is degraded to β-aminoisobutyrate, which forms succinyl CoA. The carbon skeletons of the pyrimidines, namely acetyl CoA and succinyl CoA, can be oxidized by the TCA cycle.

Anticancer drugs

These drugs inhibit the formation of nucleotides, leading to a decrease in DNA synthesis and cell growth. Cancer cells divide rapidly and have an increased demand for DNA synthesis. These drugs help to slow down the growth of cancer cells. However, they also affect normal cell replication, leading to serious side effects (Fig. 6.21).

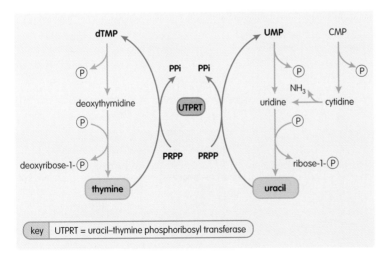

Fig. 6.19 Salvage pathway. The salvage pathways for pyrimidines are similar to those for purines. Breakdown of nucleotides releases free pyrimidines thymine and uracil. UTPRT transfers a ribose-5-phosphate unit from PRPP, to the free pyrimidine to reform the mononucleotide; for example, UMP or dTMP. Cytidine must be deaminated to uridine since it is not a substrate for UTPRT.

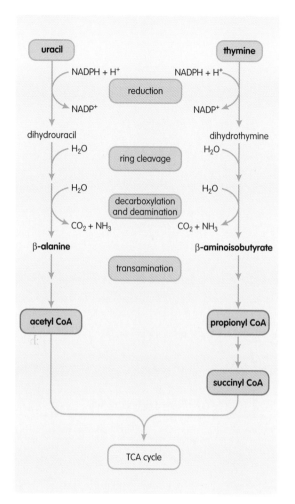

Fig. 6.20 Breakdown of pyrimidines. Purines are excreted with their ring still intact as uric acid. The pyrimidine ring, however, can be split and broken down to soluble structures such as acetyl CoA and succinyl CoA for oxidation by the TCA cycle. Note: only the main reactions and substrates are shown here.

Action of anti-cancer drugs		
Drugs	Action	Effect on pyrimidine and purine synthesis
glutamine antagonists: azaserine, diazo-oxo-norleucine	analogs of glutamine: competitively inhibit enzymes that use glutamine as substrate	↓ pyrimidine synthesis: inhibits CPS II ↓ purine synthesis: inhibits reaction 2 (PRPP amidotransferase) and reaction 5 (Fig. 6.8)
folate antagonists: methotrexate	inhibits DHF reductase leading to decreased available THF for transfer of one-carbon units	inhibits methylation of dUMP to dTMP causing ↓ dTMP synthesis ↓ purine synthesis (Fig. 6.8)
5-fluorouracil	analog of dUMP: irreversibly inhibits thymidylate synthetase	inhibits synthesis of dTMP; no effect on purine synthesis

Fig. 6.21 Action of anticancer drugs.

Most anticancer drugs affect normal cell replication and proliferation, especially cells of the bone marrow, gastrointestinal tract, gonads, skin, and hair follicles. This results in severe side effects such as anemia, neutropenia (making patients susceptibile to infection), hair loss, vomiting, infertility, impaired wound healing, and stunting of growth.

Azidothymidine and other antiviral drugs

Azidothymidine (AZT) is a nucleoside analog of thymidine in which the 3′ hydroxyl group on the ribose is replaced by an azido group (N3). AZT can be phosphorylated to the nucleotide AZTTP, which is a potent inhibitor of reverse transcriptase, the enzyme found in retroviruses that is responsible for replication of the viral genome. Therefore, AZT inhibits viral replication. AZT has been used with some success in treatment of the retrovirus HIV. Host-cell DNA polymerase is relatively insensitive to AZT.

Acyclovir or acycloguanosine is an analog of guanosine which is used in the treatment of herpesvirus infections. Humans cannot use acyclovir as a substrate, but the herpesvirus can. It can be phosphorylated by a viral enzyme and incorporated into the DNA chain, where it causes chain termination, preventing viral DNA replication.

121

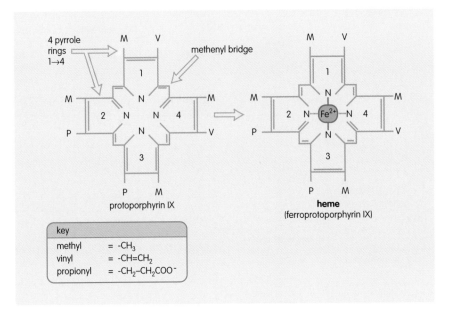

Fig. 6.22 Structure of heme. Heme consists of an Fe^{2+} atom bound in the center of protoporphyrin IX.

Heme metabolism

Structure and function of heme
Structure
It is very easy to get lost with the terminology used in heme metabolism; this is a basic "all you need to know" approach.

- The basic structure is a four-ringed cyclic structure called a porphyrin.
- Each ring is called a pyrrole ring and the rings are linked together via methenyl bridges.
- Three types of side chains can be attached to the pyrrole ring—methyl, vinyl or propionyl—and the arrangement of these is important to the activity.
- Porphyrins bind metal ions to form metalloporphyrins.

Heme is a structure containing an iron atom (as Fe^{2+}) bound in the center of a tetrapyrrole ring of protoporphyrin IX (Fig. 6.22).

Functions
Heme is the prosthetic group found in a number of proteins. The function of heme in each group can vary (Fig. 6.23). The Fe^{2+} atom (ferrous form) at the center of the heme structure can undergo oxidation to Fe^{3+} (ferric form); this is important to its function in cytochromes and enzymes, enabling it to act as a

Heme-containing proteins	
Protein	**Function of heme**
hemoglobin and myoglobin	reversibly binds O_2 for transport
peroxidases and catalase	forms part of the active site of enzyme
cylochromes [a, b, c, and P450]	electron carrier: continually oxidized and reduced, enhancing electron flow

Fig. 6.23 Main functions of heme.

recyclable electron carrier. However, in hemoglobin and myoglobin, Fe^{3+} cannot bind oxygen, and its function as an oxygen transporter is impaired (it forms methemoglobin; see Chapter 3).

Heme biosynthesis
The main locations of heme biosynthesis are:
- Bone marrow erythroid cells, where heme is used to form hemoglobin.
- Liver hepatocytes, where heme is used for cytochrome synthesis, particularly cytochrome P450 which is involved in drug metabolism.

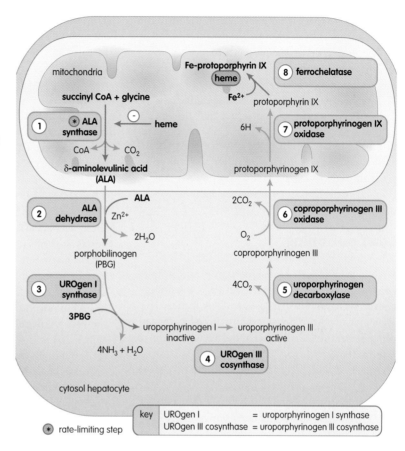

Fig. 6.24 Heme synthesis. The site of heme biosynthesis is "partitioned" between mitochondria and the cytosol. The first and last three reactions occur in the mitochondria, the rest are in the cytosol. ALA synthase catalyzes the condensation of glycine and succinyl CoA to form ALA. Two molecules of ALA condense to form PBG. Four molecules of PBG then condense to form uroporphyrinogen I, which is activated by uroporphyrinogen (UROgen) III cosynthase, converting it to the asymmetrical active form, uroporphyrinogen III. The rest of the reactions modify the side chains and degree of saturation of the porphyrin ring. Ferrochelatase inserts the Fe^{2+} ion to form heme in the mitochondria (numbers are explained in the text).

Humans make 40–50 mg/day of heme, about 80–85% of which is used for hemoglobin synthesis. Mature RBCs lack mitochondria; therefore, they cannot make heme.

Site

Heme biosynthesis is partitioned between mitochondria and the cytosol (Fig. 6.24).

An overview of the pathway

- There are eight reactions; the first and last three occur in mitochondria, the rest are in the cytosol.
- Protoporphyrin IX is derived totally from glycine and succinyl CoA.
- Eight moles of each are required to form eight moles of δ-aminolevulinic acid (ALA), which condenses to form four moles of porphobilinogen (PBG). These, in turn, condense to form one mole of uroporphyrinogen I (UROgen I).
- The rest of the reactions modify the side chains.
- If the side chains on porphyrins are arranged symmetrically, then the molecules are physiologically inactive. When the side chains are

arranged asymmetrically, the molecules are active.

The steps are now considered in detail (see Fig. 6.24).

1. The synthesis of ALA. ALA synthase catalyzes the condensation of glycine and succinyl CoA in mitochondria. The reaction requires pyridoxal phosphate (PLP) as a cofactor. This is the irreversible, rate-limiting step of heme synthesis.
2. The formation of porphobilinogen (PBG). ALA dehydrase catalyzes the dehydration of two molecules of ALA to form PBG. The enzyme is inhibited by heavy metals such as lead.
3. Formation of uroporphyrinogen I (UROgen I). UROgen I synthase catalyzes the condensation of four molecules of PBG to form UROgen I (inactive).
4. UROgen III cosynthase produces the asymmetrical active uroporphyrinogen III (UROgen III). The rest of the reactions alter the side chains and the degree of unsaturation of the porphyrin ring.

5. The first decarboxylation results in the formation of coproporphyrinogen III.
6. The second decarboxylation forms protoporphyrinogen IX in the mitochondria.
7. Oxidation to protoporphyrin IX.
8. Ferrochelatase inserts the Fe^{2+} ion into the ring to form heme.

Protoporphyrinogen IX is the colorless, unstable, easily oxidized precursor of porphyrin. Porphyrins are highly colored (red), stable compounds that characteristically absorb ultraviolet light at a wavelength of 400 nm.

Lead poisoning

The human body contains about 120 mg of lead. Excessive ingestion or inhalation can result from contaminated food, water or air. Lead-containing chemicals have industrial uses and can lead to excessive exposure. Lead inhibits three key enzymes of heme synthesis, resulting in the accumulation of intermediates:

- ALA dehydrase leads to the accumulation of ALA, which can be measured in urine.
- Coproporphyrinogen III oxidase leads to the accumulation of coproporphyrinogen III.
- Ferrochelatase leads to the accumulation of protoporphyrin IX in RBCs.

Clinical features and diagnosis of lead poisoning	
Clinical features	Diagnosis
acute exposure: • severe weakness, vomiting, abdominal pain, anorexia and constipation **chronic exposure:** • causes staining of teeth and bones, myopathy, peripheral neuropathy, renal damage and sideroblastic anemia • eventually causes lead encephalopathy and seizures • may cause mental retardation in children	blood lead levels >3 mg/L indicate significant exposure urine: ↑ δ-aminolevulinic acid levels red cell: ↑ porphyrin levels and fluorescence blood film: anemia with punctate basophilia; red cells may contain small, blue deposits

Fig. 6.25 Clinical features and diagnosis of lead poisoning.

The result is the inhibition of heme synthesis and anemia. Lead also binds to bone. The main clinical features and diagnostic criteria are discussed in Fig. 6.25.

Treatment

Treatment is with lead chelators such as desferrioxamine mesilate, sodim calcium edetate, or penicillamine. They all bind lead, forming a complex, which can be excreted in the urine.

The porphyrias

This is a group of rare, inherited disorders in which there is a partial deficiency of one of the enzymes of heme synthesis (see Fig. 6.24). This results in the inhibition of heme synthesis and thus the formation of excessive quantities of either porphyrin precursors; for example, δ-aminolevulinic acid (ALA) or porphobilinogen (PBG), or porphyrins themselves, depending on which enzyme is deficient (Fig. 6.26).

The inhibition of heme synthesis leads to decreased heme formation. The key, rate-limiting enzyme of heme synthesis is ALA synthase, which is normally inhibited by heme (Fig. 6.27). In porphyrias, the absence of heme releases the inhibition (and thus the control) of ALA synthase, resulting in the increased formation of intermediates preceding the defective enzyme in each porphyria.

When porphyrin precursors are produced in excess (ALA and PBG), they cause mainly neuropsychiatric symptoms and abdominal pain (the precursors are neurotoxins). When porphyrins themselves are produced in excess, they cause skin photosensitivity (that is, the skin burns and itches on exposure to light). This is because porphyrins absorb light, which excites them and induces the formation of oxygen free-radicals. These can attack membranes, particularly lysosomal membranes, leading to the release of enzymes which damage underlying layers of skin, rendering it susceptible to the light.

Porphyrias are diagnosed on the basis of symptoms and the pattern of porphyrins and their precursors present in the blood and urine.

Porphyrias are classified as either hepatic or erythropoeitic or acute and chronic (see Fig. 6.27). They are all rare; the most common is acute intermittent porphyria. The major features of each porphyria are now considered.

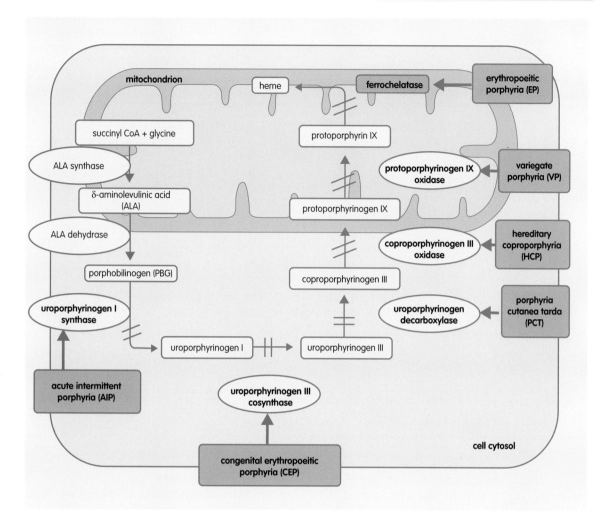

Fig. 6.26 Sites of enzyme deficiency in porphyrias.

Acute intermittent porphyria

Acute intermittent porphyria is an autosomal dominant disease with a prevalence of 1:100,000. The defect is a deficiency of uroporphyrinogen I synthase. Characteristically, acute attacks are separated by long periods of remission. The attacks are precipitated by various factors, such as alcohol, barbiturates, oral contraceptives, several anesthetic agents (including halothane), and certain antibiotics.

Clinical features

Presentation is usually in early adult life and includes:

- Acute abdominal symptoms.
- Neuropathy.
- Neuropsychiatric symptoms: depression, anxiety and even frank psychosis.

Results of laboratory tests

Increased levels of PBG and ALA can be found in the urine of these patients. The urine also darkens to a port-wine color on exposure to air, due to the presence of PBG.

Management

The treatment is with fluids, pain relief and a high carbohydrate diet, which inhibits the pathway. Avoiding precipitants is important. Therefore, it is important to ask about inherited disorders when assessing patients for surgery. Intravenous hematin can be given.

Congenital erythropoeitic porphyria

Congenital erythropoeitic porphyria is an extremely rare autosomal recessive disease that presents usually

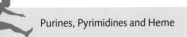
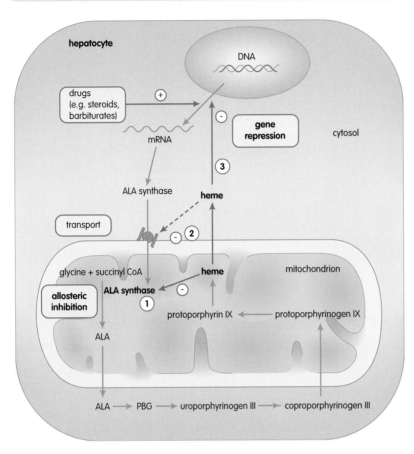

Fig. 6.27 Control of heme synthesis in the hepatocyte. In the liver, control of ALA synthase is considered at three levels:
1. Allosteric inhibition by end product, heme.
2. Inhibition of transport of newly made ALA synthase into the mitochondria by heme.
3. Heme also inhibits transcription of the ALA synthase gene.

Drugs, for example phenytoin or phenobarbitone, induce the activity of the cytochrome P450 enzymes which break heme down. This results in a decrease in the concentration of heme and thus stimulation of transcription of ALA synthase.

before 5 years of age. The defect is a deficiency of uroporphyrinogen III cosynthase. There are no neurological symptoms. In RBCs, increased levels of uroporphyrinogen I lead to severe photosensitivity. Increased levels of both uroporphyrinogen I and coproporphyrinogen I are found in the urine.

Porphyria cutanea tarda (cutaneous hepatic porphyria)

Porphyria cutanea tarda is an autosomal dominant condition. The defect is a deficiency of uroporphyrinogen decarboxylase. The condition has a high frequency in Europe and South America. There are no neurological symptoms.

Main clinical features

- Photosensitive rash.
- Skin fragility.
- Hyperpigmentation.

Precipitants are alcohol, estrogens, iron, and the autoimmune condition systemic lupus erythematosus.

Main biochemical changes

- Increased uroporphyrinogen I and III in the urine.
- Increased fecal coproporphyrinogen.
- Abnormal liver function tests.
- Mild iron overload.

Hereditary coproporphyria

Hereditary coproporphyria is a very rare autosomal dominant disease. The defect is a coproporphyrinogen III oxidase deficiency. It has an acute presentation with similar features to acute intermittent or variegate porphyria. However, patients may also be photosensitive. Increased levels of coproporphyrinogen III occur in both urine and feces.

Variegate porphyria

Variegate porphyria is a rare autosomal dominant disease. The defect is a protoporphyrinogen oxidase deficiency. It presents acutely in the same way as acute intermittent porphyria but patients are also photosensitive. Increased levels of PBG and ALA are found in the urine. Increased levels of

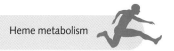

protoporphyringen IX and coproporphyrinogen III can be found in the feces.

Erythropoeitic porphyria

Erythropoeitic porphyria is an autosomal dominant condition. The defect is a deficiency of ferrochelatase, the last enzyme of the pathway.

Clinical features

These patients may present with:

- Photosensitive rash.
- Gallstones.
- Liver disease.

Results of laboratory tests

Diagnosis is made by fluorescence of peripheral RBCs because they contain free porphyrin. An increase in free protoporphyrin in RBCs, feces, and bile is also observed and may lead to mild anemia.

 Porphyrias are very rare. You will seldom see or be asked about them. Figs. 6.27 and 6.28 summarize all you will ever need to know.

Overall management

The effects of all porphyrias can be decreased by intravenous hemin which inhibits ALA synthase, the rate-controlling enzyme, regaining the control of heme synthesis. An increased dietary intake of antioxidant vitamins A, C, and E also helps to protect against free radical damage.

Regulation of heme synthesis

The key rate-limiting enzyme of heme synthesis is ALA synthase. It is an ideal control point because the enzyme undergoes rapid turnover (has a half-life of 60–70 min). ALA synthase is inhibited by high levels of the end product heme (Fe^{2+}) and also hemin (Fe^{3+}), formed by the oxidation of heme.

In the liver, control of ALA synthase by heme is considered at three levels (numbers refer to Fig. 6.28):

1. Allosteric inhibition of the enzyme by heme. However, high concentrations of heme are necessary (10^{-5} M); therefore, this is not regarded as an important control mechanism.
2. Heme also inhibits the transport of newly synthesized enzyme from cytosol into mitochondria.
3. Repression of transcription of the ALA synthase gene by heme. This is probably the most effective regulation because it works at low concentrations (10^{-7} M).

Summary of porphyrias					
Porphyria	Enzyme defect	Photosensitivity	Neurological symptoms	Biochemistry	
acute intermittent (hepatic)	uroporphyrinogen I synthase		yes	urine:	↑δ-aminolevulinic acid (ALA) and porphobilinogen (PBG)
congenital erythropoeitic	uroporphyrinogen III cosynthase	yes		red cell: ↑UROgen I urine: ↑UROgen I and COPROgen I	
cutaneous (hepatic)	uroporphyrinogen decarboxylase	yes		urine: ↑UROgen I and III feces: ↑COPROgen	
hereditary coproporphyria (hepatic)	coproporphyrinogen III oxidase	yes	yes	urine: ↑ALA, PBG and COPROgen III	
variegate (hepatic)	protoporphyrinogen IX oxidase	yes	yes	urine: ↑PBG and ALA feces: ↑PROTOgen IX, COPROgen III	
erythropoeitic	ferrochelatase	yes		red cell: ↑protoporphyrin	

Fig. 6.28 The porphyrias: summary.

In erythroid tissue, the same regulatory mechanisms apply as for the liver but, additionally, under certain conditions such as chronic hypoxia or anemia, erythropoeitin production is stimulated, leading to an increase in red cell synthesis and thus number and, therefore, an increase in heme.

Induction of ALA synthase in the liver

A number of drugs, such as steroids and barbiturates, cause an increase in the amount of hepatic ALA synthase. The mechanism proceeds as follows:

- Drugs are metabolized by microsomal cytochrome P450 enzymes, which are heme-containing proteins themselves.
- Certain drugs induce the synthesis of cytochrome P450, leading to an increase in the consumption and breakdown of heme.
- This leads to an overall decrease in the concentration of heme in the liver cells, which in turn stimulates or induces the transcription of ALA synthase and heme synthesis (see Fig. 6.28).
- Glucose blocks this induction.

Heme breakdown

About 80–85% of heme for breakdown comes from old RBCs; the rest comes from cytochrome turnover (Fig. 6.29).

Location/site

Kupffer cells and macrophages of the reticuloendothelial system (mainly liver, spleen, and bone marrow).

Pathway

The two steps in the pathway are (steps refer to Fig. 6.29):

1. Cleavage of the porphyrin ring to form biliverdin. Heme oxygenase found in microsomes splits the porphyrin ring by breaking one of the methenyl

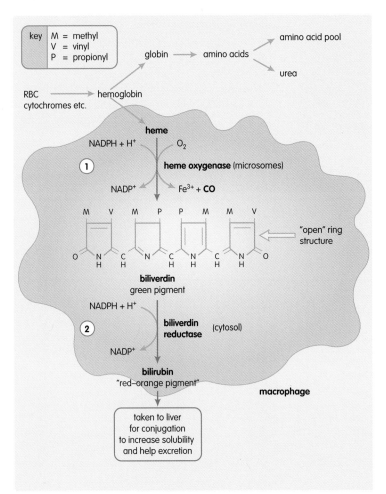

Fig. 6.29 Heme breakdown. About 80–85% of heme for breakdown comes from old red blood cells (RBCs); the rest comes from cytochrome turnover. The pathway consists of two steps: **1.** Cleavage of the porphyrin ring to form biliverdin by heme oxygenase. **2.** Reduction of biliverdin to bilirubin. Bilirubin is taken to the liver, where it is conjugated to facilitate its excretion (numbers refer to text).

bridges between two pyrrole rings. This produces biliverdin, Fe^{3+} and carbon monoxide (this is the only reaction in vivo that produces carbon monoxide).

2. The reduction of biliverdin to bilirubin in the cytosol. Bilirubin is an insoluble orange pigment, which is taken to the liver bound to albumin. In the liver it is conjugated with glucuronic acid by the enzyme bilirubin glucuronyl transferase, forming bilirubin diglucuronide. This increases its solubility, enabling its excretion in the bile.

Hemolytic anemia

Hemolytic anemia is an anemia resulting from an increase in RBC breakdown. Normally, red cell lysis releases heme for breakdown to bilirubin, which is taken to the liver to be conjugated and excreted. The liver has a large capacity to conjugate bilirubin and can cope with moderately elevated levels. However, massive red cell lysis that may occur in patients with severe hemolytic anemia, such as sickle cell anemia (during a crisis) or thalassemia, leads to a very large increase in heme breakdown and high bilirubin levels, greater than the conjugating capacity of the liver. This results in elevated plasma levels of unconjugated bilirubin, causing jaundice. In jaundice, the deposition of bilirubin leads to a yellow coloring of the skin, mucosal membranes, and the whites of the eyes (sclerae).

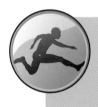

Heme breakdown occurs at sites of minor trauma underneath the skin. The changing colors of a bruise represent the different pigments produced.

- Describe the use of one-carbon units in the synthesis of amino acids.
- What is the significance of the methyl-folate trap to both folate and vitamin B_{12} metabolism?
- What are the structures and the main functions of adenine and guanine?
- Name the stages involved in *de novo* purine synthesis and the four regulatory enzymes.
- Describe the main functions of the salvage pathways.
- What use do xanthine oxidase inhibitors have?
- Describe the main clinical features of gout.
- How do anticancer drugs affect purine and pyrimidine synthesis?
- What are the similarities and differences between the mechanism of action of AZT and acyclovir?
- What clinical features would lead you to suspect acute lead poisoning?
- Why is it important to ask about porphyrias during preoperative assessment for surgery?
- Explain the biochemical basis for the signs and symptoms of hemolytic anemia.
- What investigations would you use to diagnose lead poisoning?
- What are the main locations and sites of heme biosynthesis?
- What is the effect of lead poisoning on heme synthesis?

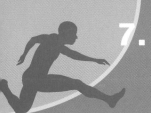

7. Glucose Homeostasis

The states of glucose homeostasis

Glucose homeostasis can be conveniently discussed by looking at three basic states: the fed, fasted (postabsorptive) and starved state (Fig. 7.1). The starved state can be further subdivided into early and late, since different fuels are available depending on the degree of starvation (Fig. 7.2).

It is important to realize that glucose homeostasis is a dynamic process. There are no well-defined boundaries between the states; instead, there is some degree of overlap between them, as the availability of substrates and hormonal influences are continually changing.

The fed state

This is the period 0–4 hours after a meal and is summarized in Fig. 7.3. During the fed state (numbers refer to Fig. 7.3):

1. An increase in plasma glucose results in the release of insulin from the beta cells in the pancreas. The availability of substrate and the increase in insulin stimulates glycogen, triacylglycerol (triglyceride), and protein synthesis by tissues; this is an anabolic state.
2. Glucose is the sole fuel for the brain; its uptake is insulin-independent.
3. Muscle and adipose tissue also use glucose; uptake by these tissues is insulin-dependent.

An increase in glucose and insulin activates glucokinase in the liver. Glucokinase, unlike hexokinase, is not inhibited by glucose-6-phosphate, enabling the liver to respond to the high blood glucose levels that occur after a meal. Glucokinase phosphorylates glucose, which can be used for synthesis of liver glycogen, therefore preventing hyperglycemia (see Chapter 2).

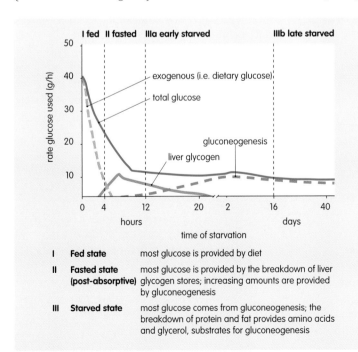

I	Fed state	most glucose is provided by diet
II	Fasted state (post-absorptive)	most glucose is provided by the breakdown of liver glycogen stores; increasing amounts are provided by gluconeogenesis
III	Starved state	most glucose comes from gluconeogenesis; the breakdown of protein and fat provides amino acids and glycerol, substrates for gluconeogenesis

Fig. 7.1 Three states of glucose homeostasis. Glucose homeostasis can be classified conveniently into three states: the fed, fasted (postabsorptive), and starved states. The starved state can be subdivided into early and late starvation.

Three stages of glucose homeostasis			
State	Time course	Major fuels used	Hormonal control
I fed	0–4 h following a meal	most tissues use glucose	↑ insulin results in: ↑ glucose uptake by peripheral tissues ↑ glycogen, TG, and protein synthesis
II fasted (post-absorptive)	4–12 h after a meal	brain: glucose muscle and liver: fatty acids	↑ glucagon and NE stimulates breakdown of liver glycogen and TG ↓ insulin
IIIa starved: early	12 h → 16 days without food	brain: glucose and some ketone bodies liver: fatty acids muscle: mainly fatty acids andsome ketone bodies	↑ glucagon and NE → ↑ TG hydrolysis and ketogenesis ↑ cortisol → breakdown of muscle protein, releasing amino acids for gluconeogenesis
IIIb starved: late	>16 days without food	brain: uses more ketone bodies and less glucose to preserve body protein muscle: only fatty acids	↑ glucagon and NE

Fig. 7.2 Three states of glucose homeostasis (NE, norepinephrine; TG, triacylglycerol).

Hexokinase, present in most cells, is maximally operational when the concentration of glucose in the blood is low.

The fasted state

This is the period 4–12 hours after a meal, also called the postabsorptive state (Fig. 7.4). During the fasted state (numbers refer to Fig. 7.4):

1. The breakdown of liver glycogen stores provides glucose for oxidation by the brain. These stores are sufficient to last only between 12 and 24 hours.
2. The hydrolysis of triacylglycerol from stores releases fatty acids, which are used preferentially as a fuel by muscle and liver.
3. Muscle can also use its own glycogen as a fuel.

All these processes involved are activated by the increase in the ratio of glucagon to insulin. This activates glycogen phosphorylase and hormone-sensitive lipase by phosphorylation. This in turn stimulates glycogen breakdown and lipolysis.

The starved state
Early starved state

Once the liver glycogen has been used up, an alternative substrate is required to provide glucose (Fig. 7.5). In early starvation (numbers refer to Fig. 7.5):

1. Glucagon and later cortisol activate protein breakdown in muscle which releases amino acids, particularly alanine and glutamine.
2. Hydrolysis of triacylglycerol stores (adipose tissue) releases glycerol. Both amino acids and glycerol are used by the liver for gluconeogenesis.
3. The glucose produced is used by the brain.
4. The fatty acids released from triacylglycerol are also used by the liver to make ketone bodies, which can be used by peripheral tissues as well as the brain.

Late starved state

This is the period of starvation of longer than 16 days up until death. In prolonged starvation the breakdown of muscle protein slows down. This is because there is less need for glucose via gluconeogenesis as the brain adapts to using more ketone bodies. This is further helped by muscle using fatty acids almost exclusively as fuel.

A comparison of the fed and the fasted state is probably the most commonly examined "metabolic" question, because it requires overall knowledge of protein, fat, and carbohydrate metabolism and their regulation. The way to answer this for each state is to think: time-course; hormonal influences; main pathways active and substrates available; any special tissue requirements.

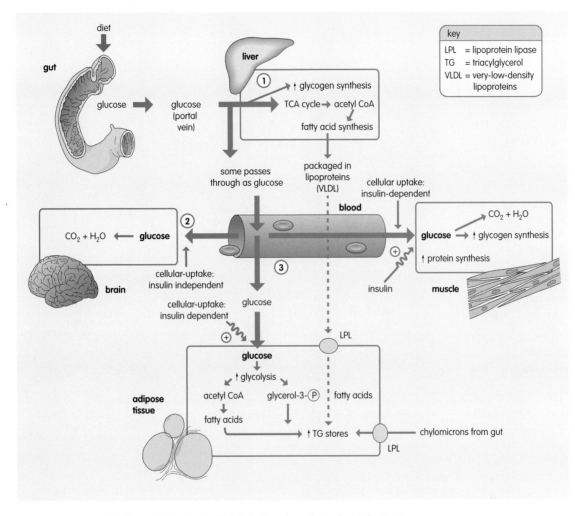

Fig. 7.3 Summary of fuel metabolism in the fed state (numbers 1–3 refer to the text).

Gluconeogenesis

Gluconeogenesis starts about 6–12 hours after a meal and is the major source of glucose once the glycogen stores are depleted. The main role of gluconeogenesis is the maintenance of blood glucose and the provision of glucose for the brain and red blood cells (RBCs) during fasting. An increased glucagon:insulin ratio activates gluconeogenesis and causes the reciprocal inhibition of glycolysis (see Chapter 5). In muscle, cortisol activates protein breakdown, releasing, in particular, alanine and glutamine—substrates for gluconeogenesis.

Ketogenesis

Ketone body synthesis begins during the first few days of starvation and increases as the brain adapts to using ketone bodies as its major fuel, therefore reducing the need for glucose. Once significant ketone body synthesis occurs, a fall in the level of gluconeogenesis from amino acids is seen. This results in a reduction in the breakdown of muscle protein, thus sparing protein.

After 2–3 weeks of starvation, muscle reduces its use of ketone bodies and uses fatty acids almost exclusively, leading to an increase in available ketone bodies for the brain.

Both ketogenesis and gluconeogenesis are balanced to ensure the efficient use of metabolic fuels during starvation. Gluconeogenesis activates ketogenesis by depleting oxaloacetate which therefore ensures that the concentration of acetyl CoA exceeds the oxidative capacity of the TCA

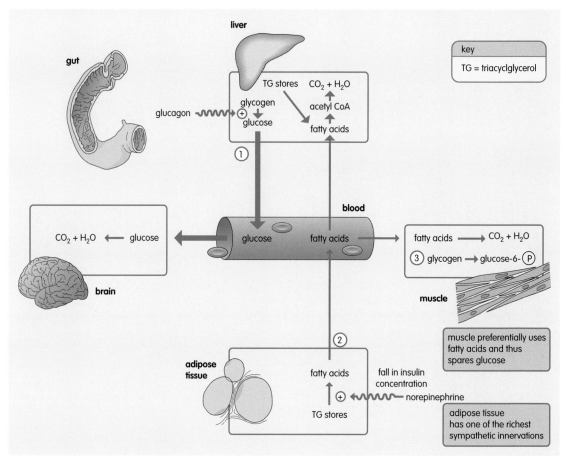

Fig. 7.4 Summary of fuel metabolism in the fasted state; that is, 4–12 hours after a meal. A high glucagon to insulin ratio activates the breakdown of liver glycogen, which provides glucose for the brain. Both the fall in insulin concentration and norepinehrine promote hydrolysis of triacylglycerol stores, releasing fatty acids which can be used as a fuel by muscle and liver. Muscle uses its own glycogen as fuel (numbers refer to text).

cycle. Acetyl CoA can therefore be used for ketone body synthesis.

Hormonal control of glucose homeostasis

Insulin is an anabolic hormone and it therefore increases the uptake and synthesis of glycogen, triacylglycerol and protein. Glucagon, norepinephrine, epinephrine, and cortisol are all catabolic hormones. The main effects of glucagon are summarized in Fig. 7.6. Norepinephrine and epinephrine (stress, or fight-and-flight hormones) have some similar effects to glucagon:
- They increase glycogen breakdown (in muscle only).
- They increase lipolysis in adipose tissue.
- They stimulate protein breakdown.

Glucose homeostasis in exercise
Sprinters
Sprinting is an anaerobic excercise.
- In muscle during intense activity there is only time for anaerobic glycolysis, resulting in the build-up of lactate.
- Lactate diffuses out of muscle and is taken to the liver, where it is oxidized to pyruvate, which can then be converted back to glucose via gluconeogenesis.
- The glucose formed diffuses out of the liver and can return to the muscle to be further used as a fuel.

134

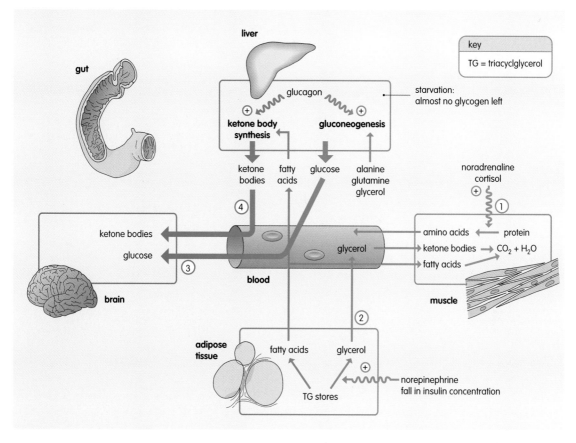

Fig. 7.5 Summary of fuel metabolism in early starvation. Norepinephrine and cortisol activate the breakdown of muscle protein to release amino acids, particularly alanine and glutamine. Norepinephrine also activates hydrolysis of triacylglycerol to release glycerol. Glycerol, alanine, and glutamine are taken to the liver, where they enter gluconeogenesis and are oxidized to glucose. Glucose is used mainly by the brain. Fatty acids released from hydrolysis of triacylglycerol can be taken to the liver and used to generate ketone bodies, which can be used by brain and other tissues (numbers refer to text).

This series of reactions, which shifts the metabolic burden from the muscle to the liver, is known as the Cori cycle (Fig. 7.7) (Compare it with the glucose–alanine cycle; see Fig. 5.31).

Long-distance running

Long-distance running is aerobic.

The body does not store enough glycogen to provide the energy necessary to run long distances. If the respiratory quotient (RQ), the ratio of the amount of O_2 consumed to the amount of CO_2 released, is measured during a run, initially it is about 1.0, indicating that mainly carbohydrate is being used. However, the RQ falls during running to give a value of about 0.77 after about 1 hr, indicating that mainly fats are being oxidized.

The type and amount of substrate used vary with the intensity and duration of exercise, in a similar way to starvation. As glycogen stores are depleted, an increase in glucagon, norepinephrine and epinephrine stimulates lipolysis, releasing fatty acids for muscle to use in order to try to conserve glucose. An increase in these hormones, along with an increase in cortisol, leads to stimulation of gluconeogenesis and protein degradation in muscle. These changes are similar to those of the fasting state, but the difference is that the level of ketone bodies in the blood is low. It is not clear whether this is because they are not being synthesized or if they are being oxidized as soon as they are formed.

135

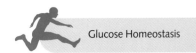
Summary of the main effects of insulin and glucagon		
Pathway	Insulin: anabolic	Glucagon: catabolic
carbohydrate metabolism		
glycogen	increases glycogen synthesis in muscle and liver	increases glycogen breakdown in liver only (NE and epinephrine increase breakdown in muscle) decreases glycogen synthesis
glycolysis/ gluconeogenesis	increases glycolysis inhibits gluconeogenesis	Increases gluconeogenesis inhibits glycolysis
glucose uptake	increases uptake by peripheral tissues, not liver	no effect
pentose phosphate pathway	increases PPP, producing NADPH for lipogenesis	
Lipid metabolism		
lipolysis and β oxidation	inhibits	activates
ketone body synthesis	inhibits	activates
lipogenesis	activates	inhibits
Protein metabolism		
uptake of amino acids by tissues	increases uptake by most tissues	increases uptake by the liver for gluconeogenesis
protein synthesis	increases rate by most tissues	decreases
protein breakdown	decreases rate	stimulates breakdown

Fig. 7.6 Summary of the main effects of insulin and glucagon (NE, norepinephrine; PPP, pentose phosphate pathway).

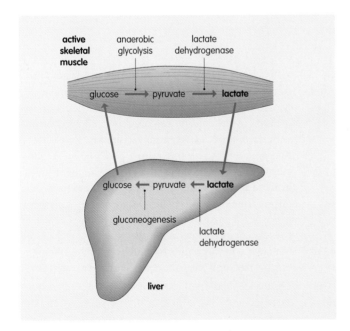

Fig. 7.7 Cori cycle distributes the metabolic burden between the muscle and the liver. Lactate, which builds up in muscle during intense activity, is taken to the liver to be converted back to glucose via gluconeogenesis. This replenishes fuel for the muscle and prevents lactic acidosis.

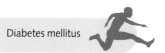

Diabetes mellitus

Classification

Diabetes mellitus is a syndrome caused by the lack, or diminished effectiveness, of insulin. It results in a raised blood glucose, hyperglycemia. There are two main types:

- Type 1: insulin-dependent diabetes mellitus (IDDM), in which there is an absolute failure of the pancreas to produce insulin.
- Type 2: non-insulin-dependent diabetes mellitus (NIDDM), in which there is a failure of the tissues to respond normally to insulin.

Type 1: Insulin-dependent diabetes mellitus (IDDM)

Insulin-dependent diabetes mellitus was often referred to as juvenile-onset diabetes because it typically presents in childhood or puberty. It accounts for only 10–20% of the total number of people with diabetes and has an incidence rate of about 1 in 3000.

The etiology of the disease is a complete deficiency of insulin that can only be corrected by life-long insulin treatment. There are three theories as to its cause:

- Autoimmune destruction of the beta cells in the islets of Langerhans in the pancreas by islet cell autoantibodies, resulting in insulin deficiency.
- Genetic factors. The evidence for a genetic cause is that, firstly, there is a 50% concordance between identical twins, which implies a mixture of both genetic and environmental factors. Secondly, there is a positive family history in approximately 10% of patients. Thirdly, more than 90% of patients with type 1 diabetes carry HLA DR3 and DR4 antigens, compared with 40% of the general population.
- A viral cause (e.g., mumps or Coxsackie B) has also been considered. However, it is likely that viral infections provide the stimulus for auto-immune destruction rather than actually initiating diabetes.

Therefore, the cause is probably a mixture of all three: an autoimmune destruction of the beta cells in genetically susceptible patients which may be precipitated by a viral infection.

The presentation of the disease is usually of rapid onset: weeks or days with the characteristic symptoms of polyuria, polydipsia and weight loss.

Type 2: Non-insulin-dependent diabetes mellitus (NIDDM)

This was also known as adult-onset diabetes, because it typically presents after the age of 35 years. The incidence is more common, and it accounts for 80–90% of the total number of people with diabetes.

Type 2 diabetes is caused by:

- Impaired insulin secretion from the β cells, that is, they fail to secrete enough insulin to correct the blood glucose level.
- Insulin resistance in the tissues, that is, cells fail to respond adequately to insulin.

Genetic factors are very important; there is almost 100% concordance between identical twins and about 30% of patients have a first-degree relative with type 2 diabetes. There is no autoimmune or viral involvement.

The presentation is of an insidious onset and more than 80% of patients are obese. Sufferers are not normally prone to ketoacidosis but it can develop under stress.

Other types of diabetes

There are a number of other types of diabetes, which usually occur secondary to a predisposing factor, for example:

- Gestational diabetes that has its onset during pregnancy.
- Secondary diabetes: this may be the result of damage to the pancreas itself, as in chronic pancreatitis or hemochromatosis, when iron may be deposited in the pancreas (see Chapter 8). It may also occur secondary to the excessive secretion of catabolic hormones, resulting in hyperglycemia and insulin resistance. For example, in acromegaly, where there is oversecretion of growth hormone; in Cushing's syndrome, where there are high levels of glucocorticoids such as cortisol; and in poorly monitored long-term steroid therapy.

These other types of diabetes are covered in more detail in endocrinology or clinical medicine textbooks.

In every examination you will ever have in medicine, there will be a question on diabetes.
Know the effects of an increased glucagon/insulin ratio—the rest is easy and can be worked out!

Metabolic effects of diabetes mellitus

Type 1 diabetes

Insulin normally facilitates the uptake of glucose by peripheral tissues. In its absence, glucose remains in the blood, resulting in a low tissue availability of glucose but a high plasma concentration of glucose. The phrase "starvation in the midst of plenty" is frequently used to describe this state. As there is a low concentration of insulin, the metabolic effects of glucagon and the other catabolic hormones are unopposed (see Fig. 7.6). This results in the predominance of catabolic processes, that is, the breakdown of carbohydrate, protein, and fat (see Fig. 7.8). This leads to hyperglycemia, ketoacidosis, hypertriglyceridemia, and also dehydration (because of osmotic diuresis caused by large amounts of glucose entering the urine). The ketoacidosis can be life-threatening. As cells cannot obtain glucose from the diet they have to obtain it by the breakdown of body stores or by synthesizing it from non-carbohydrate precursors (gluconeogenesis).

Hyperglycemia is caused by:
- A decreased uptake of glucose by the tissues, leading to a large increase in blood glucose.
- Glucagon increases the breakdown of liver glycogen and stimulates gluconeogenesis, leading to an increased hepatic output of glucose.

Ketoacidosis is caused by:
- An increase in triacylglycerol hydrolysis in adipose tissue, releasing fatty acids.
- An increase in ketone body synthesis in liver.

The release of fatty acids is much greater than in starvation; therefore, the rate of formation of ketone bodies is much greater than the rate of use, leading to ketoacidosis (see Chapter 4).

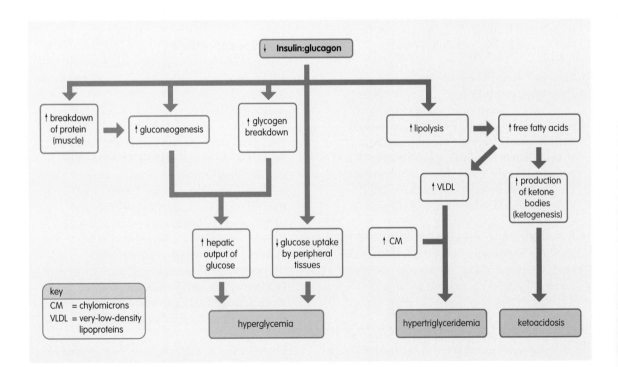

Fig. 7.8 Effect of an increased glucagon to insulin ratio in diabetes.

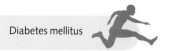

Hypertriglyceridemia is an increase in the triacylglycerol concentration in plasma. (Please note that in clinical medicine triacylglycerol is usually referred to as triglyceride.) It is caused by:

- Some of the fatty acids released from triacylglycerol being packaged in the liver as very-low-density lipoproteins (VLDL). Dietary triacylglycerol is assembled into chylomicrons.
- In the absence of insulin, the activity of lipoprotein lipase decreases, and the VLDLs and chylomicrons remain in the plasma, causing hypertriglyceridemia (see Fig. 7.8).

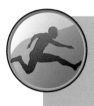

A lot of people liken diabetes to starvation, but there are some very important differences that can lead to fatal consequences for a diabetic patient (Fig. 7.9).

Type 2 diabetes

The metabolic effects are essentially the same as for type 1, but usually they are milder because insulin is present. However:

- The amount of insulin secreted from the pancreas may be inadequate to cope with the blood glucose level.
- Tissues or target organs fail to respond correctly to insulin; that is, they become resistant to it.

In type 2 diabetes, insulin resistance may be due to a number of defects; for example, an abnormal insulin receptor or a defect in a glucose transporter. Insulin resistance in the liver results in uncontrolled glucose production and a decreased uptake by the peripheral tissues. Both contribute to hyperglycemia. Hyperglycemia leads to increased insulin secretion by the pancreas. Type 2 diabetes is typically associated with older age of onset and obesity.

Regarding obesity, it is thought that overeating leads to a constantly elevated blood glucose, which overstimulates insulin secretion. The elevated levels of insulin downregulate the number of insulin receptors on adipose cells and thus cause a decreased response to insulin. In fact, the number of insulin receptors has been shown to increase again if weight is lost, but this is only a proposed mechanism. Ketoacidosis is normally absent in Type 2 diabetes, but it may develop under stress.

Differences between Type 1 diabetes and starvation		
Feature	Type 1 diabetes mellitus	Starvation
Insulin	Absent or very low due to disruption of synthesis	Insulin produced but present at low level
Blood glucose	Hyperglycemia	Normal blood glucose concentration maintained
Ketone body formation	Large increase in production of ketone bodies where rate of formation exceeds rate of use; can lead to life-threatening ketoacidosis	Increased concentration, but usually rate of formation equals rate of use

Fig. 7.9 Important differences between type 1 diabetes mellitus and starvation.

Clinical features
Type 1 diabetes

The clinical features and diagnosis of type 1 diabetes are listed in Fig. 7.10.

The treatment consists of:

- Diet, ensuring the correct content and timing of meals. The diet should be high in fiber and unrefined carbohydrate, low in saturated fat and refined carbohydrate.
- Insulin. There are three main types of insulin: short-acting, which is soluble and used in emergencies, intermediate-acting; and long-acting. The duration of action of insulin is increased by forming a complex with a protamine salt and/or varying the size of the crystals.
- Education. It is crucial that patients understand their disease, and the short- and long-term benefits of treatment.

There are a number of methods for monitoring the control of diabetes and these are covered in detail in Chapter 11. They include:

- Measuring blood glucose levels, using reagent strips based on the glucose oxidase reaction, or portable glucose meters.
- Monitoring the level of glycosylated hemoglobin (HbA_{1c}). This provides a measure of the average blood glucose control over the past 6–8 weeks.

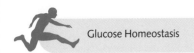

Clinical features and diagnosis of type 1 (insulin-dependent) diabetes	
Main clinical features	**Diagnostic criteria**
classically: • acute onset of symptoms (2–4 weeks) polyuria, polydipsia, accompanied by weight loss and tiredness • ketoacidosis: may present in diabetic coma	presence of symptoms raised random blood glucose, >11.1 mmol/L fasting blood glucose: venous plasma ≥7.0 mmol/L or whole blood ≥6.7 mmol/L (oral glucose tolerance test is not necessary—reserved for borderline cases; glycosuria is not diagnostic due to variation in renal threshold for glucose)

Fig. 7.10 Clinical features and diagnosis of type 1 (insulin-dependent) diabetes mellitus.

- The detection of ketones in urine (and blood), important for the detection of developing ketoacidosis.
- Long-term monitoring for chronic complications.

Type 2 diabetes
The diagnosis, management, and treatment of type 2 diabetes are covered in Fig. 7.11.

Complications of diabetes
These arise when diabetes is poorly controlled.

Acute complications
- **Hypoglycemia.** The aim of treatment of type 1 diabetes with insulin is to maintain a normal blood glucose level, which decreases the long-term effects of diabetes. However, too much insulin or infrequent "top ups" of blood glucose because of insufficient intake of carbohydrate lead to a low blood glucose (hypoglycemia). Hypoglycemia causes unpleasant autonomic symptoms, such as sweating, nausea, and palpitations, and more severe neuroglycopenic symptoms as a result of a decrease in glucose supply to the brain: drowsiness, unsteadiness, confusion, and coma (these patients may look drunk). This is a **very serious** condition and must be treated without delay with an intravenous 50% dextrose infusion. Mild hypoglycemia can be treated with sugar or sweet drinks.

Diagnosis, management, and treatment of type 2 (non-insulin-dependent diabetes)	
Clinical features	**Management**
• insidious onset: tiredness, polyuria, thirst, weight loss • patients usually older and typically obese • may be asymptomatic—detection of ↑ blood glucose on routine check-up **diagnosis:** as for type 1—symptoms usually less severe	**diet:** often the only treatment necessary **oral hypoglycemic drugs:** 2 main types: • sulphonylureas, e.g. glibenclamide: ↑ insulin secretion by islet cells (inhibits ATP-sensitive K⁺ channels in β cell membranes) • biguanides, e.g. metformin: ↑ glucose uptake by peripheral tissues and ↓ glucose production by liver N.B. acarbose inhibits intestinal enzyme, glucosidase and therefore delays the digestion of starch **insulin** is sometimes necessary when type 2 diabetes poorly controlled

Fig. 7.11 Diagnosis, management and treatment of type 2 diabetes (non-insulin-dependent diabetes, NIDDM).

- **Diabetic ketoacidosis.** In the absence of insulin, effects of glucagon are unopposed. Decreased uptake of glucose by tissues, coupled with an increased hepatic glucose production, leads to hyperglycemia. This causes an osmotic diuresis, and the resulting loss of fluid and electrolytes results in dehydration. An increase in lipolysis leads to increased ketogenesis and a metabolic acidosis. Respiratory compensation results in hyperventilation. Failure to treat a patient in ketoacidosis may result in coma and death. Both dehydration and hyperglycemia must be corrected (Fig. 7.12).

Chronic complications
Patients with diabetes have a decreased life expectancy. Patients diagnosed before the age of 20 have only a 60–70% chance of living past the age of 50. The excess deaths appear to be due mainly to diabetic nephropathy. Heart disease, peripheral

Fig. 7.12 Diabetic ketoacidosis. In the absence of insulin, hyperglycemia causes an osmotic diuresis. The loss of fluid and electrolytes results in dehydration. Increased ketogenesis causes metabolic acidosis. Respiratory compensation results in hyperventilation. Both dehydration and hyperglycemia must be corrected in parallel with insulin treatment.

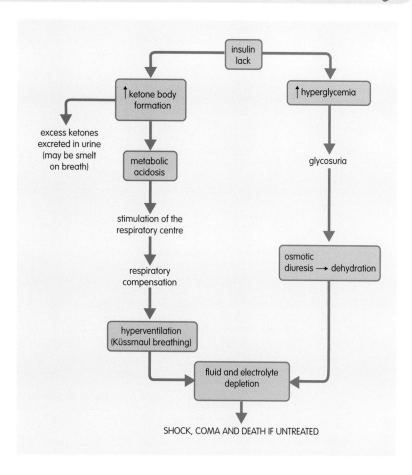

vascular disease and stroke are the major causes of death in patients over the age of 50.

Well-controlled diabetes (that is, when the blood glucose is close to normal) decreases the frequency and progression of microangiopathy (but apparently not macroangiopathy) (Fig. 7.13).

The WHO criteria for diagnosis of diabetes are as follows: fasting venous plasma glucose = 7 mmol/L. A glucose level of 6–7 mmol/L is defined as impaired fasting glucose (IFG). If the patient has no diabetic symptoms, diagnosis should not be based on a single glucose value.

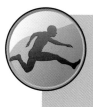

"Compare type 1 diabetes mellitus (IDDM) with type 2 (NIDDM)" is a commonly asked exam question. Fig. 7.14 should help.

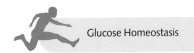

Some long-term complications of diabetes mellitus

Complications	Proposed mechanisms
diabetic microangiopathy affects small blood vessels: in eyes: causes retinopathy and cataracts kidneys: causes nephropathy peripheral and autonomic nervous system: causes neuropathy	**1. sorbitol (polyol) pathway** (see Fig. 2.43): glucose is converted to sorbitol by aldose reductase found particularly in lens, retina, Schwann cells of peripheral nerves and kidney in diabetes, hyperglycemia leads to increased sorbitol formation in these tissues as they do not require insulin for glucose entry sorbitol cannot be metabolized further or leave these cells and therefore it accumulates; it exerts a strong osmotic effect causing cells to swell, causing damage **2. glycation of proteins** hemoglobin is nonenzymatically glycosylated to form HbA_{1c} other proteins may also be glycated, which may mediate some of the damage as glycation may increase their oxidative potential
diabetic macroangiopathy affects large blood vessels causing accelerated atherosclerosis	precise mechanism is unknown the risk of cardiovascular disease in people with diabetes is 2–3 times higher than the risk of non-diabetic persons

Fig. 7.13 Some long-term complications of diabetes mellitus.

Comparison of type 1 and type 2 diabetes

	Type 1	Type 2
usual age of onset	young <25 years	>35 years
auto-immune factors	yes	no
genetic factors	risk associated with certain HLA types	yes—polygenic inheritance
concordance identical twins	50%	almost 100%
symptoms	polyuria, polydipsia, weight loss	similar but usually less severe presentation
signs	wasting, dehydration, loss of consciousness	obesity
ketosis	prone	rarely; precipitated by stress
obesity	infrequent	frequent

Fig. 7.14 Comparison of type 1 and type 2 diabetes mellitus.

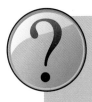

- Compare the fed and fasted states.
- Describe the main effects of insulin and glucagon on carbohydrate, protein and lipid metabolism.
- Contrast the use of fuels during sprinting and long-distance running.
- Why is lactic acidosis not an everyday occurrence?
- What is the significance of the slowdown in muscle breakdown in the late starved state?
- Describe the long-term complications of diabetes.
- What are the main metabolic effects of diabetes?
- How does the presentation of type 1 differ from type 2 diabetes?
- Why do patients with diabetic ketoacidosis hyperventilate?
- What role does genetic influence play on the aetiologies of type 1 and type 2 diabetes?

8. Nutrition

Basic principles of human nutrition

Some useful definitions
Nutrients
Nutrients are essential dietary factors, such as vitamins, minerals, essential amino acids, and essential fatty acids, that cannot be synthesized by the body at a sufficient rate. Sources of energy are not classed as nutrients; neither is water or dietary fiber.

Staple foods
Staple foods are the principal sources of energy in the diet. They are specific to a particular country. For example, in parts of Africa and Asia cereals provide more than 70% of the energy in the diet. As countries become more prosperous, the percentage of energy derived from a single staple food declines. For example, in the U.S. flour and flour products provide only about 25% of food energy.

Methods of estimating an individual's dietary intake
There are three main methods for estimating an individual's dietary intake:
- **Dietary recall.** Simply, ask the patient what he or she has eaten. This is the least accurate because it relies on the patient's recall and willingness to cooperate.
- **Food diary.** This is slightly more accurate. To improve the accuracy, a 24-hour urine nitrogen measurement can be performed. This measures the amount of nitrogen excreted in the urine in 24 hours. From this the protein excretion can be calculated to see if it balances with the protein intake as recorded in the diary.
- **Complete chemical analysis.** This is the most expensive but also the most accurate method.

Dietary reference intakes
The following definitions are in keeping with the dietary reference intakes (DRIs; Fig. 8.1) for food energy and nutrients for the U.S., as recommended by the Food and Nutrition Board of the National Research Council of the National Academy of Sciences:
- **Estimated average requirement** (EAR). This is the average requirement of a group of people for energy or a nutrient (protein, vitamin or mineral). About 50% of the population will need less than the EAR and 50% will need more.
- **Recommended daily amount** (RDA). This is the amount of nutrient that is enough or more than enough for about 97% of people in the group (EAR + 2SD).
- **Adequate intake** (AI). The AI is the mean intake for healthy breastfed infants.
- **Tolerable upper intake level** (UL) is the amount of nutrient enough for almost everyone, but not so much as to cause undesirable effects.

Energy balance

Food energy
The total energy content of food is the amount of energy released when food is completely burnt in air to CO_2 and H_2O; that is, the heat of combustion (Fig. 8.2). The total energy is equal to the sum of the digestible energy and the nondigestible energy (Fig. 8.3).
- Digestible energy is the amount of energy that can be absorbed from food and usually accounts for about 95% of the average Western diet.
- Nondigestible energy is the energy in food (e.g., in cellulose) that we cannot break down and is lost in feces.

Metabolizable energy is the energy available to the body for use. It has three fates:
- 50% is lost as heat.
- 5–10% of energy is released during the digestion, absorption, and transport of food. This is known as either the thermic effect of food, diet-induced

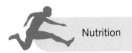

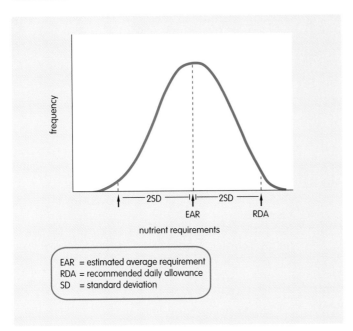

Fig. 8.1 Dietary reference values for food energy and nutrients in the U.S.

EAR = estimated average requirement
RDA = recommended daily allowance
SD = standard deviation

Major sources of energy in the diet		
Energy source	Total energy/g	
	kcal	kJ
fat: essential for absorption of fat-soluble vitamins [A, D, E and K]	9.2	38.6
carbohydrate: as either starch, sugar or non-starch polysaccharide (NSP), i.e. fiber	4.0	16.8
protein:	5.4	22.7
alcohol: "empty calories"	7.0	29.4

Fig. 8.2 Major sources of energy in the diet.

thermogenesis, or postprandial thermogenesis (they all mean the same thing).
- Only about 25–40% of the energy is trapped as ATP; that is, the body is only 25–40% efficient.

From Fig. 8.2, it can be seen that protein has a higher total energy content than carbohydrate. However, protein is not as efficiently oxidized (it forms urea and requires ATP for this [see Chapter 5]), and only about 4 kcal/g are available for the body to use as metabolizable energy. Carbohydrate is oxidized completely to CO_2 and H_2O and therefore all the available energy is obtained for use; that is, the metabolizable energy is also 4 kcal/g.

Body composition
An average 72-kg man is composed of:
- 15% fat.
- 85% fat-free mass.

Fat-free mass or lean body mass (LBM) is made up of:
- 72% water.
- 20% protein.
- 8% bone mineral.

Women generally have a higher fat content than men; typically they consist of about 25% fat. Fat content tends to increase with age. An average 72-kg man can

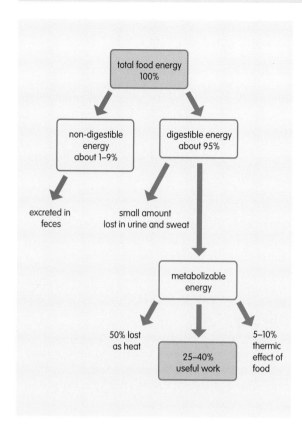

Fig. 8.3 Food energy utilization.

survive on his energy stores for about 50–60 days, provided he is given water. This is mostly due to fat reserves; glycogen stores last only 12–24 hours. Fig. 8.4 summarizes the methods available to measure body composition. However, most of the methods, with the exception of anthropometry, are rarely used in clinical practice.

Energy requirements

Energy is used by the body for three main processes.

Basal metabolic rate

The basal metabolic rate (BMR) is the energy used to carry out normal body functions such as blood flow, breathing, and so on; that is, it is the energy expended doing nothing! The units of BMR are kJ/h/kg of body weight. To calculate the BMR the patient must be:

- At rest, lying down but not asleep.
- The temperature of the environment must be moderate and constant.
- Assessed about 12 hours after the last meal or any exercise.

The BMR is usually measured first thing in the morning. It is proportional to LBM. Therefore, men have a higher BMR than women. Women have a greater percentage of fat, which is less metabolically active. The BMR usually accounts for 50–70% of the total energy expended.

Thermic effect of food

This is the energy required for the digestion and absorption of food and accounts for 5–10% of the energy expenditure.

Physical activity

The amount of energy consumed depends on the duration and intensity of exercise. The physical activity ratio (PAR) can be measured for situations in which activity is expressed as a multiple of the BMR (i.e., BMR = 1).

The PAR = metabolic rate during exercise ÷ BMR.

For example:

Lying	1.0 (equal to BMR)
Sitting	1.2
Standing	1.7
Football	7.0

The physical activity level (PAL) can also be calculated. This is equal to the total energy expenditure in 1 day divided by the BMR.

Other factors can also affect energy requirements. For example:

- Environmental temperature changes. This is a very small effect unless the temperature is either extremely high or low.
- Pregnancy and lactation. For the first 6 months of pregnancy no extra energy is necessary, but for the last 3 months an extra 0.8 MJ (200 kcal) are needed each day. During lactation, an extra 2.0 MJ (500 kcal) are required each day.
- Growth. The energy requirement in the first year of life is double that of adulthood.
- Age. The BMR decreases after the age of about 20 years.

How do we measure energy requirements?
Indirect calorimetry

The measurement of O_2 consumption allows the indirect measurement of the metabolic rate. This is because 1 L (1 liter) of O_2 consumed at rest is equal to 20 kJ of energy expenditure.

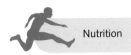

Measurement of body composition	
Measurement	Method
body density	weigh in air to give fat content (density = 0.9 mg/mL); weigh in water to give lean body mass (density = 1.1 mg/mL)
body water	the patient is injected with a known volume of tritiated water its concentration of equilibrium is measured this is representative of lean body mass
total body potassium	$^{40}K^+$ is injected and its distribution assessed this is a measure of lean body mass as there is no potassium in fat
body fat	the uptake of a fat-soluble gas, e.g. xenon or cyclopropane is measured biopsy to measure concentration
anthropometry	measure: • weight and height • mid-arm circumference (biceps and triceps) • skin-fold thickness (subscapular and suprailiac) compare with normograms for weight and height

Fig. 8.4 Measurement of body composition. Some of these methods are a little drastic and, therefore, seldom used. Anthropometry is the most widely used method.

Indirect mass spectrophotometry

The incorporation of doubly labeled water ($^2H_2{}^{18}O$) into body fluids and its loss in the urine can be measured. ^2H is incorporated only into H_2O, but ^{18}O is incorporated into both H_2O and CO_2. The difference between them is equal to the CO_2 produced.

Regulation of food intake

A number of systems are thought to participate in the regulation of food intake.

Overall control is thought to be at the level of the hypothalamus

There are two important areas for the control of food intake:

• The hunger or "feeding" center in the lateral hypothalamic area.
• The satiety center in the ventromedial nucleus.

Lesions in the hunger center have been shown to inhibit appetite and thus feeding and to lead to anorexia. Lesions in the satiety center cause overeating and obesity.

Gastric distention and gut hormones

Cholecystokinin (CCK) and calcitonin are known to decrease appetite. CCK slows gastric emptying, thus maintaining gastric distension, which is thought to be an important satiety signal.

Plasma concentration of glucose, insulin, and glucagon

Originally it was thought that low plasma glucose levels had a direct stimulatory effect on the hunger center. Now it is believed that it is the increased availability of glucose to tissues that produces satiety (the glucostat hypothesis). Insulin, therefore, promotes satiety by stimulating the uptake of glucose by peripheral tissues.

Obesity

If energy intake is equal to energy expenditure, there is no change in body mass. Obesity results from an imbalance between the input, storage, and expenditure of energy; that is, energy intake is greater than energy expenditure.

Definition

Obesity can be defined or graded in terms of the body mass index (BMI).

$$BMI\,(kg/m^2) = weight/(height)^2$$

The grading for BMI is:

20–25 Ideal weight
25–30 Obesity grade I (overweight)
30–35 Obesity grade II (obese)
35+   Obesity grade III

Obesity grades II and III are associated with an increased risk of various clinical disorders. A BMI of 20–25 is considered to be within the range for ideal weight. However, these ideal weights are obtained from tables compiled by a life insurance company in New York and are based on data obtained from upper middle class Caucasians; therefore, they are not accurate for everybody! The tables give ranges of ideal weights for height. As most people get older, they develop some degree of obesity.

In the U.S., 45% of men and 36% of women are overweight. Of these, about 8% of men and 12% of women are obese. These numbers appear to be increasing.

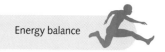

Etiology

Fig. 8.5 discusses some of the proposed theories for obesity. Twin studies suggest a genetic factor, and this is now backed up by recent evidence identifying a gene for obesity. However, genetic factors are clearly greatly influenced by environmental and socioeconomic factors. Poor education, high alcohol intake, and less energy expenditure increase the incidence of obesity. The increase in obesity seen in the lower social classes may be related to the type of food consumed, which is largely governed by financial status. The most obvious cause for obesity is an imbalance between energy input and expenditure. The reasons for overeating are usually complex and may be psychological in origin (e.g., related to stress or a life event), but generally they are not metabolic causes.

Clinical consequences

The effects of obesity are clearly recognizable. In obese patients, there is an increased morbidity and mortality, mainly from heart disease, stroke and diabetes. Therefore obesity is associated with an increased risk of:

Causes of obesity		
Cause	**Evidence**	**Comments**
excessive intake of calories	due to psychological factors, stress or social reasons	most common cause
genetic	identical twins are not always the same weight adopted children resemble their new family weightwise	likely genetic predisposition but also modified by environmental factors (diet, social-economic status) recent evidence suggests that there is a "gene" for obesity
socio-economic	in the West, low socio-economic class → obesity in the East, high socio-economic class → obesity	surveys in Finland and Scotland showed obesity is associated with: • low education • high alcohol intake • giving up smoking • getting married!
endocrine	adrenal hyper function (Cushing's syndrome), hypothyroidism, and Type 2 diabetes mellitus are all associated with obesity	but most obese people do not have endocrine problems
energy expenditure	DIT is greater in lean people (N.B. basal metabolic rate is not lower in obese people!) 80% of obese teenagers become obese adults hypothesis is that standard weight is set in infancy when fat people develop a greater number of fat cells than thin people Note the recently increasing rate of child and adolescent obesity	maybe obese people are better at conserving energy not true!

Fig. 8.5 Causes of obesity. There are a number of proposed causes of obesity: excessive calorie intake, genetic, endocrine, etc. However, evidence suggests that the major cause of obesity is excessive calorie intake, usually due to an underlying social or socio-economic cause.

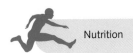

- Coronary heart disease. There is a linear increase in morbidity and mortality caused by coronary heart disease with obesity. It may be that other risk factors are more likely to be present in obese patients.
- Hypertension.
- Type 2 diabetes. Obesity results in persistently high insulin levels, leading to a downregulation of insulin receptors and thus insulin resistance by the tissues.
- Respiratory problems.
- Stroke.
- Gallstones. Especially if fat, female, forty, and fertile!
- Osteoarthritis and back pain.
- Gout.

Treatment

Treatment of obesity is generally unsatisfactory. Possibilities include:

- Reduction of energy intake. The main treatment of an obese patient is an appropriate diet, with plenty of support and encouragement from a doctor. Lots of different weight-reducing diets have been formulated; most do not work! For example, a low-carbohydrate diet, where bread, potatoes, cakes and any starch-containing foods are cut out of the diet. Initially, weight loss is fast (0.5 kg/day) but most of the loss is water. Protein is also broken down to maintain the blood glucose, but is replaced as soon as the diet is stopped. However, the loss of fat is the same as for a normal mixed diet.
  Most diets allow an intake of 1000 kcal/day. This must be a balanced intake of protein, carbohydrate and fat (i.e., a mixed diet). Why is it that 80–100% of obese people regain lost weight? During starvation, the metabolic rate falls by 15–30%. Therefore, after dieting, to remain at a lower weight a lower energy intake must be maintained, otherwise the weight will be put straight back on. The only way to lose weight is a prolonged moderation of intake and then a permanent change in eating habits to maintain the weight loss.
- Increase energy expenditure in a way appropriate to age and health.
- Drug therapy is not generally recommended. Orlistat, a pancreatic lipase inhibitor, is the most commonly used drug. It is licensed for use in conjunction with a mildly hypocaloric diet in those with a body mass index of greater than 30 kg/m^2. Part of its effect may be related to the reduction of fat intake necessary to avoid severe gastrointestinal effects such as steatorrhea. Appetite suppressants such as phentermine (a catecholaminergic drug with minor sympathomimetic and stimulant effects) are not presently used. Leptins are central nervous system proteins believed to be important in the neurotransmission of a sense of satiation. These and other molecules of the central nervous system are the subject of intensive study for use in obesity.
- Surgery. This is extreme and performed in selected cases only. Examples include jaw wiring, gastric plication (stapling the walls of the stomach together to form a smaller stomach), bypass of the small intestine, and gastric distention.

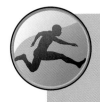

The main cause of obesity is probably an excessive intake of calories, usually accompanied by a decrease in energy expenditure.

Morbidity is the incidence or prevalence of disease in a population.
Mortality is the number of deaths from disease in a population.

Protein nutrition

More definitions
Reference proteins

Reference proteins contain all the amino acids in the exact proportions needed for protein synthesis. Albumin (found in egg white) and casein (milk) are closest to the ideal. Other proteins are compared with these reference or "perfect" proteins.

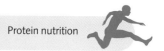

Limiting amino acids

A limiting amino acid is the essential amino acid present in a protein in the lowest amount relative to its requirement for protein synthesis. Examples of protein-containing foods and their limiting amino acids are:

- Wheat, limited by lysine.
- Meat and fish, limited by methionine and cysteine.
- Maize, limited by tryptophan.

Combining different protein-containing foods, such as meat and the pulses, ensures an adequate intake of all the amino acids, that is, protein complementation. This is particularly important in vegetarian diets. A diet of beans on toast provides adequate amounts of protein (you may not have many friends though!).

Protein quality

The quality of any protein can be assessed using a rating system based on a number of variables.

Chemical score

The chemical score is the ratio of the amount of limiting amino acid to its requirement, expressed as percentage points. For example, if the amount of limiting amino acid in a test protein is 2% and the amount of limiting amino acid in the reference protein is 5%, the chemical score is therefore 40%.

Biologic value

The biologic value is the proportion of the absorbed protein which is retained by the body for protein synthesis.

Net protein utilization

The net protein utilization (NPU) is the proportion of dietary protein which is retained by the body for protein synthesis. For example:

- For a typical mixed Western diet, NPU is 70%, meaning that 70% of the dietary protein is retained for protein synthesis.
- For a diet of mainly meat, NPU would be 75%.
- For a diet of cereals, NPU would be 50–60%.
- For a diet of eggs, NPU would be 100%.

Net dietary protein as a percentage of energy

Net dietary protein as a percentage of energy (NDPE%) is the proportion of total dietary energy provided by fully "usable" protein. This method provides a way of comparing different diets. For example:

- Cereal-based diets provide 5–6%.
- Western diets provide 10–12%.
- In India, the diet provides 10%.

Children require an NDPE% of greater than 8%; that is, at least 8% of their diet must come from usable protein. Adults require an NDPE% of greater than 5%. In areas where the staple food is starch (e.g., yam, cassava), the diet provides only low levels of protein. It would be physically impossible to consume the amount of food necessary to satisfy the protein requirement, especially for children, and this leads to protein deficiency states. Cereal-based diets are adequate for adults but not for children.

Protein requirement

Diet should provide the essential amino acids and enough amino-acid nitrogen to synthesize the nonessential amino acids. These are required for:

- The maintenance of tissue proteins in adults.
- The formation of body proteins during periods of growth, pregnancy, lactation, infection, and after major trauma or illness such as cancer.

The recommended protein requirement for an adult in the U.S. is 0.8 g/kg/day of protein and should not be greater than 1.5 g/kg/day.

The RDA for protein is 55 g/day for men and 44 g/day for women.

Protein–energy deficiency states

Protein–energy malnutrition (PEM) arises when the body's need for protein or energy, or both, is not met by the diet. The physiologic effects of severe prolonged malnutrition are discussed in Fig. 8.6. It is most commonly seen in developing countries.

Causes of PEM

These can be one or a combination of the following:

- Decreased dietary intake.
- Malabsorption.
- Increased requirement; for example, in preterm infants, infection (septic state increases catabolism), major trauma, or surgery.
- Psychological; for example, depression or anorexia nervosa.

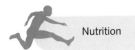

The bulk of excess protein is oxidized via gluconeogenesis to glycogen or fat and stored by the body. Therefore protein is not a slimming food.

A famous diet is made of protein-supplemented modified fast (PSMF) which is hydrolyzed gelatine and collagen; that is, it is cheap! However, in the hydrolysis process a lot of electrolytes are lost, including potassium, which may lead to serious problems.

In developing countries, PEM manifests as two conditions in children:
- Marasmus: lack of protein and energy (i.e. starvation).
- Kwashiorkor: lack of protein only—energy supply is adequate.

Incidence

In developing countries, 20–75% of children below 5 years of age have some form of malnutrition. Five million children die every year because of malnutrition.

Etiology and mechanisms of pathogenesis
Marasmus

Marasmus is the childhood form of starvation (Figs 8.7 and 8.8). Both protein and energy are limited, leading to a low concentration of insulin but increased levels of glucagon and cortisol, that is, a starved state (see Chapter 7). As no fuel is available for the body, muscle protein and fat are broken down to provide energy, which leads to wasting. Muscle protein is broken down to amino acids which are used for the synthesis of albumin by the liver; therefore, this prevents edema.

Kwashiorkor

Translated, this means the "disease the first child gets when the second child is born." In kwashiorkor

Physiological effects of severe prolonged malnutrition	
Effect	**Consequence**
decreased brain development	permanent damage to both physical and mental development
defective immune system	decreased cell-mediated response immunoglobulin production is maintained: this can have harmful effects as it depletes production of other proteins
loss of protein	firstly from muscle, then viscera → death
electrolyte losses	may effect Na^+/K^+ pump and the maintenance of ion gradients across cells
low hemoglobin	anemia
low serum albumin (only kwashiorkor)	→ edema
impaired gastrointestinal function	bacterial overgrowth and malabsorption
fatty liver	fat accumulates since its transport requires apolipoproteins that are deficient (not seen in marasmus)

Fig. 8.6 The physiologic effects of severe prolonged malnutrition.

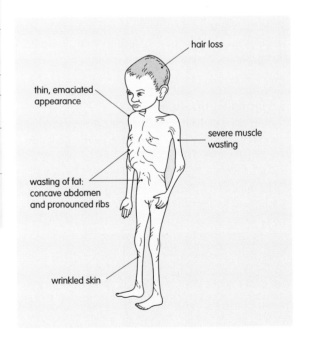

Fig. 8.7 Marasmus.

- hair loss
- thin, emaciated appearance
- severe muscle wasting
- wasting of fat: concave abdomen and pronounced ribs
- wrinkled skin

The features of marasmus

very thin, wasted appearance
obvious muscle wasting and loss of body fat; <60% normal body weight
age: usually <18 months
no edema
wrinkled skin, hair loss and apathy
plasma albumin is usually **normal**
diarrhoea and infection may be present
electrolyte disturbances: low potassium and sodium common
anemia

Fig. 8.8 The clinical features of marasmus.

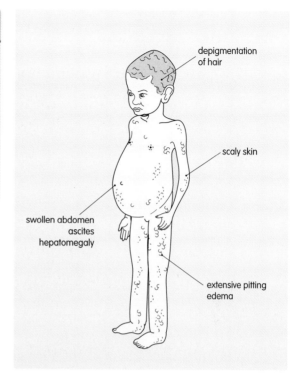

Fig. 8.9 Kwashiorkor.

severe protein deficiency occurs, but energy is maintained (Figs 8.9 and 8.10). It usually occurs when a young child is weaned from breast feeding because of the arrival of a new baby. The first child is fed a low-protein, high-starch diet instead. Kwashiorkor often develops after an acute infection, such as measles or gastroenteritis, when the demand for protein is increased.

As energy is not limiting, there is a high insulin-to-glucagon and a high insulin-to-cortisol ratio. Amino acids are taken up by muscle for protein synthesis. This diverts amino acids from the liver, so fewer are available for albumin synthesis. The resulting low albumin levels reduce the plasma oncotic pressure, causing edema. The edema causes a deceptively fat appearance, and such children are known as water or "sugar" babies. It is possible there may also be some degree of energy loss in kwashiorkor; therefore, other factors may contribute to, or cause, the edema. For example:

- Excessive generation of free radicals causing membrane damage and edema.
- Infection diverts protein synthesis from albumin to the synthesis of immunoglobulins and acute-phase proteins (e.g., C-reactive protein).

A comparison of kwashiorkor and marasmus is given in Fig. 8.11.

Management and treatment of PEM

It is important to restore fluid and electrolyte balance first. Following this:

- Any infection, hypothermia, or hypoglycemia present can be treated.

The features of kwashiorkor

edema: "hides" severe wasting of underlying tissues
age: usually 2–4 years
scaly skin: "flaky point" rash with hyperkeratosis
depigmentation of hair
distended abdomen caused by ascites and enlarged fatty liver
hypothermia and bradycardia
apathy
anemia: due to folate, iron or copper metabolism disturbances
low plasma albumin
usually diarrhoea and/or infection
low potassium, sodium, glucose, and other electrolyte disturbances

Fig. 8.10 The clinical features of kwashiorkor.

- Refeed initially, just enough to maintain a steady state to satisfy the normal daily requirement. Milk is often given with flour or maize, slowly and regularly.
- Eventually, high-energy foods are given to restore weight and also any necessary vitamin and mineral supplements.

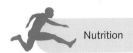

A comparison of marasmus and kwashiorkor		
Feature	Marasmus	Kwashiorkor
deficiency	protein and energy	protein only
age	usually <18 months	older: 1–5 years
edema	absent severe wasting of body protein and fat	present edema hides wasting of body protein
body weight	<60% normal	60–80% normal
cause	severe malnutrition	malnutrition infection
features	wrinkled skin hair loss thin and emaciated	scaly skin and dermatitis sparse, depigmented hair distended abdomen hepatomegaly

Fig. 8.11 A comparison of marasmus and kwashiorkor.

Prognosis

Mortality rates for children with severe malnutrition are about 50%. The rate is so high because adequate treatment is usually not available.

Consequences of prolonged PEM

Malnourished children are less active and more apathetic; these behavioral abnormalities are usually reversed by refeeding. However, severe, prolonged malnutrition causes much reduced brain growth and permanent damage to both physical and mental development. Immunity is impaired, leading to delayed wound healing; protein loss from muscle may eventually include the diaphragm, leading to death. The physiologic effects of severe prolonged malnutrition are listed in Fig. 8.6.

Prevention

Prevention of childhood malnutrition is a World Health Organization priority. The main targets are to provide:
- Food supplements and additional vitamins to at risk groups.
- Family planning.
- Immunization programs.

However, the occurrence of drought, famine, and war in affected countries makes these targets practically impossible to achieve.

In Western countries, a degree of PEM may be seen in hospitalized patients with the following conditions:
- Anorexia.
- Trauma, severe infection, major surgery, or burns.
- Cancer.

That is, anything that causes a negative nitrogen balance (see Chapter 5).

Malnutrition in adults in developing countries has symptoms similar to those seen in children, but the results are not as devastating. This is because adults are already physically and mentally mature and are thus more resilient.

Vitamins

Definition

A complex organic substance required in the diet in small amounts compared with other components such as protein, carbohydrate or fat, and the absence of which leads to a deficiency disease.

Vitamins can be divided into two main groups: fat-soluble vitamins and water-soluble vitamins.

Fat-soluble vitamins

Vitamins A, D, E, and K. These are:
- Stored in the liver.
- Not absorbed or excreted easily.
- Sometimes toxic in excess (particularly A and D).

Water-soluble vitamins

The B-group vitamins and vitamin C. These are:
- Not stored extensively.
- Required regularly in the diet.
- Generally nontoxic in excess (within reason).

All B vitamins are coenzymes in metabolic pathways.

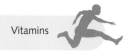

Fat-soluble vitamins
Vitamin A (retinol)
RDA
1000 µg RE equivalents/day for men; 860 µg RE equivalents/day for women.

Sources
Animal sources are butter, whole milk, egg yolk, liver, and fish liver oils; they contain retinol.

Plant sources are most green, yellow or orange vegetables; they contain β-carotene, the precursor of retinol.

Absorption and transport of vitamin A
Retinol is absorbed in the intestinal mucosa and esterified to long-chain fatty acids, forming retinyl esters. These are packaged in chylomicrons and transported to the liver for storage. When required, retinol is released and transported bound to retinol-binding protein. Retinol can be oxidized to other active forms, namely retinoic acid and retinal. β-Carotene is absorbed in the intestine and converted into retinal.

Functions
There are three active forms of vitamin A:
- Retinoic acid, which acts as a typical steroid hormone. It binds to chromatin to increase the synthesis of proteins controlling cell growth and differentiation of epithelial cells. Therefore, it increases epithelial cell turnover.
- Retinal. 11-*cis* Retinal binds to opsin to form rhodopsin, the visual pigment of the rod cells in the retina involved in vision and dark adaptation to light. Low light intensity (scotopic vision) activates a series of photochemical reactions that bleach rhodopsin, converting it to all-*trans* retinal, which triggers a nerve impulse in the optic nerve to the brain (Fig. 8.12).
- β-Carotene is an antioxidant. The role of antioxidants, particularly vitamins C, E, and β-carotene in the prevention of heart disease and lung cancer is being studied intensively but has not yet produced any conclusive results.

Clinical manifestations of a deficiency or excess
Fig. 8.13 lists the symptoms of a deficiency and an excess of vitamin A.

Deficiency
Incidence　Vitamin A deficiency is rarely seen in developed countries because liver stores are sufficient to last 3–4 years. It is commonly found in children in developing countries such as India and parts of Southeast Asia, where about 500,000

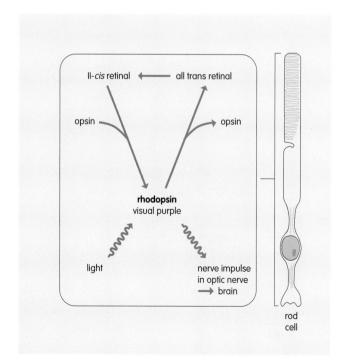

Fig. 8.12 Role of vitamin A in vision. 11-*cis* Retinal binds to opsin, converting it to rhodopsin, the visual pigment of the rod cells in the retina involved in vision and dark adaptation to light. Low light intensity (scotopic vision) activates a series of photochemical reactions that bleach rhodopsin, converting it to all-*trans* retinal, which triggers a nerve impulse in the optic nerve to the brain.

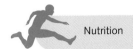
Deficiency and excess of vitamin A	
Deficiency	**Excess**
initially causes impaired adaptation to darkness and night blindness	excessive intake leads to a toxic syndrome called hypervitaminosis A
increased epithelial keratinization of the comea leads to xerophthalmia	teratogenic
progresses to keratomalacia and cataracts	

Fig. 8.13 Deficiency and excess of vitamin A.

Uses of vitamin A in the treatment of skin disorders	
Condition	**Treatment**
moderate acne	topical retinoic acid (all *trans* retinoic acid)
severe disfiguring acne	isotretinoin (13-*cis* retinoic acid) orally
psoriasis	acitretin
	(both are contraindicated in pregnancy as they are teratogenic)

Fig. 8.14 Uses of vitamin A in the treatment of skin disorders.

children each year are blinded as a result of vitamin A deficiency.

Causes   Vitamin A deficiency may be caused by a decreased dietary intake; however, this is usually only seen in very severe malnutrition. It may also occur secondary to fat malabsorption.

Clinical features   In the eye, the symptoms are progressive:
- Initially, deficiency causes impaired dark adaptation and night blindness. This is reversible.
- Severe prolonged deficiency results in xerophthalmia: a dryness of the cornea and conjunctiva due to progressive epithelial keratinization. Bitôt's spots may be seen, which are white plaques of keratinized epithelial cells on the conjunctiva.
- If untreated, keratomalacia develops, causing corneal ulceration and the formation of opaque scar tissue (cataracts). This causes irreversible blindness.

In the skin, decreased epithelial cell turnover produces:
- Thickening and dryness of skin due to hyperkeratosis.
- Impaired mucosal function.

Diagnosis and treatment   Diagnosis and treatment are usually on the basis of the above clinical features. The following can also be measured:
- The plasma concentration of vitamin A and retinol binding protein.
- The response to replacement therapy.

Urgent treatment with vitamin A (as retinol palmitate) orally or intramuscularly prevents blindness. If the deficiency is severe and has already caused keratomalacia, eyesight cannot be restored. It is interesting to note that vitamin A is also used successfully to treat a number of skin problems, including acne (Fig. 8.14).

Toxicity
Hypervitaminosis A   Hypervitaminosis A is a serious toxic syndrome. Excessive intake of vitamin A causes:
- Dry, itchy skin: dermatitis.
- Mucous membrane defects and hair loss.
- Hepatomegaly.
- Thinning and fracture of the long bones.
- Increased intracranial pressure.

Toxicity is very unlikely with normal sources but must be taken into account when prescribing high doses of retinoic acid for severe acne sufferers.

Teratogenicity   Pregnant women must not take more than 3.3 mg/day because vitamin A causes congenital defects. Therefore, they must avoid vitamin A supplements or eating liver because it contains about 13–40 mg of vitamin A per 100 g. Isotretinoin treatment for acne is absolutely contraindicated in pregnancy.

Vitamin D₃ (cholecalciferol)
RDA
10 µg/day for adults.

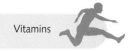

Sources

The sources of vitamin D include:
- Diet. In fish liver oils as cholecalciferol.
- Endogenous synthesis: most vitamin D is made by the body.

Vitamin D is a derivative of cholesterol and is therefore not present in plants; vegetarians must make their own.

Synthesis

Vitamin D is manufactured in the skin by the action of sunlight of wavelength 290–310 nm (Fig. 8.15). In areas where there is little radiation of this length during winter months, the body relies on stores made during summer.

Cholecalciferol undergoes two hydroxylation reactions, the first in the liver and the second in the kidney to form the active form, 1,25-dihydroxycholecalciferol (see Fig. 8.15). Vitamin D is mostly stored as 25-hydroxycholecalciferol in the liver.

Functions

The main role of vitamin D is in calcium homeostasis, which it controls in three ways:
- Increases uptake of calcium (and inorganic phosphate) from the intestine (main role).
- Increases the reabsorption of calcium from the kidney (minor role).
- Increases resorption of bone (when necessary) so that calcium is released.

Therefore, vitamin D increases the plasma concentration of calcium ions.

Mechanism of action

The active form, 1,25-dihydroxycholecalciferol, is a steroid hormone. In intestinal cells it binds to a cytosolic receptor. The resulting complex enters the nucleus and binds to chromatin at a specific site (enhancer region or response element) to increase the synthesis of a calcium-binding protein, calbindin, resulting in increased calcium reabsorption in the intestine.

Clinical manifestations of a deficiency or excess

Fig. 8.16 lists the symptoms of a deficiency and an excess of vitamin D.

Deficiency

Causes
- Decreased dietary intake of vitamin D.
- Inadequate exposure to sunlight of the correct wavelength.
- Renal disease leads to inadequate formation of the active form 1,25-dihydroxycholecalciferol.
- Liver disease leads to decreased formation of 25-hydroxycholecalciferol (precursor to active form).
- Fat malabsorption, for example, due to celiac disease or after surgery (gut resection).

Groups at risk of deficiency are:
- Children and women of Asian origin in sunlight-poor areas.
- Elderly and housebound individuals.
- Babies breast-fed in winter because light of the correct wavelength for production of vitamin D is not available for mothers.
- Vegans (vitamin D is not present in food of plant origin).

Clinical features and pathogenesis Vitamin D deficiency disrupts bone mineralization (Fig. 8.17). In children, this causes rickets; in adults, it causes osteomalacia. These disorders are covered later in this chapter with calcium deficiency.

A disruption of calcium homeostasis also causes hypocalcemia and hypophosphatemia (low plasma calcium and phosphate). This may cause symptoms of neuromuscular irritability, numbness, parasthesiae, tetany and, possibly, seizures.

Toxicity

Vitamin D is the most toxic of all vitamins. It is fat-soluble, stored in the body, and slowly metabolized. Normally, it is well tolerated but, in high doses over a period of time, it can cause hypervitaminosis D. This condition presents with nausea, vomiting, and muscle weakness. Very high levels of vitamin D result in greatly increased rates of calcium absorption and bone resorption, causing hypercalcemia and calcium deposition in tissues, particularly the arteries, heart, liver, kidneys, and pancreas. This is known as metastatic calcification and may interfere with the correct functioning of the organs, possibly causing renal stones, calcification of other arteries, and heart failure.

Vitamin E (tocopherol)

Vitamin E consists of eight naturally occurring tocopherols; α-tocopherol is the most active.

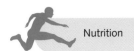

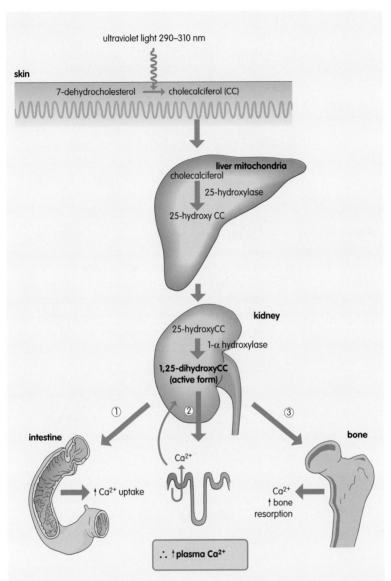

Fig. 8.15 Synthesis, metabolism, and functions of vitamin D. The active form, 1,25-dihydroxycholecalciferol, has three main effects that increase the plasma calcium concentration:
1. Increases uptake of Ca^{2+} from the intestine.
2. Increases reabsorbtion of calcium from the kidney.
3. Increases resorption of bone.

Deficiency and excess of vitamin D	
Deficiency	**Toxicity**
low plasma Ca^{2+} and impaired bone mineralization	most toxic of all vitamins
if severe, children develop rickets, adults develop osteomalacia	high levels lead to a large increase in calcium absorption and bone resorption resulting in **hypercalcemia** and Ca^{2+} deposition in organs

Fig. 8.16 Deficiency and excess of vitamin D.

The diagnosis and treatment of vitamin D deficiency	
Diagnosis	**Treatment**
low or normal serum calcium	exposure to sunlight
low phosphate	daily oral vitamin D supplements
increased serum alkaline phosphatase	
bone X-rays show defective mineralization	

Fig. 8.17 Diagnosis and treatment of vitamin D deficiency.

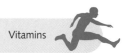

RDA
10 mg/day for men; 8 mg/day for women
(δ-tocopherol equivalents).

Sources
Vegetable oils, especially wheat germ oil, nuts, and green vegetables.

Absorption and transport
Tocopherol is found "dissolved" in dietary fat and is therefore absorbed with it. It is transported in the blood by lipoproteins, initially in chylomicrons which deliver dietary vitamin E to the tissues. Vitamin E is transported from the liver with very-low-density lipoproteins (VLDL) and is stored in adipose tissue. Thus a defect in lipoprotein and fat metabolism may lead to a deficiency of vitamin E.

Functions
The functions of vitamin E are listed in Fig. 8.18. Its mechanism of action is described in Fig. 8.19.

Clinical manifestations of a deficiency or excess
Note that deficiency is very rare (see Fig. 8.18). No adverse effects are seen with doses as high as 3.2 g/day!

Deficiency
Incidence   In humans, vitamin E deficiency is very rare and is seen virtually only in:
- Premature infants, causing hemolytic anemia of the newborn. Vitamin E crosses the placenta in the last trimester of pregnancy; therefore, premature infants have only small vitamin E stores. Their red blood cell (RBC) membranes are fragile and are susceptible to free radical damage, leading to lysis of RBCs. Vitamin E supplements are given to pregnant mothers to prevent this.
- Children and adults, secondary to severe fat malabsorption. For example, biliary atresia, cholestatic liver disease, or a lipoprotein deficiency (e.g. abetalipoproteinemia).

Clinical features   Vitamin E deficiency causes muscle weakness, peripheral neuropathy, ataxia, and nystagmus. In children with abetalipoproteinemia, vitamin E therapy can prevent the occurrence of severe spinocerebellar degeneration and gross ataxia. Animal studies with rats have shown that vitamin E deficiency causes muscular dystrophy and sterility; this is not true in humans.

Toxicity
Vitamin E is the least toxic of all the fat-soluble vitamins. The use of vitamin E supplements may help to protect against the development of heart disease

Functions of vitamin E	
Functions	**Deficiency**
• naturally occurring antioxidant which prevents oxidation of cell components by free radicals, e.g. PUFA present in cell membranes • may protect against the development of heart disease by preventing LDL oxidation	very rare except in premature infants in whom it can cause hemolytic anemia of newborn

Fig. 8.18 Vitamin E: function and effects of deficiency. PUFA, polyunsaturated fatty acid; LDL, low-density lipoprotein.

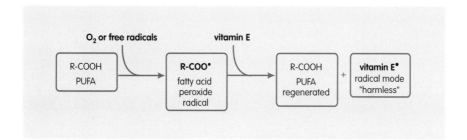

Fig. 8.19 Vitamin E as an antioxidant. Free radicals attack double bonds in polyunsaturated fatty acids to form a highly reactive fatty acid peroxide radical. This can attack other fatty acids, disrupting membrane structure and cell integrity. Vitamin E "scavenges" fatty acid peroxide radicals to form a free radical itself. It is regenerated by other antioxidant nutrients (vitamins A and C). PUFA, polyunsaturated fatty acids.

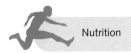
by protecting low-density lipoproteins (LDL) from oxidation by free radicals.

Vitamin K

RDA
Varies with age; 45–80 µg/day.

Sources
The sources of vitamin K include:
- Diet: especially green vegetables, egg yolk, liver and cereals.
- It is made mostly by the normal bacterial flora of jejunum and ileum.
- Human milk contains only a small amount.

Functions
Vitamin K is a coenzyme required for the γ-carboxylation of clotting factors II, VII, IX, and X, activating them and thus the clotting cascade. The functions and clinical manifestations of a deficiency of vitamin K are listed in Fig. 8.20.

Deficiency
A true deficiency is rare because most of the body's vitamin K is synthesized by bacteria in the gut.

Causes
The main causes of vitamin K deficiency are:
- A decreased level of bacteria in the gut, due, for example, to long-term antibiotic therapy.
- A decrease in dietary intake.
- Newborn babies have sterile guts and therefore cannot initially make vitamin K.

- Oral anticoagulant drugs (e.g., warfarin) are vitamin K antagonists (Fig. 8.21).

Mechanism
A deficiency of vitamin K results in low levels of the vitamin K-dependent clotting factors II, VII, IX, and X and thus inhibition of the clotting cascade. Patients will have an increased tendency to bleed and to bruise.

Diagnosis and treatment
The diagnosis and treatment of vitamin K deficiency are covered in Fig. 8.22.

Deficiency in newborn babies
Newborn babies have sterile gut and thus have no bacteria to make vitamin K. Since human milk is a very poor source, babies are particularly susceptible to deficiency. Vitamin K deficiency causes hemorrhagic disease of the newborn, which can occur either in the first week of life or between weeks 1 and 8. Usually, the bleeding is minor, but it can result in major bleeds, leading to intracranial

Functions and deficiency of vitamin K	
Functions	**Deficiency**
vitamin K is a coenzyme for the carboxylation of glutamate residues of blood clotting factors II, VII, IX and X	true deficiency is rare because bacteria in the gut usually produce enough
carboxylation activates clotting factors and thus clotting cascade	long-term antibiotic therapy leads to ↓ bacteria and ↓ vitamin K, resulting in poor blood clotting and bleeding disorders
anticoagulants warfarin and dicoumarol inhibit vitamin K	may result in hemorrhagic disease of the newborn

Fig. 8.20 Functions and deficiency of vitamin K.

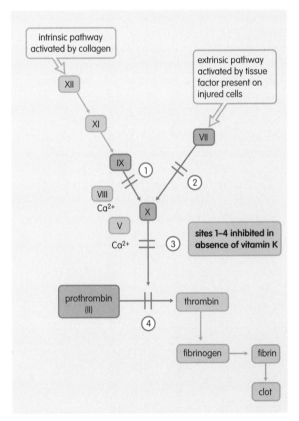

Fig. 8.21 Vitamin K deficiency: inhibition of the clotting cascade.

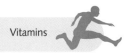

The diagnosis and treatment of vitamin K deficiency	
Diagnosis	**Treatment**
clinical features: bruising and bleeding, e.g. hematuria or bleeding from the GI tract	vitamin K supplements
increased prothrombin time (PTT)	
increased activated partial thromboplastin time (APTT) less marked than PTT	

Fig. 8.22 Diagnosis and treatment of vitamin K deficiency.

hemorrhage. About 50% of children with major bleeds end up permanently disabled or die. Therefore, every newborn baby in the U.S. is given prophylactic intramuscular or oral vitamin K.

Water-soluble vitamins
Vitamin B₁ (thiamin)
RDA
1.5 mg/day for men; 1.1 mg/day for women.

Sources
Whole grain cereals, liver, pork, yeast, dairy produce, and legumes.

Active form
Thiamin pyrophosphate (TPP), which is formed by the transfer of a pyrophosphate group from ATP to thiamin.

Functions
The functions of thiamin are listed in Fig. 8.23, with its mechanism of action described in Fig. 8.24.

Deficiency diseases
A deficiency of thiamin causes:
- Beriberi. This occurs in two forms: wet beriberi, which results in edema, cardiovascular symptoms, and heart failure, and dry beriberi, which causes muscle wasting and peripheral neuropathy.
- Wernicke's encephalopathy, which is associated with alcoholism (alcohol is thought to impair the absorption of thiamin).
- Korsakoff's psychosis.

Beriberi
Incidence Beriberi (Fig. 8.25) is now seen only in the poorest areas of South-East Asia, where the

Functions and effect of thiamin deficiency	
Functions	**Deficiency**
Thiamine pyrophosphate is cofactor for **four key enzymes**:	
• pyruvate dehydrogenase • α-ketoglutarate dehydrogenase (TCA cycle) • branched-chain amino acid α-ketoacid dehydrogenase	decreased activity of pyruvate dehydrogenase and α-ketoglutarate dehydrogenase causes: • accumulation of pyruvate and lactate • decreased acetyl CoA and ATP formation and thus decreased acetylcholine and central nervous system activity
• transketolase (pentose phosphate pathway)	decreased activity of pentose phosphate pathway results in low levels of NADPH necessary for fatty acid synthesis; therefore this leads to a decrease in synthesis of myelin, which may cause peripheral neuropathy

Fig. 8.23 Thiamin: functions and effects of deficiency.

staple food is polished rice; that is, the husk that contains most of the vitamins, including thiamin, has been removed.

Diagnosis Diagnosis is by measurement of the transketolase activity in RBCs, before and after the addition of TPP. A greater than 30% increase in activity with TPP indicates a deficiency.

Treatment Treatment is initially with intramuscular injections of thiamin for approximately 3 days (varies according to severity), followed by daily oral supplements of thiamin. For wet beriberi, treatment results in a dramatic decrease in edema and a quick improvement of symptoms. For dry beriberi, there is a slower improvement.

Wernicke–Korsakoff syndrome
Incidence As thiamin is present in most foods, a dietary deficiency is rare in developed countries. The deficiency manifests itself as Wernicke's encephalopathy (Fig. 8.26). In the U.S., a low thiamin intake is seen in:

159

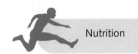

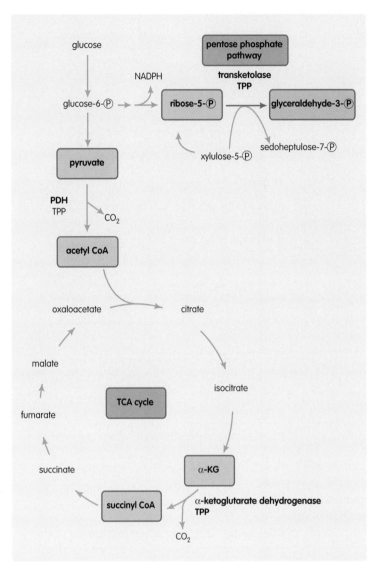

Fig. 8.24 Mechanism of action of thiamin. Thiamin pyrophosphate (TPP), the active form of thiamin, acts as coenzyme for pyruvate dehydrogenase and α-ketoglutarate dehydrogenase reactions in the TCA cycle and for transketolase in the pentose phosphate pathway.

- Chronic alcoholics: alcohol inhibits the uptake of thiamin.
- The elderly.
- People with diseases of the upper gastrointestinal tract (e.g., gastric cancer).

Toxicity
Toxicity is rare, but an excess causes headaches, insomnia, and dermatitis.

Vitamin B₂ (riboflavin)
RDA
1.7 mg/day for men; 1.3 mg/day for women.

Sources
Milk, eggs, liver. Riboflavin is readily destroyed by ultraviolet light.

Active forms
Riboflavin occurs in two active forms:
- Flavin mononucleotide (FMN).
- Flavin adenine dinucleotide (FAD).

Functions and deficiency
The functions and clinical manifestations of a deficiency of riboflavin are listed in Fig. 8.27. Riboflavin is not toxic in excess.

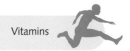

Types of beriberi		
	Clinical features	**Signs**
wet beriberi	edema: spreads to involve the whole body → ascites and pleural effusions congestive heart failure	raised JVP tachycardia and tachypnea
infantile beriberi	a form of wet beriberi that occurs in breastfed babies whose mothers are thiamin deficient	acute onset: anorexia and edema that can involve the larynx → aphonia tachycardia and tachypnea develop → death
dry beriberi	gradual, symmetrical, ascending peripheral neuropathy resulting in progressive paralysis	initially, stiffness of legs → weakness, numbness, and "pins and needles" ascends to involve trunk, arms and eventually brain

Fig. 8.25 Types of beriberi.

Functions and deficiency of riboflavin	
Functions	**Deficiency**
FAD and FMN are coenzymes for a number of oxidases and dehydrogenases	rare except in elderly or alcoholic individuals
they can accept two hydrogens to form $FADH_2$ and $FMNH_2$ respectively and take part in redox reactions, e.g. electron transport chain or act as antioxidants	symptoms of deficiency: • angular stomatitis (inflammation at sides of mouth) • cheilosis (fissures at corners of mouth) • cataracts • glossitis (inflamed tongue)

Fig. 8.27 Riboflavin: functions and effects of deficiency.

Wernicke's encephalopathy and Korsakoff's psychosis	
Clinical features	**Causes**
Wernicke's encephalopathy:	alcohol
• acute confusional state	ischemic damage to brainstem
• ataxia; cerebellar signs	
• ophthalmoplegia and nystagmus	major cause of dementia in developed countries
• peripheral neuropathy	
diagnosis: made on clinical grounds; condition is reversible with immediate thiamin therapy	
if untreated it may develop into **Korsakoff's psychosis:** a severe irreversible syndrome characterized by loss of short-term memory	progression from untreated Wernicke's encephalopathy

Fig. 8.26 Clinical features of Wernicke's encephalopathy and Korsakoff's psychosis.

Niacin or nicotinic acid

RDA
19 mg/day for men; 15 mg/day for women.

Sources
Whole grain cereals, meat, fish, and the amino acid tryptophan.

Synthesis of niacin from tryptophan
The synthesis of niacin from trytophan is a very inefficient process: as much as 60 mg of tryptophan is needed to make 1 mg of niacin. Synthesis requires thiamin, riboflavin, and pyridoxine as cofactors and occurs only after the needs of protein synthesis are met. This means, in theory, that niacin deficiency can be treated with a high protein diet, but lots would be needed!

Active forms
NAD^+ and $NADP^+$.

Functions and deficiency
The functions and clinical manifestations of a deficiency of niacin are listed in Fig. 8.28.

161

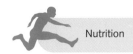

Functions and deficiency of niacin	
Functions	**Deficiency**
NAD^+ and $NADP^+$ are coenzymes for many dehydrogenases in redox reactions	pellagra
	symptoms, the **3Ds**:
NAD is required for repair of UV light-damaged DNA in areas of exposed skin (nothing to do with redox state)	**d**ermatitis **d**iarrhea **d**ementia leading to death
nicotinic acid is used for treatment of certain dyslipidemias because it inhibits lipolysis, leading to decreased VLDL synthesis (see Chapter 4)	

Fig. 8.28 Niacin: functions and effects of deficiency.

Clinical features of pellagra	
Clinical features	**Symptoms**
3Ds: **dermatitis**; deficiency of, NAD inhibits DNA repair of sun-damaged skin (Fig. 8.17)	photosensitive symmetrical skin rash occurs when skin is exposed to sunlight: • skin may crack and ulcerate • on neck, extent depends on area of skin exposed
diarrhea	may also see glossitis and angular stomatitis
dementia	dementia occurs in chronic disease and is usually irreversible; may develop tremor and encephalopathy

Fig. 8.29 Clinical features and symptoms of pellagra.

Pellagra
Defintion A disease of the skin, gastrointestinal tract, and central nervous system.

Incidence Pellagra is rare and is found in areas where maize is the staple food. It is now seen only in certain parts of Africa. Maize contains niacin in a biologically unavailable form, niacytin. Niacin can be removed from the maize only by alkali treatment (Mexicans soak maize in lime juice to release the niacin). Pellagra (Fig. 8.29) can also occur in conditions in which large amounts of tryptophan are metabolized; for example, carcinoid syndrome, which is also rare.

Causes The causes of pellegra are:
• A dietary deficiency of niacin.
• A deficiency of protein (as niacin is made from tryptophan).
• Vitamin B_6 and thus pyridoxal phosphate deficiency (pyridoxal phosphate is a cofactor for niacin synthesis from tryptophan).
• Hartnup's disease: a failure to absorb tryptophan from the diet (see Fig. 5.27).
• Isoniazid treatment for tuberculosis inhibits vitamin B_6, causing a decrease in tryptophan synthesis.

Diagnosis Diagnosis is by the measurement of niacin or its metabolites (N-methylnicotinamide or 2-pyridone) in the urine.

Treatment As niacin can be formed from tryptophan, treatment involves:
• High-dose niacin supplements.
• A high protein diet.

Mild cases are reversible. Dementia usually is not and may lead to death.

Toxicity
A high intake upsets liver function, carbohydrate tolerance, and urate metabolism. More than 200 mg/day will cause vasodilatation and flushing.

Vitamin B$_6$
Vitamin B_6 exists in three forms: pyridoxine, pyridoxal, and pyridoxamine.

RDA
2.0 mg/day for men; 1.6 mg/day for women.

Sources
Whole grains (wheat or corn), meat, fish, and poultry.

Active form
All three forms can be converted to the coenzyme pyridoxal phosphate (PLP).

Functions and deficiency
The functions and clinical manifestations of a deficiency of vitamin B_6 are listed in Fig. 8.30.

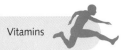

Functions and deficiency of vitamin B$_6$	
Functions	**Deficiency**
• pyridoxal phosphate is a co-enzyme for many enzymes:	→ primary deficiency is very rare
• in amino acid metabolism: aminotransferases and serine dehydratase	→ abnormal amino acid metabolism
• in heme synthesis, ALA synthase (catalyzes rate-limiting step)	→ hypochromic, microcytic anemia
• glycogen phosphorylase	
• conversion of tryptophan to niacin	→ secondary pellagra
• indirect role in serotonin and noradrenaline synthesis as they are derived from amino acids	→ convulsions and depression

Fig. 8.30 Vitamin B$_6$: functions and effects of deficiency.

Functions and deficiency of pantothenic acid	
Functions	**Deficiency**
as coenzyme A, it is involved in the transfer of acyl groups, e.g. acetyl CoA, succinyl CoA, fatty acyl CoA	very rare; causes "burning foot syndrome"
it is also a component of fatty acid synthase: acyl carrier protein (see Chapter 4)	N.B. can induce a deficiency in rats, which causes depigmentation of fur, i.e. it turns gray; this is widely exploited by the shampoo industry; not toxic in excess

Fig. 8.31 Functions and effects of deficiency of pantothenic acid.

Pyridoxine deficiency

Causes   Dietary deficiency is extremely rare but may be seen in:
• Newborn babies fed formula milk.
• Elderly people and alcoholics.
• Women taking oral contraceptives.
• Patients on isoniazid therapy for treatment of tuberculosis.

Isoniazid binds to pyridoxal phosphate to form an inactive hydrazone derivative, which is rapidly excreted, thus causing the deficiency.

Clinical features   The main features include:
• Hypochromic, microcytic anemia.
• Secondary pellagra.
• Convulsions and depression.

Treatment   Vitamin B$_6$ supplements are given to all patients on isoniazid therapy. A deficiency caused by an increased requirement due to either a physiologic or pathologic state or due to the action of an antagonistic compound (e.g., isoniazid mentioned above) is called a "vitamin-dependency" state.

Toxicity

Toxicity is rare. In fact vitamin B$_6$ is actually used in the treatment of premenstrual tension (PMT). An excess is, however, associated with the development of a sensory neuropathy.

Pantothenic acid
Sources

Most foods but eggs, liver, and yeast are very good sources.

Active form

Component of coenzyme A (see Chapter 2).

Functions and deficiency

The functions and manifestations of a deficiency of pantothenic acid are listed in Fig. 8.31. Panthothenic acid is not toxic in excess.

Biotin
Sources

Most foods, especially egg yolk, offal, yeast, and nuts. A significant amount is synthesized by bacteria in the intestine.

Active form

As a coenzyme for carboxylation reactions, biotin binds to a lysine residue in carboxylase enzymes (Fig. 8.32).

Functions and deficiency

The functions and clinical manifestations of a deficiency of biotin are listed in Fig. 8.33.

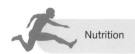
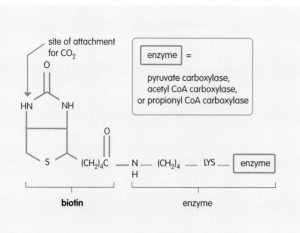

Fig. 8.32 Biotin is a coenzyme for carboxylation reactions. It binds to a lysine residue in carboxylase enzyme molecules.

Functions and deficiency of biotin	
Functions	**Deficiency**
it is an activated carrier of CO_2	very rare on a normal diet, may cause dermatitis
it is a coenzyme for: • pyruvate carboxylase in gluconeogenesis (see Chapter 5) • acetyl CoA carboxylase in fatty acid synthesis (see Chapter 4) • propionyl CoA carboxylase in β oxidation of odd-numbered fatty acids (see Fig. 8.35) • branched-chain amino acid metabolism	can be induced by: • eating lots of raw egg whites, rich in a glycoprotein, avidin, that binds to biotin in the intestine preventing its absorption • long-term antibiotic therapy, which kills intestinal bacteria

Fig. 8.33 Biotin: functions and deficiency.

Vitamin B$_{12}$ (cobalamin)

RDA

2.0 mg/day.

Sources

Only animal sources: liver, meat, dairy foods. Therefore, vegans are at risk of deficiency.

Active forms

Two active forms: deoxyadenosylcobalamin and methylcobalamin.

Absorption and transport

The absorption and transport of vitamin B$_{12}$ occurs in several steps (numbers refer to Fig. 8.34):

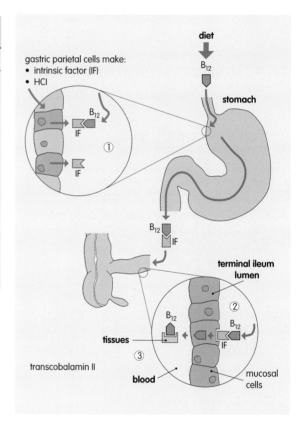

Fig. 8.34 The absorption and transport of vitamin B$_{12}$ (numbers refer to the text).

1. Vitamin B$_{12}$, released from food in the stomach, becomes bound to a glycoprotein carrier, intrinsic factor (IF), produced by gastric parietal cells (see Fig. 8.34).
2. The complex of B$_{12}$ and intrinsic factor binds to receptors on the mucosal cells of the terminal ileum.

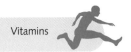

3. B_{12} is absorbed and transported to tissues, attached to transcobalamin II. About 2–3 mg of B_{12} are stored by the body, mainly in the liver. This is relatively large compared with its daily requirement.

Functions

Vitamin B_{12} is a carrier of methyl groups. It is the coenzyme for two enzymes:

- Methylmalonyl CoA mutase, as deoxyadenosylcobalamin, to assist in the breakdown of odd-numbered fatty acids (Fig. 8.35).
- Homocysteine methyltransferase, as methylcobalamin, to assist in the synthesis of methionine. This reaction also reverses the methylfolate trap, regenerating tetrahydrofolate (THF) from methyl-THF (discussed below with folate).

Deficiency and toxicity

A significant amount of vitamin B_{12} is stored; therefore, it takes about 2 years for symptoms of deficiency to develop. Deficiency can cause two main problems:

- The accumulation of abnormal odd-numbered fatty acids, which may be incorporated into the cell membranes of nerves, resulting in neurologic symptoms, inadequate myelin synthesis and nerve degeneration.
- Secondary "artificial" folate deficiency since folate is "trapped" as methyl-THF. This causes a decrease in nucleotide synthesis, resulting in megaloblastic anemia.

The most common cause of vitamin B_{12} deficiency is pernicious anemia, an autoimmune condition in which antibodies are made by the body to intrinsic factor.

The toxicity of vitamin B_{12} is low.

Causes of deficiency

Reduced intake (e.g., by vegans) because vitamin B_{12} is found only in animal-derived foods. Reduced absorption caused by:

- A lack of intrinsic factor, for example in pernicious anemia.
- Diseases of the terminal ileum (the site of B_{12} absorption); for example, Crohn's disease or tuberculosis.
- Bypass of the B_{12} absorption site; for example, fistulas or surgical resection of gut.
- Blind-loop syndrome: parasites compete for B_{12}.

Body stores (mainly in the liver) are large relative to the daily requirement; therefore, a reduced intake alone takes about 2–3 years to cause a deficiency.

Pernicious anemia

Pernicious anemia is the most common cause of vitamin B_{12} deficiency.

Incidence   It is more common in older women and is often associated with fair-haired and blue-eyed individuals and also the presence of other autoimmune disorders (e.g., thyroid disease and Addison's disease).

Pathogenesis   Pernicious anemia is an autoimmune disorder in which antibodies are made to either:

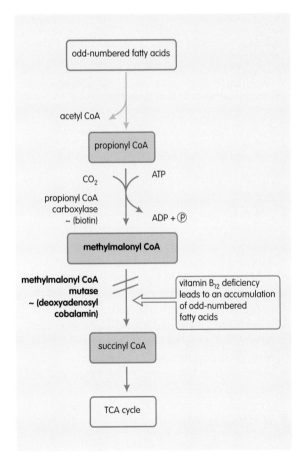

Fig. 8.35 β Oxidation of odd-numbered fatty acids. B_{12} is a carrier of methyl groups. It is the coenzyme for methylmalonyl CoA mutase, assisting in the breakdown of odd-numbered fatty acids.

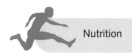

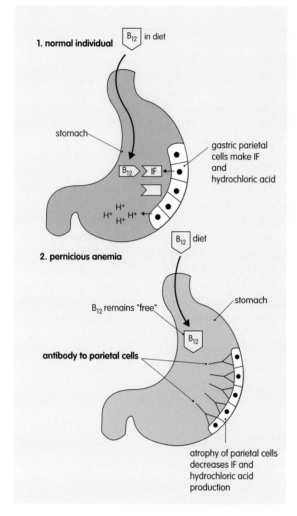

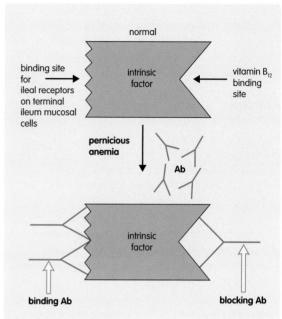

Fig. 8.36B Antibodies to intrinsic factor. Intrinsic factor contains two binding sites—one for vitamin B_{12} and a second one for ileal receptors in the terminal ileum, its site of absorption. In pernicious anemia, antibodies produced may bind to either or both of these sites.

Fig. 8.36A Antibodies in pernicious anemia.
1. In normal individuals, vitamin B_{12} released from food in the stomach becomes bound to intrinsic factor (IF) produced by gastric parietal cells.
2. In individuals with pernicious anemia, antibodies to the gastric parietal cells cause wasting of the cells and thus prevent production of intrinisc factor by them. Vitamin B_{12} is therefore not absorbed, resulting in B_{12} deficiency.

- Gastric parietal cells, causing atrophy or wasting of the cells, thus preventing the production of intrinsic factor and stomach acid (Fig. 8.36A).
- Intrinsic factor itself (Fig. 8.36B). The antibodies bind to the intrinsic factor, preventing it from either binding to vitamin B_{12} (blocking antibodies) or binding to the receptors in the terminal ileum (binding antibodies). A lack of intrinsic factor leads to a decreased uptake of vitamin B_{12}.

The clinical features of pernicious anemia are discussed in Fig. 8.37.

Diagnosis Diagnosis is performed by analysis of the blood film and bone marrow specimens and by the Schilling test, which measures the absorption of vitamin B_{12}:
- Radioactive vitamin B_{12} is given orally.
- A 24-hour urine collection is performed to measure the percentage of the dose of radioactive vitamin B_{12} excreted in the urine.
- If the subject is vitamin B_{12}-deficient, less than 10% will be excreted because the vitamin B_{12} is being used to replenish depleted stores.
- If the result is abnormal, the test is repeated with the addition of intrinsic factor.
- If excretion is now normal, the diagnosis is pernicious anemia.

Treatment The treatment of vitamin B_{12} deficiency is intramuscular injections of hydroxycobalamin for life. Initially, these are more frequent to fill the stores. Pernicious anemia carries a slightly increased risk of carcinoma of the stomach.

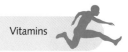

The clinical features and mechanism of pernicious anemia	
Clinical features	**Mechanism**
megablastic anemia: blood film: macrocytes (MCV >100 fL)	B_{12} deficiency causes secondary folate deficiency, which leads to decreased production of DNA and defective cell division
bone marrow: megaloblasts (developing red cells where nuclei mature more slowly than the cytoplasm)	
neurological abnormalities peripheral neuropathy affecting sensory neurons of posterior and lateral columns of spinal cord; leads to subacute combined degeneration of spinal cord	pathogenesis of CNS damage unknown impairment of CNS amino acid and fatty acid metabolism has been implicated
lemon yellow color	combination of jaundice from red cell lysis and pallor because of anemia
glossitis, diarrhea, and weight loss	
gastric atrophy and achlorhydria ($\downarrow$ hydrochloric acid production)	antibodies to gastric parietal cells

Fig. 8.37 Clinical features and mechanism of pernicious anemia.

Folate

RDA
200 mg/day.

Sources
Green vegetables, liver, and whole grain cereals.

Active form
5,6,7,8-THF, which is involved in the transfer of one-carbon units (see Chapter 6).

Absorption and storage
Folate is absorbed in the duodenum and jejunum. About 10 mg of folate is stored, mainly in the liver.

The store is small relative to the daily requirement; therefore, deficiency can occur quickly, usually within about 2–3 months.

The role of folate and vitamin B_{12}
All one-carbon THF units are interconvertible except N^5-methyl-THF; the THF cannot be released from it and is trapped, forming the "methyl-folate trap" (see Chapter 6). The only way to re-form THF is via vitamin B_{12}-dependent synthesis of methionine: the methionine salvage pathway (Fig. 8.38).

Even if plenty of folate is present in the diet, if there is a deficiency in vitamin B_{12}, this will lead to secondary folate deficiency.

Functions and deficiency
The functions and clinical manifestations of a deficiency of folate are listed in Fig. 8.39. The stores of folate are small relative to the daily requirement, therefore a deficiency state can develop in only weeks, particularly if it is associated with a period of rapid growth.

Causes of folate deficiency
- Decreased intake: a poor diet is the most common cause; for example, in dieters, elderly people, and alcoholics.
- Increased requirement: during periods of rapid cell growth, such as pregnancy, infancy, or adolescence; in patients with cancer, inflammatory states, or recovering from illness; and in patients with hemolytic anemias.
- Malabsorption: occurring, for example, in celiac disease or gut resection.
- Drugs, such as anticonvulsants (e.g., phenytoin and phenobarbitone), which impair absorption; dihydrofolate reductase inhibitors (e.g., methotrexate); antimalarial drugs (e.g., pyrimethamine).
- Secondary to B_{12} deficiency. Vitamin B_{12} is essential to maintain an adequate supply of the active form of folate, that is, 5,6,7,8-tetrahydrofolate. Specifically, it regenerates THF from N^5-methyl-THF in the methionine salvage pathway (see Fig. 6.2). Even if there are adequate amounts of folate in the diet, in the absence of vitamin B_{12} folate deficiency arises.

Clinical features and diagnosis of folate deficiency
The clinical features and diagnosis of folate deficiency are covered in Fig. 8.40.

Treatment
The treatment of folate deficiency is daily oral folate supplementation.

Folate deficiency in pregnancy
It is known that the development of the neural tube in the fetus is dependent on the presence of folic

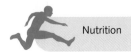
Fig. 8.38 Role of folate and B$_{12}$. The only way to reform tetrahydrofolate is via vitamin B$_{12}$-dependent synthesis of methionine: the methionine salvage pathway.

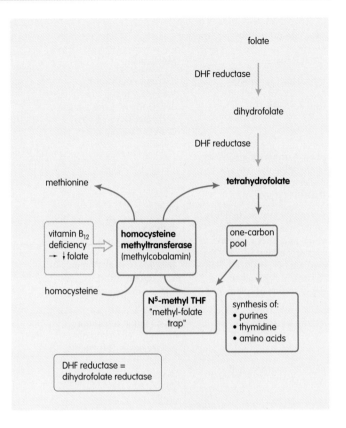

Functions and deficiency of folate	
Functions	**Deficiency**
synthesis of: • amino acids, e.g. glycine and methionine • purines, AMP, and, GMP (see Chapter 6) • thymidine (see Chapter 6)	**megaloblastic anemia:** • decrease in purines and pyrimidines leads to a decrease in nucleic acid synthesis and cell division • shows up mostly in cells that are rapidly dividing, e.g. bone marrow and gut • large, immature red blood cells are present

Fig. 8.39 Folate: function and deficiency.

The clinical features and diagnosis of folate deficiency	
Clinical features	**Diagnosis**
megablastic anemia: this is identical to vitamin B$_{12}$ deficiency (see Fig. 8.37) growth failure N.B. peripheral neuropathy and neurological symptoms do not occur in folate deficiency	blood film: macrocytes (MCV >100 fL) megaloblasts in bone marrow low serum folate red cell folate is a better test of folate stores normal = 135–750 mg/mL must always consider and eliminate vitamin B$_{12}$ deficiency and malignancy

Fig. 8.40 Clinical features and diagnosis of folate deficiency.

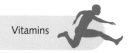

Vitamin B$_{12}$ deficiency compared with folate deficiency		
Characteristics	Vitamin B$_{12}$	Folate
most common cause	pernicious anemia	↓ dietary intake
onset	slow, 2–3 years	develops over weeks
neurological symptoms	frequent + severe	never
drug-related	no: vitamin B$_{12}$ deficiency usually causes secondary folate deficiency	yes: anticonvulsants, dihydrofolate reductase inhibitors

folate deficiency occurs frequently on its own because of ↓ intake or ↑ demand |

Fig. 8.41 A comparison of vitamin B$_{12}$ and folate deficiency: main differences.

Functions and deficiency of ascorbate	
Functions	Deficiency
co-enzyme in hydroxylation: reactions
• proline and lysine hydroxylases in collagen synthesis
• dopamine β-hydroxylase in adrenaline and noradrenaline synthesis

powerful reducing agent:
• reduces dietary Fe^{3+} to Fe^{2+} in the gut, allowing its absorption (therefore deficiency can lead to anemia)

antioxidant and free-radical "scavenger"
• inactivates free oxygen radicals which damage lipid membranes, proteins and DNA
• also protects other antioxidant vitamins A and E | **scurvy** most symptoms are due to a decrease in collagen synthesis, leading to poor connective tissue formation and wound healing |

Fig. 8.42 Ascorbate: function and deficiency.

acid. All women planning a pregnancy should take prophylactic folate supplements to reduce the risk of neural tube defects such as spina bifida or anencephaly. The critical time is the first few weeks after conception: women, therefore, should start supplements before conception to cover this period. A woman who has already had a baby with a neural tube defect has about a 1:20 risk of a second affected baby; the use of folate supplements has been shown to reduce this risk.

A comparison of folate and vitamin B$_{12}$ deficiencies

A comparison of folate and vitamin B$_{12}$ deficiencies is given in Fig. 8.41. A deficiency of either can cause a macrocytic, megaloblastic anemia. Patients suspected of having either deficiency must always be investigated for both folate and B$_{12}$ deficiency, since the administration of folic acid corrects the anemia but masks a B$_{12}$ deficiency. Therefore, folate should never be given alone in treatment of pernicious anemia and other B$_{12}$ deficiency states because it may precipitate an irreversible, peripheral neuropathy.

Vitamin C (ascorbate)
RDA
60 mg/day.

Sources
Citrus fruits, tomatoes, berries, and green vegetables.

Active form
Ascorbate.

Functions and deficiency
The functions and clinical manifestations of a deficiency of ascorbate are listed in Fig. 8.42.

Vitamin C deficiency: scurvy
A long time ago this used to be common among sailors who spent weeks at sea without any fresh fruit or vegetables.

Causes   Scurvy is caused by a poor dietary intake of fresh fruit and vegetables. In the U.S. it is seen in elderly people, alcoholics, and smokers. Smokers require twice the normal intake of vitamin C (80 mg/day). Humans have about 6 months' store of vitamin C.

Clinical features   The clinical features of scurvy are described in Fig. 8.43.

Treatment   The treatment of vitamin C deficiency is 1 g daily of ascorbate and lots of fresh fruit and vegetables in the diet.

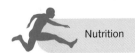

Clinical features of scurvy	
Clinical features	**Diagnosis**
• swollen, sore, spongy gums with bleeding; loose teeth	hypochromic, microcytic anemia caused by secondary iron deficiency
• spontaneous bruising and petechial hemorrhages	low plasma ascorbate level (not very accurate)
• anemia	the measurement of ascorbate concentration in white blood cells provides an assessment of tissue stores
• poor wound healing	
• swollen joints and muscle pain	

Fig. 8.43 Clinical features of scurvy.

The megadose hypothesis

Some people believe that large doses of vitamin C cure many illnesses, such as the common cold and certain immune-mediated diseases, and even help in cancer prevention and promote fertility. The benefits of large doses are unresolved and under review. It is thought that 1–4 g/day of vitamin C can decrease the severity of symptoms of colds but not the incidence. Vitamin C is an antioxidant, and it is thought that, along with vitamins A and E, it might decrease the incidence of coronary heart disease and certain cancers by scavenging free radicals, thus preventing oxidative damage to cells and their components. This theory is still being investigated.

Toxicity

A high intake of vitamin C may lead to the formation of kidney stones or diarrhea and also cause systemic conditioning; that is, requirements increase as the body adapts to metabolizing more.

The role of ascorbate in hydroxylation reactions: Hydroxylase enzymes contain iron, which exists in two oxidation states: Fe^{3+}, which is inactive, and Fe^{2+}, which is reduced and active. Ascorbate is necessary to maintain iron in its reduced and active state (Fe^{2+}).

The best way to learn this sort of information is to take a large piece of paper and for each vitamin list only the main points mentioned above. Examiners (unfortunately) love to ask about deficiency diseases.

You must know about Wernicke–Korsakoff syndrome, pernicious anemia, folate deficiency, and scurvy, because these topics are commonly examined.

Minerals

Classification of minerals

There are 103 known elements. Living organisms are composed mainly of 11 of these: carbon, hydrogen, oxygen, nitrogen, and the seven major minerals:
- Calcium, phosphorus, and magnesium, which are used mainly in bone.
- Sodium, potassium, and chloride, which are electrolytes.
- Sulphur, which is used mainly in amino acids.

The RNI is greater than 100 mg/day for each of these (the exception is sulphur, for which no RNI is published).

In addition, there are at least 12 other elements that are required in the diet in smaller quantities. These are known as the essential trace elements, for which the RNI is less than 100 mg/day: iron, zinc, copper, cobalt, iodine, chromium, manganese, molybdenum, selenium, vanadium, nickel, and silicon.

Calcium

Calcium is the most abundant mineral in the human body. There is about 1.2 kg of calcium in the average 70-kg adult, of which 99% is in bone.

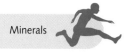

RDA

The RDA of calcium is 1200 mg/day; it is higher during periods of growth, pregnancy, lactation and after the menopause.

Sources

Milk and milk products; a lot of foods are fortified with calcium (e.g., bread).

Absorption

Absorption of calcium from the diet is variable, usually $32 \pm 14\%$. Factors affecting absorption:
- Lactose and basic amino acids increase absorption because they form complexes with calcium.
- Fiber decreases absorption; therefore, vegans need a lot more calcium.

Active forms

The ionized form, Ca^{2+}.

Main functions

The main functions of calcium are listed in Fig. 8.44.

Regulation of calcium

Calcium levels are controlled by three hormones which also regulate plasma phosphate levels:
- Parathyroid hormone, which increases plasma calcium but decreases levels of inorganic phosphate.
- Vitamin D, which increases both plasma calcium and inorganic phosphate levels.
- Calcitonin, which decreases both plasma calcium and inorganic phosphate levels.

For further information refer to an endocrinology text.

Deficiency and toxicity

The clinical manifestations of a deficiency and excess of calcium are listed in Fig. 8.45.

Calcium deficiency

In children, calcium deficiency causes rickets (derived from the old English word "wrickken," meaning to twist). In adults, calcium deficiency causes osteomalacia. Both may result:
- From dietary deficiency of calcium, seen particularly in developing countries.
- Secondary to vitamin D deficiency. Vitamin D is necessary for the intestinal absorption of calcium and phosphate (see Fig. 8.15).
- From malabsorption; for example, due to celiac disease.

Pathogenesis   Both rickets and osteomalacia are the result of inadequate mineralization of bone, resulting in a reduction in its normal strength, leading to soft, easily deformed bones. The difference is that they occur at different stages of bone development. In rickets the production of undermineralized bone results in a failure of adequate growth, whereas, in osteomalacia, demineralization of existing bones leads to an increased risk of fractures.
- **Rickets**. The characteristics of rickets are listed in Figs. 8.46 and 8.47. Treatment is with calcium

Main functions of calcium	
Function	Examples
structural role	bone and teeth calcium is present as calcium phosphate (hydroxyapatite) crystals
muscle contraction	calcium binds to troponin C
nerve impulse transmission	calcium is released in response to hormones and neurotransmitters
blood clotting	coenzyme for coagulation factors
ion transport and cell signaling	intracellular second messenger

Fig. 8.44 Main functions of calcium.

Deficiency and excess of calcium	
Deficiency (e.g. vitamin D deficiency, thyroid/parathyroid surgery, renal failure with high phosphate)	Excess (e.g. malignancy, primary hyperparathyroidism, sarcoidosis)
in children leads to rickets in adults leads to osteomalacia, that is defective mineralization of bone	hypercalcemia Ca^{2+} is deposited in many organs, particularly arteries, heart, liver, and kidneys, leading to tissue calcification
in post-menopausal women it may contribute to osteoporosis, i.e. loss of bone mass	this may interfere with organ function and, in the kidney, results in the formation of renal stones

Fig. 8.45 Effects of calcium deficiency and excess.

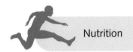
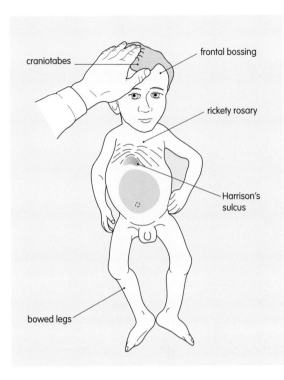

Fig. 8.46 Characteristic deformities of rickets.

Clinical features of rickets	
Clinical features	**Diagnosis**
bowed legs, short stature and failure to thrive	↓ serum calcium and phosphorus
craniotabes: skull bones easily indented by finger pressure	↑ alkaline phosphatase: secreted by osteoblasts to compensate and ↑ bone formation
rickety rosary: expansion or swelling at costochondral junctions	
Harrison sulcus: indrawing of softened ribs along attachment of diaphragm → "hollowing"	X-rays show defective mineralization of pelvis, long bones and ribs
expansion of metaphyses especially at wrist	N.B. low calcium results in ↓ neuromuscular transmission; therefore infant may present with seizures
delayed dentition	

Fig. 8.47 The clinical features and diagnosis of rickets.

Clinical features of osteomalacia	
Clinical features	**Diagnosis**
spontaneous, incomplete (sub-clinical) fractures, often in long bones or pelvis	low serum calcium
bone pain	bone biopsy shows increase in non-mineralized bone matrix
weakness of proximal muscles causing a proximal myopathy with a characteristic waddling gait	X-rays show defective mineralization of long bones and pelvis

Fig. 8.48 Clinical features of osteomalacia.

supplements and education about a balanced diet. Vitamin D supplements may also be required.

- **Osteomalacia.** This disease of adults is seen particularly in elderly people and is usually secondary to vitamin D deficiency. The characteristics of osteomalacia are listed in Fig. 8.48.
- **Osteoporosis.** This is the progressive reduction of total bone mass, usually due to the effects of estrogen deficiency after menopause. It is prevented by the use of hormone replacement therapy, but calcium is also thought to have a role in its prevention. It is thought that adequate calcium nutrition, when young, helps to achieve a peak bone mass. This decreases the effects of loss and osteoporosis in later life. Calcium supplements, both before and after menopause, usually with vitamin D, are recommended.

Calcium overload: hypercalcemia

Causes The major causes of hypercalcemia are primary hyperparathyroidism and malignant disease. They have nothing to do with nutrition and are therefore beyond the scope of this book. Very rarely, hypercalcemia is associated with the excessive ingestion of milk and antacids for the control of indigestion. This decreases the renal excretion of calcium: milk–alkali syndrome.

Clinical features Calcium ions are normally found in cells, but calcium salts are restricted to bones and teeth. In overload, calcium salts are deposited in normal tissues, leading to tissue "metastatic calcification" and impaired function. This may cause renal stones, arrhythmias, heart failure, and calcification of the arteries. Muscle weakness,

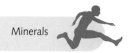

tiredness, anorexia, constipation, and a sluggish nervous response may also be seen.

Phosphorus
RDA
1200 mg/day.

Sources
Most foods; a dietary deficiency has not been described.

Functions
Phosphorus works in conjunction with vitamin D and calcium:
- It has a structural role in bones and teeth.
- Required for the production of ATP and other phosphorylated metabolic intermediates. It is therefore fundamental to the maintenance of the function of all the cells of the body.

Deficiency and toxicity
The clinical manifestations of a deficiency and excess of phosphorus are listed in Fig. 8.49.

Magnesium
RDA
350 mg/day.

Sources
Most foods, especially green vegetables.

Functions
The functions of magnesium are:
- Structural role in bones and teeth.
- Cofactor for more than 300 enzymes in the body, that is, those enzymes that catalyze ATP-

dependent reactions. Magnesium binds to ATP, forming a magnesium–ATP complex which is the substrate for enzymes such as kinases.
- Interacts with calcium to affect the permeability of excitable membranes and neuromuscular transmission.

Deficiency
Seen in alcoholics; patients with liver cirrhosis; following diuretic therapy; and in renal disease. The symptoms are:
- Muscle weakness.
- Secondary calcium deficiency.
- Confusion, hallucinations, convulsions and other neurologic symptoms.

Excess
Extremely rare.

Sodium, potassium, and chloride
Sodium, potassium, and chloride function together to regulate the osmolality of intracellular and extracellular fluids. Importantly, both high and low potassium concentration in plasma can cause severe cardiac problems. For further information refer to a physiology text. The characteristics of sodium and potassium are listed in Fig. 8.50.

Sulphur
The dietary intake of the sulphur-containing amino acid methionine is essential for synthesis of cysteine (see Fig. 5.5); both can then be incorporated into proteins and enzymes.

Iron
RDA
The daily loss of iron from the body is 0.5–1.0 mg/day and is due to:
- Gastrointestinal tract turnover, about 0.5 mg/day.
- Desquamation of intestinal mucosal cells and biliary excretion, about 0.3 mg/day.
- Sweat and desquamation of skin cells, about 0.1 mg/day.
- Urinary losses, about 0.1 mg/day.

Small daily losses are accounted for by the absorption of dietary iron in the duodenum. The demand for iron increases during growth, pregnancy, and menstruation (1 ml of blood loss is equal to 0.5 mg of iron). The recommended daily allowances are:

Deficiency and excess of phosphorus	
Deficiency	Excess
if severe (<0.3 mmol/L), will affect the function of all cells causing: • muscle weakness • in RBC leads to a decrease in formation of 2,3-bisphosphoglycerate and therefore reduces unloading of oxygen to tissues • rickets and osteomalacia	may combine with calcium to produce calcium phosphate and be deposited in tissues (see Fig. 8.45)

Fig. 8.49 The effects of phosphorus deficiency and excess.

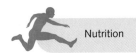

Characteristics of sodium and potassium		
	Sodium	**Potassium**
AI	2.3 g/day	4.7 g/day
sources	salt, most foods	most foods
function	principal cation of ECF: plasma concentration maintained between 135 and 145 mmol/L; necessary for: • control of ECF volume • Na$^+$/K$^+$-ATPase and uptake of solutes by cell • Na$^+$ gradient provides driving force for secondary active transport • neuromuscular transmission	principal cation of ICF: plasma concentration 3.5–5.0 mmol/L fundamental to: • Na$^+$/K$^+$-ATPase and uptake of molecules by cell • neuromuscular transmission • acid–base balance • cardiac muscle contraction
deficiency	• disturbances common in hospitalized patients; causes of loss include: vomiting, diarrhea, use of diuretics, Addison's disease, hyperglycemia (causing an osmotic diuresis) or renal failure • sodium loss is usually accompanied by water loss, leading to decrease in plasma volume and signs of circulatory failure and collapse	• loss may be secondary to vomiting and the use of diuretics, diarrhea, excess steroids, hyperaldosteronism (e.g. Conn's syndrome), Cushing's syndrome or alkalosis • high chance of cardiac arrhythmias and neuromuscular weakness • remember: intravenous insulin treatment without supplementation of potassium leads to hypokalemia
excess	role in hypertension	• the most common cause of potassium retention and hyperkalemia is renal failure • both severe hypokalemia and hyperkalemia are dangerous and require immediate treatment

Fig. 8.50 The characteristics of sodium and potassium.

- Adult male: 12.0 mg
- Child: 10.0 mg
- Menstruating woman: 15.0 mg
- Pregnant woman: 30.0 mg

Only about 10% of dietary iron is absorbed; therefore, the amount ingested daily is equal to the daily requirement ×10.

Sources

Liver, meat, green vegetables, and cereals. Dietary iron exists in two forms:
- Heme iron, which is derived from hemoglobin or myoglobin in meat and is rapidly absorbed.
- Nonheme iron, which is present in vegetables and cereals and is absorbed slowly.

Absorption, transport, and storage

A summary of the absorption, transport, and functions of iron is given in Fig. 8.51. Total body iron is about 3–5 g. About 60% is in hemoglobin and most of the rest is stored, mainly as ferritin, with a small amount as hemosiderin. Ferritin is a protein–iron complex. The protein part, apoferritin, has 22 subunits which form a hollow protein shell. It is capable of binding about 4300 Fe^{3+} ions.

Dietary iron is more readily absorbed in the Fe^{2+} state, and ascorbic acid, alcohol, and other reducing substances favor its absorption. Iron is transported in the blood bound to transferrin; each molecule of transferrin binds two Fe^{2+}ions. This transports iron from sites of absorption and hemoglobin breakdown to storage sites: mainly the reticuloendothelial cells (bone marrow, spleen), hepatocytes (liver), and muscle cells. These cells have transferrin receptors enabling iron to be taken up by receptor-mediated endocytosis. Iron is also transported to these sites for production of hemoglobin (bone marrow), myoglobin (muscle) or production of enzymes (liver). Fig. 8.52 summarizes the functions of body iron.

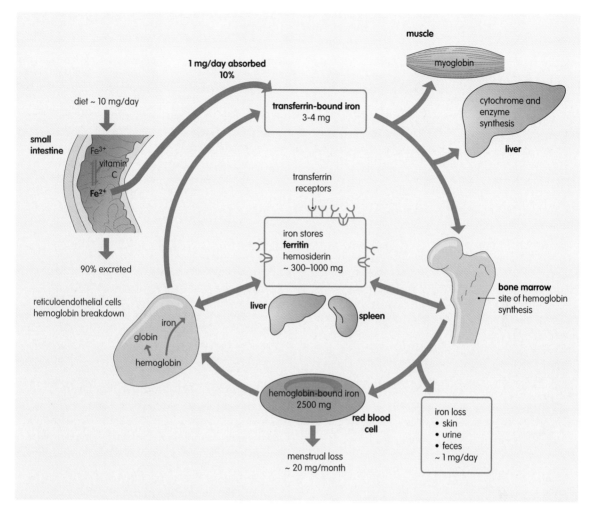

Fig. 8.51 A summary of the absorption, transport, and functions of iron. Dietary iron is more readily absorbed in the Fe^{2+} state. Only about 10% is absorbed. Iron is transported in the blood bound to transferrin, which takes iron either "newly absorbed" from the diet or released from hemoglobin breakdown to muscle, liver, bone marrow, or spleen, either for production of hemoglobin, myoglobin or other enzymes, or for storage. About 60% of total body iron is in hemoglobin.

Iron deficiency anemia
Bioavailability
Heme iron, present in meat, is readily absorbed. Inorganic (nonheme) iron, present in vegetables and cereals, is mostly in the oxidized (Fe^{3+}) state and must be reduced for absorption.

Factors affecting bioavailability:
- Absorption is favoured in the ferrous (Fe^{2+}) as opposed to the ferric (Fe^{3+}) form.
- Stomach hydrochloric acid and ascorbic acid both favor absorption by reducing iron to the ferrous form.
- Increased erythropoietic activity—due, for example, to bleeding, hemolysis, or high altitude—increases absorption.
- Alcohol increases absorption.
- Phosphates and phytates (from plants) form insoluble complexes with iron and prevent absorption.

Causes of deficiency
Inadequate intake   This is probably the most common cause of iron deficiency, particularly in a vegan diet.

Increased requirement   This occurs in premature babies, because iron is transferred to the fetus during the last trimester of pregnancy; also during infancy, adolescence, and pregnancy, that is, during periods of increased growth.

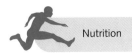
Distribution and function of total body iron			
Site	Function	Amount of iron (mg)	Percentage total body iron
total body iron		3500–5000	100
hemoglobin	oxygen transport	2500	60–70
ferritin (2/3) and hemosiderin (1/3)	iron storage: mainly liver, spleen and bone marrow	1000	27
myoglobin	oxygen transporter in muscle	130	3.5
uncharacterized iron-binding molecules	storage	80	2.2
cytochromes and other iron-containing enzymes	electron transport chain cytochrome P450 (drug metabolism) catalase (H_2O_2 breakdown) peroxidase	8	0.2
transferrin	transports iron from intestines to tissues	3	0.08

Fig. 8.52 The distribution and function of total body iron.

Bioavailability is the efficiency (%) with which any dietary nutrient is used in the body. A number of factors can influence the absorption and use of nutrients. For example:
1. The chemical form of the nutrient.
2. Antagonistic or facilitatory ligands.
3. The breakdown of the nutrient.
4. The pH and redox state.
5. Anabolic requirements, endocrine influences, infection, and so on.

Blood loss   1 mL of blood contains 0.5 mg of iron. Therefore, a small blood loss of 3–4 mL/day over a period of weeks to months can cause a chronic iron deficiency. Losses can be from:
- The gut; for example, due to peptic ulcers, hiatal hernias, cancer of the stomach or cecum, ulcerative colitis, and so on.
- Menstrual loss, if periods are particularly heavy.

Always look for causes of chronic blood loss in a person with iron deficiency anemia.

Malabsorption   Malabsorption may be due to high levels of phytates in the diet, vitamin C deficiency, or surgery (partial or total gastrectomy). Often, there is more than one cause; for example, a poor quality diet and heavy periods in an adolescent girl.

Groups in the population at risk of deficiency
Infants, toddlers, adolescents, pregnant women, menstruating women, and elderly people are all at risk of iron deficiency.

Clinical features and diagnosis of iron deficiency anemia
The clinical features and diagnosis of iron deficiency anemia are covered in Fig. 8.53.

Management and treatment
Finding the cause is essential. The treatment for iron deficiency anemia is oral iron supplements (e.g., ferrous sulphate or gluconate). If malabsorption is suspected, use intramuscular or intravenous iron. Iron supplements should be given long enough to correct the hemoglobin level; when this is normal, iron must then be continued for 3–6 months to replenish stores.

Prognosis
Pathologic changes are reversed by adequate replacement therapy.

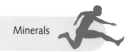

Clinical features and diagnosis of iron deficiency anemia	
Signs and symptoms	**Diagnosis**
↓ **production of hemoglobin:** less oxygen reaches the tissue, especially the brain and heart muscle, causing **pallor, tiredness, shortness of breath, giddiness, palpitations** symptoms usually occur when hemoglobin <8 g/dL	**blood tests:** • ↓ hemoglobin, serum ferritin and iron • FBC, blood film • ↑ total iron-binding capacity (TIBC) (due to increase in "free" transferrin) **gold standard** for diagnosis of iron deficiency is the absence of iron stores in the bone marrow
epithelial abnormalities: angular stomatitis (cracked corners of mouth) glossitis (sore tongue) koilonychia (spoon-shaped nails)	**blood film:** microcytic, hypochromic red blood cells (RBC), i.e. small, pale RBCs where: • MCV (mean cellular volume) <80 fL • MCH (mean cell Hb) <27 pg **N.B.** normal hemoglobin concentration is 13–18 g/dL in men, 11.5–16 g/dL in women

Fig. 8.53 Clinical features and diagnosis of iron deficiency anemia.

Iron overload

Iron overload leads to iron deposition in the tissues, which may interfere with their function (see Fig. 8.54).

Causes

There are two principal causes of iron overload. There is an inherited form, called idiopathic primary hemochromatosis, which has a prevalence in the population of 0.5% for homozygotes. Iron overload may also be acquired secondary to an increased administration of iron. This is called transfusional iron overload.

Idiopathic primary hemochromatosis

Pathogenesis. Idiopathic primary hemochromatosis is an autosomal recessive disorder characterized by the excessive absorption of iron in the small intestine. The gene defect is located on chromosome 6. Only homozygotes manifest clinical features; the accumulation of iron is gradual. It usually presents in

Sites of iron deposition	
Tissue	**Effect**
liver	liver fibrosis and pigmentation resulting in cirrhosis and eventually liver failure; may progress to hepatocellular carcinoma (30%)
pancreas	"bronze diabetes": iron damages islet cells causing diabetes mellitus
heart	heart failure
skin	gray/bronze skin color because of increased production of melanin
testes	impotence
joints	arthropathy

Fig. 8.54 Sites of iron deposition in iron overload.

the fifth decade when levels of iron are about 40–60 g compared with 3–5 g in a normal person. The disease is clinically manifested more commonly in men because women can compensate a certain amount for excessive absorption by menstrual bleeding. The course of the disease depends on the amount of dietary iron and the presence of other dietary factors, such as vitamin C or alcohol.

Clinical consequences. Iron is deposited as insoluble hemosiderin, forming yellow granules in tissues (see Fig. 8.54), which eventually interfere with tissue function. Ultimately, increased iron leads to the increased formation of free radicals, especially the hydroxyl radical. At normal iron levels, a very reactive superoxide radical O_2 is removed effectively by the enzyme superoxide dismutase, as shown in the reaction below:

$$2O_2^{\cdot} + 2H^+ \rightarrow H_2O_2 + O_2$$

However, in iron overload, Fe^{3+} reacts with the superoxide radical to form an extremely reactive hydroxyl radical, $OH^{\cdot}$. This hydroxyl radical is capable of damaging biologic molecules, particularly lipids, leading to lipid peroxidation and membrane damage (especially of lysosomal membranes).

$$2O_2^{\cdot} + Fe^{3+} \rightarrow Fe^{2+} + O_2$$
$$Fe^{2+} + H_2O_2 \rightarrow Fe^{3+} + OH^- + OH^{\cdot}$$

This results in the oxidation and destruction of cell membranes and tissues.

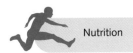

Treatment. The treatment for idiopathic primary hemochromatosis is regular venesection (i.e., removal of blood) to reduce the iron load. Usually about 500 ml are removed, once or twice a week for about 2 years (there are 250 mg of iron in one unit of blood). Plasma iron and ferritin levels are used to monitor the treatment. Once the excess iron is removed, the frequency of venesection is reduced.

Transfusional iron overload: transfusion siderosis

Causes. Repeated blood transfusions over a long period of time can cause iron overload. The ability of the reticuloendothelial cells (spleen, liver, and bone marrow) to store iron is exceeded and iron is deposited at other sites. As with primary iron overload, iron is deposited mainly in the skin, heart, liver, and pancreas. Patients with any condition requiring regular blood transfusions are regarded as at risk (e.g., thalassemia major, aplastic anemia).
Treatment. Chelation therapy with desferrioxamine is highly effective in chelating the iron, thus enabling its excretion.

Zinc

The daily zinc requirement is 2–3 mg/day, but absorption is only approximately 30% effective. Therefore, the RDA is 12–15 mg/day. Zinc can be found in most foods. The total body zinc is 2–3 g. It is found in all tissues but high concentrations are present in the liver, kidney, bone, retina, muscle, and prostate. The role of zinc in the body is described in Fig. 8.55.

Zinc deficiency
Acrodermatitis enteropathica

Acrodermatitis enteropathica is an extremely rare autosomal recessive disorder that leads to the malabsorption of zinc in the small intestine. It presents in infancy with a severe symmetrical eczematous rash around orifices and on the hands and feet. Frequently, the lesions become severely infected with *Candida* or bacterial infections, leading to death. Infants may also develop growth retardation, hypogonadism, and poor wound healing.

Treatment

The condition is completely cured by zinc therapy. Zinc deficiency is also a very rare complication of parenteral nutrition when insufficient supplementation is given.

Role of zinc in the body	
Functions	**Deficiency**
co-factor of over 100 enzymes, e.g.: • dehydrogenases, e.g. LDH • peptidases • carbonic anhydrase • enzymes of DNA and protein synthesis • superoxide dismutase transcription factors are thought to contain "zinc fingers" that enable them to bind DNA	causes: growth retardation, hypogonadism, and delayed wound healing these effects are mainly a result of decreased activity of the enzymes of DNA synthesis

Fig. 8.55 The role of zinc in the body.

Copper
RDA
0.9 mg/day.

Sources
Liver is a very good source.

Copper metabolism
The total body copper is about 75–150 mg. High copper concentrations are found in the liver, brain, heart and kidneys. Dietary copper is absorbed in the stomach and duodenum and transported to the liver loosely bound to albumin; the absorption is about 30% effective. It is incorporated into ceruloplasmin, a glycoprotein synthesized by the liver, which transports copper to the tissues where it can be used for the synthesis of other copper-containing enzymes. Normally, it is excreted in the bile (daily loss is approximately 2–3 mg/day). In the blood, 80–90% of the copper present is bound to ceruloplasmin.

Function
Copper is required for the synthesis of a number of copper-containing enzymes (Fig. 8.56).

Copper deficiency: Menkes' kinky hair syndrome
Menkes' kinky hair syndrome is a rare X-linked disease with an incidence of 1 in 50,000–100,000. It is caused by the defective absorption of copper from the intestine, leading to a decreased synthesis of copper-containing enzymes (Fig. 8.57).

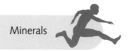

Role of copper and effects of deficiency		
Enzyme	Functional role	Effect of deficiency
ceruloplasmin	promotes absorption of iron	iron deficiency anemia
lysyl oxidase	cross-links collagen and elastin	weak-walled blood vessels
tyrosinase	melanin production	failure of pigmentation
dopamine β-hydroxylase	catecholamine production	neurological effects
cytochrome c oxidase	electron transport chain	decreased ATP formation
superoxide dismutase	scavenges the superoxide radical and prevents lipid peroxidation and membrane damage	tissue damage

Fig. 8.56 The role of copper and the effects of copper deficiency.

Clinical features of copper deficiency	
Clinical features	Explanation
depigmentation of hair "steely hair"	↓ tyrosinase and melanin production
arterial degeneration	↓ lysyl oxidase resulting in defective collagen and elastin
neuronal degeneration and mental retardation	↓ catecholamine neurotransmitters
growth failure and anemia	↓ ceruloplasmin

Fig. 8.57 Clinical features of copper deficiency.

Clinical features of copper overload	
Clinical effects of copper accumulation	Diagnosis
liver: chronic hepatitis → cirrhosis **brain:** severe, progressive neurological disability including tremor, mental deterioration and loss of co-ordination	low serum concentration of ceruloplasmin ↑ urinary copper
eyes: characteristic yellow–brown Kayser–Fleischer rings around corneal limbus	excess copper in liver biopsy

Fig. 8.58 Clinical features of copper overload.

Treatment

Copper therapy has no significant effect. The life expectancy is less than 2 years.

Copper overload: Wilson's disease
Etiology

Wilson's disease is a rare autosomal recessive disorder (incidence of 1 in 100,000). The defect has been identified on chromosome 13 and results in failure of the liver to excrete copper in the bile. Copper incorporation into ceruloplasmin is also impaired. Copper accumulates and is deposited in the liver, basal ganglia of the brain, kidneys and the eyes, causing damage (Fig. 8.58).

Treatment

Wilson's disease is treated by daily chelation therapy with d-penicillamine. This is very effective at binding copper and eliminating it in the urine. However, the resulting liver and neurologic damage is permanent.

Iodine

The human body contains only about 15–20 mg of iodine, most of which is in the thyroid gland. It is essential for the synthesis of the thyroid hormones thyroxine and triiodothyronine.

Deficiency
Endemic goiter

Endemic goiter, a generalized enlargement of the thyroid gland, occurs in areas where the soil and water lack iodine such that the daily intake is less

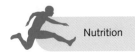
than 70 mg (usually mountainous areas). The problem has now been eliminated in most countries by the addition of iodine to table salt, and its prevalence is mostly restricted to developing countries.

Pathogenesis of goiter   Normally, iodine is used to make thyroxine and triiodothyronine. Increased levels of these hormones exert a negative feedback effect on the hypothalamus and anterior pituitary, inhibiting the further release of thyroid-releasing hormone and thyroid-stimulating hormone (Fig. 8.59), resulting in a decrease in their synthesis. However, low levels of iodine decrease thyroxine formation by the thyroid gland. This releases the negative feedback on the hypothalamic-pituitary axis, causing an uncontrolled increase in thyroid-stimulating hormone secretion. High levels of TSH overstimulate the thyroid gland, causing hyperplasia of the thyroid epithelium and generalized enlargement (Fig. 8.60). The addition of iodine to the diet should reverse this effect.

Cretinism

Pregnant mothers who are deficient in iodine may give birth to babies who are hypothyroid. Growth and mental development in these babies are severely impaired, sometimes irreversibly so. The diagnosis is made by a neonatal screening test, called the Guthrie test, which is performed on all newborn babies and looks for raised thyroid-stimulating hormone levels. The same test is used to screen for phenylketonuria. Treatment is lifelong oral replacement of thyroxine. Cretinism can be prevented by the iodination of salt in the maternal diet.

Fig. 8.59 The hypothalamic–pituitary–thyroid feedback system: normal status. In the presence of dietary iodine, thyroid hormones are produced which exert a negative feedback effect on hypothalamus and pituitary, inhibiting release of TRH and TSH.

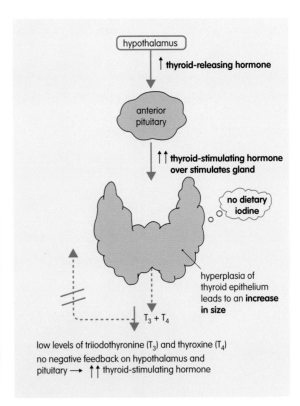

Fig. 8.60 The hypothalamic–pituitary–thyroid feedback system: dietary iodine limiting. Decreased production of thyroid hormones releases negative feedback on hypothalamus and anterior pituitary.

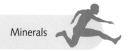

Iodine overload

Excessive dietary iodine may cause the symptoms of hyperthyroidism, that is, an overactive thyroid.

Other trace elements

The characteristics of some of the other trace elements not covered here are listed in Fig. 8.61.

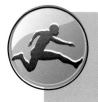

Know about iron deficiency and overload, calcium deficiency, and copper overload, because they are commonly asked about.

				Characteristics of some of the other trace elements					
Element	Iodine	Chromium	Cobalt	Manganese	Molybdenum	Selenium	Silicon	Fluoride
Source	supplemented salt RDA = 150 µg	meat, liver, yeast, whole grains	foods of animal origin			meat, green vegetables RDA = 60 µg	green vegetables	drinking water
Main function	synthesis of thyroid hormones	possibly improves glucose tolerance	constituent of vitamin B_{12} as cobalamin	cofactor for enzymes: decarboxylases, transferases, superoxide dismutase	constituent of xanthine oxidase: involved in purine breakdown	cofactor of glutathione peroxidase	bone calcification, glycosamino-glycan metabolism in connective tissue	increases hardness of teeth
Deficiency	• goiter in adults • cretinism in babies	impaired glucose tolerance (seen in patients on parenteral nutrition)	as for vitamin B_{12} deficiency	unknown	decreased uric acid synthesis	endemic in parts of China → cardiomyopathy (Keshan disease)	decrease in normal growth	low intake leads to increased dental caries
Excess	toxic goiter hyperthyroidism	non-specific: nausea, diarrhoea and irritability		inhalation poisoning leading to psychotic symptoms and parkinsonism (rare)		leads to hair loss, dermatitis, and irritability	silicosis: long-term inhalation of silicon dust leads to pulmonary fibrosis	fluorosis: where fluorine infiltrates enamel causing pitting and discoloration of teeth

Fig. 8.61 The characteristics of some of the other trace elements.

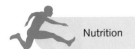
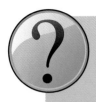

- Define the terms nutrient and staple food and give examples of each.
- Give three methods for assessing dietary intake.
- Give definitions for RDA and AI.
- What are the major energy sources in the diet?
- Discuss the terms total energy, digestible energy, and metabolizable energy.
- Name three methods for measuring body composition.
- Define the BMR, and know how to measure it and the main factors affecting it.
- Define obesity in terms of BMI.
- What are the causes of obesity and the problems of dieting?
- Explain the following terms: reference protein, limiting amino acid, protein quality, net protein utilization and net dietary protein energy ratio.
- Discuss protein requirements.
- Define protein–energy malnutrition, giving two examples.
- Discuss the physiologic effects of malnutrition.
- Name the main causes of marasmus and kwashiorkor and give at least five features of each.
- Describe the management and consequences of protein–energy malnutrition.
- What are the clinical consequences of obesity and its treatment?

For each vitamin discuss:
- Whether it is water- or fat-soluble and the implications for storage.
- The approximate RDA value and two or three examples of good sources.
- Its active form and main functions.
- The result of deficiency. Try to relate this to function.
- The effect of toxicity when relevant.

For each fat-soluble vitamin describe:
- The main causes and clinical features of their deficiency disease.
- A basic idea of the diagnosis and the treatment available.
- The effects and problems of toxicity.

For each deficiency disease describe:
- The incidence, where in the world they still occur, and two or three causes of each.
- The main clinical features, relating them to the functions of the vitamin concerned.
- The main diagnostic criteria and the treatment.

For each of the main minerals and trace elements covered here describe:
- The major sources, functions, transport, and storage forms.
- The effects of deficiency and excess.
- Have a rough idea of the RDA. Examiners usually ask about iron, copper, or calcium—know these!

For each mineral disorder describe:
- The main causes, clinical features, and criteria for diagnosis and treatment.
- Know differences between iron-deficiency anemia and pernicious anemia—this is very important.

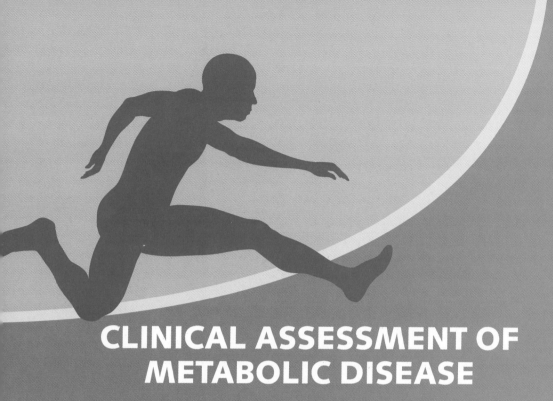

CLINICAL ASSESSMENT OF METABOLIC DISEASE

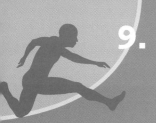

9. Presentation of Metabolic Disease

This section deals with some examples of common presenting complaints and symptoms of metabolic diseases. For each complaint, the major metabolic causes are considered.

Remember, for each symptom there are also lots of nonmetabolic causes, which are probably more common but are beyond the scope of this book. For further discussions of these refer to a clinical medicine textbook.

Fatigue

Fatigue covers a wide range of symptoms reported by patients, including tiredness, lack of energy (one of the most common general symptoms), weakness, exhaustion, sleepiness, or weariness.

Causes of fatigue

Fatigue is a very common complaint, and there are many causes. It is important to obtain a clear history of the complaint in terms of when it started, its progression, precipitating and relieving factors, and any associated symptoms that clearly help to eliminate other causes. The main metabolic causes of fatigue are described in Fig. 9.1.

Weight loss

Weight loss is a sign of a great many diseases. Only the main metabolic causes are considered here.

Working definition

A loss of 5% or more of the usual body weight over a period of 6 months.

It is essential to take a clear, well-documented history from the patient. It is often difficult to verify the true amount of weight lost, unless the patient is continually weighed and monitored over a period of time. Ask about:
- Changes in clothing or belt size.
- Verification from friend or relative.

Involuntary weight loss is often a clue that the patient has a serious underlying disease such as cancer. Fig. 9.2 lists the common metabolic causes of weight loss.

Symptoms of anemia

Anemia is defined as a low hemoglobin concentration in the blood, resulting in a reduction in oxygen supply to the tissues.

The symptoms depend on the severity of the anemia; a small reduction in hemoglobin is usually asymptomatic. Most symptoms are nonspecific and result from a decreased oxygen supply to the tissues:
- Fatigue.
- Headaches.
- Fainting.
- Breathlessness.
- Angina of effort (i.e., brought on by exercise, relieved by rest).
- Palpitations.
- Intermittent claudication.

As these symptoms are relatively nonspecific, to find out the cause of the anemia a number of laboratory tests may be performed, including:
- Complete blood count. This measures the concentration of hemoglobin, the red cell count, and other indices (e.g., mean cell volume, mean cell hemoglobin; see Fig. 11.1).
- Blood film. This provides data on the morphology of cells.
- Reticulocyte count.
- Serum iron and total iron-binding capacity (rarely measured now).
- Serum ferritin.
- B_{12} and folate levels.
- Schilling test. This is specific for pernicious anemia.

These tests and their results are discussed fully in Chapter 11.

Main metabolic causes of fatigue	
Causes	**Examples and notes**
anemia	this may be secondary to: • iron/B_{12}/folate deficiency • hemolytic anemia, e.g. G6PDH or pyruvate kinase deficiency (see Fig. 9.3 for other examples)
hypothyroidism	this may be due to an iodine deficiency or an auto-immune disease, Hashimoto's thyroiditis
malnutrition	• protein–energy malnutrition (PEM): marasmus or kwashiorkor (see Chapter 8) • general vitamin deficiencies
obesity	tiredness, glucose intolerance, risk of hypertension
diabetes mellitus	see types of diabetes (Fig. 9.4)
Ca^{2+} or vitamin D deficiency	osteomalacia (weak, easily deformed bones)
glycogen storage disorders	e.g. McArdle's syndrome (see Chapter 2)

Fig. 9.1 Main metabolic causes of fatigue.

Metabolic causes of anemia	
Cause	**Notes**
iron deficiency	decrease in heme and red blood cell production, leading to microcytic, hypochromic cells (see Chapter 8)
folate/B_{12} deficiency	macrocytic, megaloblastic anemia (see Chapter 8)
pernicious anemia	auto-immune condition in which antibodies are made to intrinsic factor, preventing vitamin B_{12} absorption; results in deficiency of B_{12} and folate (see Chapter 8)
vitamin C deficiency	vitamin C is required for absorption of Fe^{2+} (see Fig. 8.42)
hemolytic anemia	deficiency of RBC enzymes such as pyruvate kinase or G6PDH (see Chapter 2)
lead poisoning	lead inhibits three enzymes of heme synthesis, leading to anemia (see Chapter 6)

Fig. 9.3 Metabolic causes of anemia.

Common metabolic causes of weight loss	
Main cause	**Differential diagnosis**
decreased calorie intake	• malnutrition: common in developing countries, and in the U.S. may be seen in the elderly • cancer • alcoholism • anorexia nervosa • depression
increased loss or energy expenditure	• hyperthyroidism • poorly controlled diabetes • cancer

Fig. 9.2 Common metabolic causes of weight loss.

Causes of anemia

There are many causes of anemia, ranging from acute blood loss to hereditary hemolytic anemias such as sickle cell anemia. The main metabolic causes of anemia are listed in Fig. 9.3.

Symptoms of diabetes mellitus

The presentation of the symptoms of diabetes mellitus may be acute or insidious in onset (types are listed in Fig. 9.4).

Acute

Young people often present with a brief 2–4 week history of the classic symptoms, such as polyuria, polydipsia, and weight loss, accompanied by tiredness. These patients usually have type 1 diabetes.

Subacute

The onset of symptoms is usually over months to years. Patients may still present with the classical symptoms although, quite often, tiredness is the prominent symptom. These patients usually have type 2 diabetes.

Asymptomatic

Glycosuria or raised blood glucose is detected during a routine medical examination.

Types of diabetes mellitus	
Type	**Notes**
Diabetes mellitus:	overall incidence, approximately 2% in Western world
Type 1, insulin-dependent diabetes mellitus	patients are usually younger than 25 years
Type 2, non-insulin-dependent diabetes mellitus	patients are usually older than 25 years and often obese
impaired glucose tolerance	affects about 5% of population; these patients are more likely to develop diabetes when they are older
secondary diabetes	either due to pancreatic damage e.g. chronic pancreatitis, hemochromatosis or Wilson's disease, or due to endocrine disease, e.g. acromegaly, Cushing's disease
Note that a new category of impaired fasting glucose (>6 mmol/L) has been recognized recently	

Fig. 9.4 Types of diabetes mellitus.

Differential diagnosis of amino acid disorders in infants
phenylketonuria
inborn errors of carbohydrate metabolism, e.g. galactosemia, glycogen storage disorders
neurological disorders, e.g. febrile convulsions, infantile spasms
infections (common), e.g. gastroenteritis, urinary tract infection
celiac disease (1 in 2000 in the UK)
acute abdomen

Fig. 9.5 Differential diagnosis of amino acid disorders in infants.

Diabetic ketoacidosis

If the early symptoms are not recognized, patients can present with ketoacidosis (Fig. 7.12):

- Severe hyperglycemia causes an osmotic diuresis. The loss of fluid and electrolytes results in dehydration. If this is severe, the patient may be confused and be in shock. Remember to consider the diagnosis in patients presenting with abdominal pain.
- The increased production of ketone bodies results in metabolic acidosis and characteristic ketotic breath. The acidosis typically causes nausea and vomiting and further loss of fluid and electrolytes. Respiratory compensation results in hyperventilation (Kussmaul breathing). Failure to treat a patient in ketoacidosis may result in coma and death.

Complications

Patients may also present with diabetic complications such as retinopathy, neuropathy or nephropathy (see Fig. 7.13). For example, they may present after visits to the opticians (diabetic retinopathy), or with tingling and numbness in the leg, or with leg or foot ulcers (neuropathy). The diagnosis of diabetes is discussed fully in Chapter 7 but is based on measurement of the fasting plasma glucose. A confirmed fasting plasma glucose of greater than 7.0 mmol/L is diagnostic of diabetes.

Symptoms of amino acid disorders

Amino acid disorders are all rare. Most present in infancy with developmental delay, vomiting, failure to thrive, mental retardation and seizures. The symptoms are all non-specific, making the differential diagnosis complex. All neonates are now screened for phenylketonuria at a few days of age using the Guthrie test. The other amino acid disorders must be considered and eliminated when infants present with these symptoms without other adequate explanation; for example, in the absence of infection (Fig. 9.5). Their diagnosis depends on the measurement of metabolites in the blood and urine.

Symptoms of porphyrias

There are two main types of symptoms (Fig. 9.6).

- Neuropsychiatric symptoms with abdominal pain. These present acutely and there is usually some obvious precipitating factor, for example drugs, infection, stress. Acute attacks are separated by long periods of remission.
- Photosensitivity. This is a nonacute presentation in which the skin burns or itches on exposure to

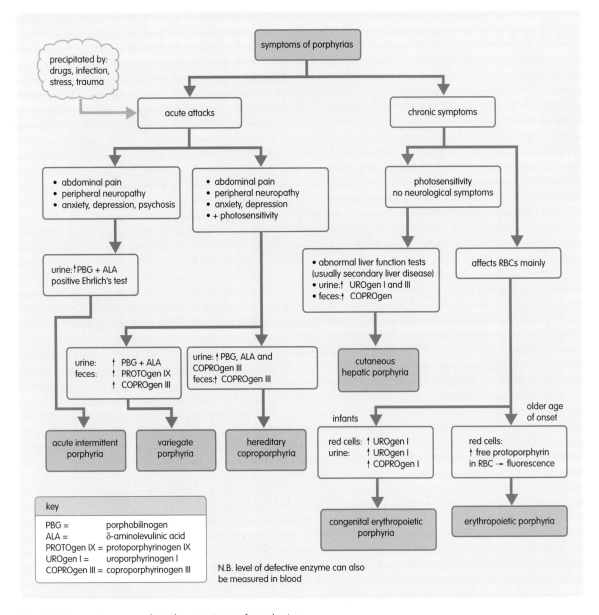

Fig. 9.6 Diagnostic approach to the symptoms of porphyrias.

light. Usually no neurological symptoms are observed.

The diagnosis is based on:
- Clinical features.
- The presence of increased levels of porphyrins and their precursors in the blood, urine and feces.
- All six porphyrias are very rare (roughly 1 in 100,000).

Symptoms of gout

Gout initially presents as recurrent, acute attacks of arthritis, usually affecting only one joint (monoarthropathy). The patient complains of a warm, swollen, and very tender joint, usually a big toe. Eventually, the attacks fail to resolve completely and persistent symptoms occur because of the permanent deposition of urate crystals, leading to chronic tophaceous gout. Persistent symptoms may also be due to the presence of kidney stones, which can cause abdominal pain or renal colic. The most common differential diagnoses for the acute symptoms of gout are trauma and infection (Fig. 9.7).

Symptoms of vitamin deficiencies
Fat-soluble vitamins: A, D, E, and K
The symptoms and signs of each individual vitamin deficiency are covered fully in Chapter 8 and therefore will be covered only briefly here (Fig. 9.8).

General causes of deficiency are:

- Decreased intake, which may either be due to: generalized malnutrition, mainly seen in developing countries; poor diet, commonly seen in the elderly and the housebound in developed countries; or a vegan diet with specifically no vitamin D.
- Fat malabsorption; for example due to liver and biliary tract disease or obstruction, meaning that no bile salts are available to facilitate absorption.

Vitamin E deficiency is very rare.

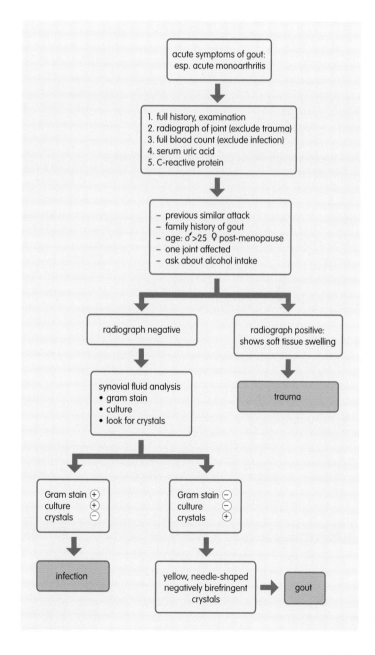

Fig. 9.7 Simplified diagnostic approach to gout.

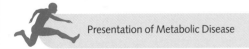
Differential diagnosis of fat-soluble vitamin deficiency diseases	
Vitamin deficiency	**Differential diagnosis**
vitamin A: night blindness and keratomalacia	other causes of degenerative eye changes, e.g. infections such as syphilis, gonorrhea, chlamydia in neonates (rare)
vitamin D: rickets or osteomalacia	• Ca^{2+} deficiency • renal disease—causing ↓ activity of 1-α hydroxylase • liver disease: causing ↓ activity of 25-α hydroxylase
vitamin K: increased bleeding produces clotting problems (in newborn babies, causes hemorrhagic disease of the newborn)	• inherited coagulation disorders, e.g. hemophilia, von Willebrand's disease • anticoagulant therapy: warfarin/dicoumarol • antibiotic therapy which destroys vitamin K-producing bacteria in gut

Fig. 9.8 Differential diagnosis of fat-soluble vitamin deficiency diseases.

Symptoms of mineral deficiencies	
Symptoms	**Cause**
iron deficiency: anemia (symptoms of anemia have been covered earlier)	may be due to: ↓ dietary intake ↓ absorption caused by: ↑ phosphates and phytates in diet or vitamin C deficiency ↑ blood loss: either acute or chronic ↑ requirement: periods of growth
calcium: (and phosphate) **deficiency:** • in children: rickets; present with soft, easily deformed bones, short stature and failure to thrive • in adults: osteomalacia "brittle bones"	• ↓ dietary intake • secondary to vitamin D deficiency: vitamin D is necessary for intestinal absorption of calcium and phosphate (see Chapter 8) • Intestinal malabsorption • renal failure • hypothyroidism
iodine deficiency: goiter can lead to symptoms of hypothyroidism: tiredness, weight gain, anorexia, cold intolerance, constipation	• auto-immune: Hashimoto's thyroiditis • after surgery for hyperthyroidism

Fig. 9.10 Symptoms of mineral deficiencies.

Symptoms of water-soluble vitamin deficiencies	
Vitamin deficiency	**Main symptoms**
vitamin B₁—thiamin wet beriberi	edema tachycardia, shortness of breath and other signs of heart failure (see Fig. 8.25)
dry beriberi	ascending peripheral neuropathy: initially weakness and numbness of legs that ascends to involve trunk, arms and eventually brain
Wernicke-Korsakoff syndrome	confusion, ataxia, ophthalmoplegia and peripheral neuropathy
niacin deficiency: pellagra	3 D's: dermatitis, dementia and diarrhea
vitamin B₆: secondary pellagra	very rare
vitamin B₁₂: megaloblastic, macrocytic anemia	see "symptoms of anemia" earlier
folate: megaloblastic, macrocytic anemia	see "symptoms of anemia" earlier
vitamin C: scurvy	failure of wound healing hypochromic, microcytic anemia swollen, sore, spongy gums with bleeding

Fig. 9.9 Symptoms of water-soluble vitamin deficiencies.

Water-soluble vitamins (B and C)

The symptoms of a deficiency of vitamins B and C are listed in Fig. 9.9.

Symptoms of mineral deficiencies

The symptoms and signs of each individual mineral deficiency are covered in detail in Chapter 8. The symptoms of the more important mineral deficiency disorders are listed in Fig. 9.10. The differential diagnosis is biased towards metabolic causes.

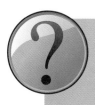

- What clinical symptoms would cause you to suspect anemia?
- A 55-year-old obese man developed diabetes 2 years ago. It is now controlled with insulin injections. What type of diabetes does he have?
- Describe five clinical signs associated with thyroid underactivity.
- What are the causes of osteomalacia?
- How would you investigate an acutely swollen joint in the foot?

10. History and Examination

Things to remember when taking a history

The purpose of this section is to remind you of the main points involved in taking a history from a patient.

The history is usually the most important part of the consultation.

Before you start:
- Always introduce yourself and shake hands. Make sure that the patient is comfortable and that, if possible, there are no large obstacles (e.g., a desk) between the two of you.
- Stand back and look around the bedside for clues. Is the patient being monitored (e.g., for blood pressure, oxygen saturation, blood glucose)? Look for oxygen masks, inhalers, sputum cups, drains, walking sticks or frames. All of these provide indicators to the patient's condition.
- Observe the patient. Is he or she agitated or distressed, either physically or emotionally? Are there any obvious signs (e.g., tremor, squint, pallor, hyperactivity)?

Structure of a history

This is a basic plan designed for you to photocopy and take with you when you first start clerking patients.

Personal information
- Name and sex.
- Age/date of birth.
- Occupation.

Presenting complaint (PC)

This should be a short statement of the symptoms of which the patient is complaining, in his or her own words. For example: pain, thirst, poor appetite, tiredness, weight loss, vomiting, and so on. Remember, look for symptoms, not diagnoses: patients do not complain of coronary heart disease, diabetes, or acute intermittent porphyria!

History of presenting complaint (HPC)

Try to get the patient to tell the story in his or her own words from when he or she thought it began. For most symptoms you will need to know:
- What is the time course? When did the problem start, or when did the patient first feel unwell?
- Was the onset rapid or slow?
- What is the nature of the complaint? If it is pain: site, radiation and so on. If it is vomiting: how much? what color? Is there any blood in the vomitus?
- Is there a pattern? Is the complaint continuous, intermittent, or continuous with acute exacerbations?
- Are there any precipitating or relieving factors? For example, is the complaint related to meals, type of food eaten, or stress? Is it helped by painkillers?
- Are there any other relevant or associated symptoms? For example, for chest pain, ask about palpitations, sweating, and nausea.
- Has it happened before? Ask about any previous treatment or investigations for the complaint.

Make an effort to use simple terms and avoid medical jargon. Ask additional questions to see whether your key points were understood.

For any pain, you need to know the site, radiation, onset, timing, character (e.g., sharp, dull, colicky), precipitating and relieving factors, and associated symptoms.

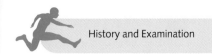

Previous medical history (PMH)

Ask the patient about previous illnesses, operations, and investigations, with dates. You may find the mnemonic **MTHREADS** helpful: **m**yocardial infarction, **t**uberculosis, **h**ypertension, **r**heumatic fever, **e**pilepsy, **a**sthma, **d**iabetes, **s**troke. You should always ask specifically about these conditions as well as anemia and jaundice.

Ask about the patient's nutritional history, if you think it is relevant. A lot of metabolic and nutritional diseases present in infancy. When dealing with children, ask the parents specifically about problems during the pregnancy or birth or when their child was a neonate; for example, problems with feeding, bowels, or a failure to thrive. Inquire about developmental milestones: smiling, sitting, walking, talking, playing.

Drug history (DH)

Is the patient taking any medication at present, either over the counter or prescription? Are there any problems with tolerating drugs? Is the patient taking his or her drugs regularly?

Allergies

Is the patient allergic to any medicines or foods that they know of? Ask specifically about penicillin.

Smoking

How many cigarettes per day and how long ago did the patient start? If the patient says that he or she has quit, you must also ask when—it will often be yesterday! Ask whether the patient really wants to stop.

Alcohol

How many drinks or units each week? If lager or beer, is it a high-strength variety?

Family history (FH)

Ask about any known illnesses in first-degree relatives, particularly diabetes and heart disease. Remember to ask specifically about premature heart disease ("Has there been any talk in the family about a lot of people having heart disease at a young age?"). It may help you to make a quick sketch of the family tree.

A number of inborn errors of metabolism are inherited as autosomal recessive disorders and have a high incidence among races in which marriages between first cousins are quite common (e.g., Ashkenazi Jews).

Social history (SH)

Ask about marital status, number of children, and type of accommodation. Ask about the patient's occupational history: current and previous jobs, exposure to chemicals or asbestos and any time off work due to illness. Ask about financial and personal worries and any risk-related behavior (e.g., illegal drugs or any history of risky homosexual or heterosexual contacts).

Review of systems

Some of these symptoms may have already been covered in the history of the presenting complaint. You need to use your discretion about the extent of this enquiry.

Cardiovascular system, ask specifically about:
- Chest discomfort and pain.
- Palpitations.
- Exercise tolerance ("If you and I were to climb three flights of stairs, how would you feel about it?").
- Shortness of breath (SOB) at rest, when lying down flat (orthopnea), or waking up at night breathless (paroxysmal nocturnal dyspnea, PND).
- Claudication (calf pain on walking).
- Leg pain at rest.

Respiratory system, ask specifically about:
- Persistent cough or wheeze.
- Sputum: amount, color.
- Hemoptysis (coughing up blood).
- Shortness of breath.

Gastrointestinal system, ask specifically about:
- Appetite or weight loss.
- Change in weight.
- Nausea or vomiting.
- Difficulty swallowing (dysphagia).
- Heartburn or indigestion.
- Change in bowel habit: diarrhea, constipation, frequency, consistency, color.

Urinary system, ask specifically about:
- Frequency.
- Nocturia.
- Urine stream: hesitancy, dribbling.
- Dysuria (pain on passing water).
- Hematuria.
- Incontinence.

Skin, ask specifically about:
- Rashes or sensitive skin.
- Dermatitis.
- Eczema/psoriasis.
- Remember that skin is frequently affected by materials encountered at work and in the home.

Musculoskeletal system, ask specifically about:
- Painful joints.
- Stiffness.
- Swelling.
- Arthritis.
- Remember that inflammatory pain is typically worse in the morning and osteoarthritic pain worse in the evening.

Nervous system, ask specifically about:
- Headaches or migraines.
- Fits or faints.
- Changes in vision, hearing, speech or memory.
- Anxiety, depression or suicidal thoughts.
- Sleep.

Menstruation and obstetric history
This should only be taken when relevant.

Summary
This should be a brief recall of the main points. For example: Jonathan Brown, a 4-year-old boy referred by his general practitioner, presenting with a 6-week history of increasing thirst, polyuria, and weight loss. His mother has insulin-dependent diabetes mellitus. On examination...

- When talking to patients, try to maintain appropriate eye contact throughout and look (be) interested.
- Take brief notes and write them up afterward—you will be surprised at how much you can remember!

Communication skills

Many medical schools place great emphasis on communication skills, reflecting its importance in the practice of medicine. Do not be tempted to dismiss this teaching as less important than the more factual elements of the course. Newly qualified doctors often comment that this training was one of the most immediately useful things they learnt in medical school.

Most medical school examinations now feature some form of structured clinical examination (e.g., USMLE 2-CS). You should remember some important points in relation to these:
- None of us are as good at communicating as we like to think we are.
- A lot of this material seems to be stating the obvious—but the obvious can be easy to forget under pressure, and reminding ourselves of the basics is a useful exercise.
- Communication skills account for nearly half the marks in the clinical exams—even in the system examination stations there are marks for your approach to the patient.
- Practicing a few communication scenarios with friends before the exam is an easy way to pick up a lot of extra marks.
- If you get on the right side of the patient or actor in a clinical exam, he or she is likely to divulge information much more easily.

Obstacles to communication
There are many factors that can make it difficult to talk with patients and colleagues. It is important to be aware of these factors and to address the ones that you can do something about, while making allowances for those you cannot. For example:
- Noisy environment and lack of privacy—try to find a quiet room or cubicle in which to see the patient if possible.
- Nervousness—both yours and the patient's. You can help yourself with practice. The patient can be put more at ease by a sensitive approach (more about this later).
- Pain—does the patient need analgesia now rather than after the history?
- Other medical factors—breathlessness, hearing impairment, and confusion (acute or chronic) can all make communication difficult. Patience and persistence are required in these situations.
- Language and cultural barriers—if you encounter problems, try to take the history with a member of the family who can interpret. If this is not possible, it may be possible to obtain the help of an interpreter. In an acute situation, you may have to make do with smiles, drawings, and gestures to

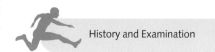

establish the important points, such as the presence and site of pain.

- Hostility—some people may feel (rightly or wrongly) aggrieved by some aspect of the treatment they have already received. It is vital that you do not take this personally or be drawn into a confrontation. Try to remain calm and civil, empathize with the patient, and apologize if appropriate. If all else fails, politely explain that you don't feel anything is being achieved and come back later.

Nonverbal communication skills

A large proportion of our communication "bandwidth" is nonverbal. This includes body posture, facial expression, eye movements, and gestures; we are conscious of some of these things, but most are subconscious. Nonverbal cues are very important in a clinical setting, both in achieving a rapport with patients and in gaining insight into their condition.

The following points may be helpful during a consultation:

- Sit with the patient so that your eyes are on roughly the same level, preferably without a desk as a barrier between you. Maintain a comfortable distance, and try to face the patient while you are talking. It is also useful to make sure you have a comfortable position to write when you are taking a history—kneeling by the bedside is sometimes the best option!
- Maintain good eye contact, even if the patient doesn't.
- Use nonverbal cues to show you are listening, and encourage the patient: nodding, smiling, and even appropriate laughter can help to put the patient at ease. Smiling is particularly important!
- It is worth having practice sessions with friends before you go into an exam, as they can point out any nervous habits that you might be unaware of.

Verbal communication skills

The things we say and how we say them. It is important to put the patient at ease during a consultation, although this is often easier said than done, as people are often understandably concerned in the clinical situation. The following are important skills:

- *Always* begin by checking the patient's identity, explaining who you are, and gaining consent from the patient to take a history.

- Empathize with the patient: this means understanding the patient's point of view and is not the same as sympathy. It is perfectly good practice to use such phrases as "I understand" or "That must have been very frightening" when a patient is relating the details of the history.
- Use open questions at first, such as: "What made you come to see a doctor today?" or "Have you any other problems that have been worrying you?" Always ask the old doctor's question: "How do you feel generally?" You will be surprised how many things you will learn. It is a good idea to let the patient talk freely for the first minute or so, before you focus the history with closed questions such as: "Does the pain catch you when you breathe in?"
- Avoid "leading" questions, which direct the patient as to what to say. For example compare "Does the pain go anywhere?" with "Does the pain shoot down your left arm?"
- Use verbal cues such as "I see" or "I understand" to help the flow of conversation.
- Check that you have understood what the patient has told you by repeating a summary back to him or her.
- Use plain English and avoid medical jargon. Reflect the terminology your patient uses for symptoms and diagnoses as appropriate.

Objectives in the consultation

It is important to have a mental checklist of objectives when you go into a consultation with a patient—especially when this is part of an exam. Once again, the key is practice, preferably on the wards, but you can also run through mock scenarios in a study group if you are short of time. You may also need to produce this kind of list in a short-answer exam paper or viva. For example:

- Introduce yourself and establish a rapport with the patient.
- Find out why the patient has presented to you.
- Find out what the patient understands about the problem, and if the patient has a theory as to what has caused it.
- What are the patient's expectations of this consultation—what does the patient want from you?
- Explore the problem with history and examination, and formulate a plan for further management—investigations, treatment, etc.

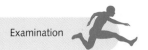

- Explain your findings and plan to the patient as clearly as possible.
- Give the patient time to react to new information.
- Check that the patient understands what you have told him.
- Ask the patient if he or she is unhappy with anything.
- Literature—provide leaflets or write things down for the patient to take away.
- Follow-up—make sure the patient knows what the next point of contact will be (e.g., an outpatient appointment).
- The last four points can be remembered with the mnemonic **CALF** (check–ask–literature–follow-up) and are a good way to use the last few minutes of a USMLE 2-CS station to your advantage.

The following section deals with the main signs caused by an underlying metabolic disease, which may be observed on examination of a patient. It is not a comprehensive guide to clinical assessment. Some of the signs mentioned are relatively nonspecific and may be related to several types of disease, which may indeed be a lot more common than the metabolic cause. Others may be specific to, and in fact diagnostic of, a metabolic disease. Just remember: a lot of metabolic diseases are very rare and you may go through all your working life without seeing them, as many a clinician will tell you. It also provides some guidelines about how to examine certain parts or areas of the body and the best or simplest way to elicit signs.

Examination

General inspection

This section considers the main signs, observed on general inspection, that are indicative of an underlying metabolic cause. These signs are reasonably nonspecific and therefore there may be other possible, nonmetabolic causes that must be considered and eliminated in the differential diagnosis. In any clinical examination it is important that you are seen to generally inspect the patient. Stand at the foot of the bed and observe the patient taking a breath in and out.

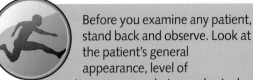

Before you examine any patient, stand back and observe. Look at the patient's general appearance, level of consciousness, any obvious color (pale or jaundiced), and whether he or she looks tired or distressed. These comments earn you extra points.

The **main signs** you need to look for are detailed below.

Wasting, cachexia, and obesity

The term "wasting" is usually used to describe a mild to moderate generalized loss of muscle and thus weight. Cachexia, however, is reserved for severe, generalized muscle wasting, which usually implies a serious underlying cause (e.g., cancer or AIDS). An assessment of wasting and obesity in patients and the underlying metabolic causes is set out in Fig. 10.1.

Pallor or jaundice

Pallor is usually associated with anemia. Jaundice refers to the yellow pigmentation of skin or sclerae of the eyes due to a raised plasma bilirubin level. Jaundice has many causes, which are often classified into three main ones: prehepatic jaundice, in which there is excess bilirubin (e.g., due to increased hemolysis); hepatic jaundice, in which there is diminished liver cell function (e.g., due to a viral infection); and posthepatic or obstructive jaundice. Both pallor and jaundice are common signs, which have a number of possible causes (Fig. 10.2). However, the best way to observe them is by observation of the eyes (see Fig. 10.9).

Respiratory distress

This is often best assessed by inspection (Fig. 10.3).

Tremors

The four common tremors are (Fig. 10.4):
- Essential or physiologic tremor.
- Flapping tremor (CO_2 retention/chronic liver disease).
- Resting, "pill-rolling" tremor of parkinsonism.
- Intention tremor of cerebellar disease.

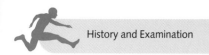

Assessment of wasting and obesity in patients, with their underlying metabolic causes		
Physical examination	**Symptoms and signs**	**Possible diagnosis**
wasting: look for generalized muscle wasting	• when severe, patient has a thin emaciated appearance, almost skeletal, and it is referred to as cachexia • skin is wrinkled and there may be hair loss (see Fig. 8.7)	• implies serious disease, principally cancer • in developing countries: probably due to malnutrition caused by marasmus • in children also consider malabsorption, e.g. celiac disease
obesity: observe; can also: • measure weight and height and calculate body mass index (BMI) • compare with tables of ideal weight for height (mid-arm circumference and skin-fold thickness are rarely useful in practice)	• when severe it is obvious on inspection • BMI > 30 kg/m² is regarded as obese (see Chapter 8)	usually energy input is greater than energy output obesity is also seen in: • Cushing's syndrome • hypothyroidism • drug-induced, e.g. corticosteroids • consider the possibility of Type 2 diabetes mellitus

Fig. 10.1 An assessment of wasting and obesity in patients, with their underlying metabolic causes.

Assessment of pallor and jaundice in patients, and their underlying metabolic causes		
Physical examination	**Symptoms and signs**	**Possible diagnosis**
pallor: observe skin color N.B. best way to assess pallor is to observe conjunctivae of eyes (see Fig. 10.9)	• normal skin color varies according to skin thickness, circulation and pigmentation • paleness may be normal for patient or indicative of anemia N.B. poor indicator of anemia	• iron deficiency anemia • B₁₂/folate deficiency often secondary to pernicious anemia causes pale-lemon skin as result of anemia and increased hemolysis
jaundice: observe skin color N.B. best way to assess jaundice is to observe sclerae of eyes (see Fig. 10.9)	• yellow color of skin is fairly insensitive indicator of mild to moderate jaundice • with severe jaundice, skin is yellow-green	three basic causes of jaundice: • pre-hepatic: hemolytic anemia, e.g. G6PDH deficiency • hepatocellular: problem with liver itself, e.g. viral hepatitis, paracetamol overdose • obstructive: obstruction of bile duct because of gallstones or carcinoma gallstones or carcinoma of head of pancreas

Fig. 10.2 Assessment of pallor and jaundice in patients, with their underlying metabolic causes.

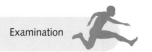
Fig. 10.3 Assessment of respiratory distress and its metabolic significance to diabetes.

Assessment of respiratory distress and its metabolic significance to diabetes		
Physical examination	**Symptoms and signs**	**Possible diagnosis**
respiratory rate, rhythm, and depth of breathing are observed	• hyperventilation • "Kussmaul respiration": deep, sighing breathing with rapid respiratory rate • smell of ketones on breath heightens suspicion	• accumulation of ketone bodies → metabolic acidosis • respiratory compensation → hyperventilation • untreated → severe diabetic ketoacidosis (see Chapter 7) • also seen in uremia

Fig. 10.4 Assessment of tremors in patients and their significance to metabolic disease.

Assessment of tremors in patients and their significance to metabolic disease		
Physical examination	**Symptoms and signs**	**Possible diagnosis**
patient holds arms outstretched in front of them with hands flat place a piece of paper on them	look for fluttering of paper → tremor present	**essential tremor:** normal tremor associated with anxiety, ↑ caffeine and ↑ exercise also seen in: hypoglycemia alcoholics, hyperthyroid (thyrotoxic) patients, and Wilson's disease
ask patient to hold arms outstretched with wrists hyperextended	observe flapping motion of hands	**flapping tremor:** CO_2 retention caused by hyperventilation may be seen in people with diabetes
finger-nose test	tremor arises on movement associated with cerebellar lesions	**intention tremor:** seen in chronic alcoholics with Wernicke-Korsakoff syndrome

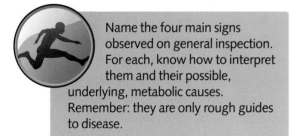

Name the four main signs observed on general inspection. For each, know how to interpret them and their possible, underlying, metabolic causes. Remember: they are only rough guides to disease.

Limbs
Hands
There are a number of signs on the hands and nails indicative of underlying metabolic disease. They are often subtle (Fig. 10.5). Clubbing, shown in Fig. 10.6, may be indicative of liver cirrhosis due to a number of causes, some of which are listed in Fig. 10.5. However, it is most commonly caused by suppurative lung disease or infective endocarditis; therefore, these must always be uppermost in your differential diagnosis. It may also be congenital. Remember tendon xanthomas in familial hypercholesterolemia (see below).

Arms and legs
Examination of the limbs for underlying metabolic disease can be conveniently divided into assessment of vascular supply (Fig. 10.7) and skin and joint problems associated with metabolic disease (Fig.

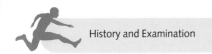
Main metabolic signs observed on examination of the hands		
Physical examination	**Symptoms and signs**	**Possible diagnosis**
nails:	**clubbing:** • loss of the angle between the nail and nail-bed • underlying nail feels soft, fluctuant and "boggy" • increased curvature in all directions	liver cirrhosis caused by: • hemochromatosis ($\uparrow$ iron) • Wilson's disease ($\uparrow$ copper) • glycogen storage disorders (very rare) • alcohol
	koilonychia spoon-shaped brittle nails, may be ridges	iron-deficiency anemia
palms:	**palmar erythema** reddening of palms indicative of a hyperdynamic circulation	liver cirrhosis caused by: • increase in either alcohol, iron or copper • thyrotoxicosis

Fig. 10.5 Main metabolic signs observed on examination of the hands.

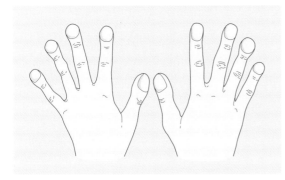

Fig. 10.6 Clubbing of the nails observed in liver cirrhosis, suppurative lung disease, or infective endocarditis.

10.8). It is important to remember to check peripheral pulses.

Main metabolic problems to consider in examination of the limbs
Diabetic patients
Look specifically for ischemic and neuropathic damage leading to ulceration and deformity of limbs (see Chapter 9).

Patients with peripheral vascular disease secondary to hyperlipidemias
Look for arterial ulceration and, in extreme disease, gangrene.

Skin manifestations of hyperlipidemias
Tendon xanthoma, which are observed usually on the Achilles tendon or extensor tendons on the back of the hand, are often diagnostic of hyperlipidemias.

Gout
Gout can affect any joint in the body. In an acute attack, look for a red, inflamed, painful joint. In chronic gout, look for gouty tophi: deposits of urate crystals around joints, tendons and the cartilage of ear lobes, causing yellow discoloration of the overlying skin.

Examination of the limbs should include:
• Assessment of the vascular supply. The quickest way to do this is to feel the pulses (see Fig. 10.7). You should also observe color, assess capillary filling time, feel temperature, and look for edema.
• Skin. Look for any obvious lesions (see Fig. 10.8).
• Neurologic assessment. Both motor and sensory systems are particularly important in patients with diabetes.

Main metabolic signs observed on examination of the limbs		
Physical examination	**Symptoms and signs**	**Possible diagnosis**
arm pulses: • radial: assess rate, rhythm and volume • brachial	↑ rate: tachycardia	• anemia, acute blood loss/shock • thyrotoxicosis • hypoglycemia
	↓ rate: bradycardia	• hypothermia • hypothyroid
	irregular rhythm	atrial fibrillation: hyperthyroidism
legs pulses: • femoral • popliteal • posterior tibial • dorsalis pedis	↓ or absent peripheral pulses (may also hear bruit over the femoral artery, indicating turbulent blood flow caused by stenosis of arteries)	peripheral vascular disease seen in diabetes or patients with dyslipidemias
blood pressure (b.p.)	high	may occur secondary to endocrine or renal disease or to obesity in 95% of cases, cause of high b.p. is unknown, "essential" hypertension
	low	• severe anemia, acute blood loss/shock • diabetic ketoacidosis • hypothyroidism

Fig. 10.7 Main metabolic signs observed on examination of the limbs. Peripheral pulses provide a quick assessment of vascular supply.

Head and neck

Face

A number of metabolic and nutritional diseases result in clinical signs evident on the face. For ease, the signs observed are divided into those affecting either the eyes (Fig. 10.9) or the lips and mouth.

Neck

With the exception of iodine deficiency and thyroid disease, there are very few metabolic or nutritional diseases that manifest as signs in the neck.

Thyroid disease

Look at the patient's neck and ask the patient to swallow. You will often observe a prominent goiter (a diffuse enlargement of the thyroid gland). Goiters, however, can also be seen in other thyroid diseases such as Graves' disease and Hashimoto's thyroiditis.

All thyroid lumps ascend on swallowing because they are attached to the trachea.

In your clinical career you will encounter "lumps" on examination of every body system. It is crucial that you know the characteristics to elicit for any lump from benign hernias to malignant cancer. For every lump define the site, size, shape, surface, color, temperature, tenderness, edge, composition, reducibility, and state of overlying and adjacent tissues.

Thorax

The thorax is divided into the respiratory and cardiovascular systems.

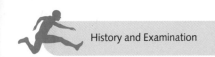

Main metabolic signs observed on examination of the limbs		
Physical examination	**Symptoms and signs**	**Possible diagnosis**
skin lesions: • ischemic skin ulcers • note position, size, tenderness, edge of ulcer and note any discharge	• usually found over pressure areas: tips of toes/fingers • painful • discharge, usually serum or pus, rarely blood-stained because of impaired blood supply • surrounding tissues pale and cold	ischemic damage seen in: • diabetes • atherosclerosis
neuropathic ulcers	• usually found over pressure areas • painless (as lack of sensation) • surrounding tissues are healthy because of good blood supply	peripheral nerve lesions: chronic complication of diabetes
gangrene-dead tissue	• brown/black tissue usually found on extremities and pressure points • painless and senseless	ischemic damage
tendon xanthomata: look especially on Achilles tendon and finger extensors on back of hand	• fatty deposits on tendons leading to thickening • may see fat deposition in palmar creases of hand called palmar xanthomata	characteristic of dyslipidemias (see Chapter 4)
gouty tophi	• deposits of urate crystals around joints, tendons and cartilage of ear lobes • cause yellow discoloration of overlying skin	gout
joint problems: • arthropathy • observe joints for signs of inflammation, especially big toe	painful, red, hot, inflamed joint acute onset	acute gout pseudogout

Fig. 10.8 Main metabolic signs observed on examination of the limbs: skin and joint problems associated with metabolic disease.

Respiratory system

Very few metabolic diseases result in obvious respiratory signs. Therefore, only a brief discussion is included here for completion.

Check list for examination of the respiratory system

This is only a brief list to help you get started:
• Introduce yourself.
• The patient should be undressed to the waist so that the appropriate part of the body is exposed.
• Position the patient so that he or she is comfortable and at the correct angle for examination (45° for respiratory and cardiovascular examinations).
• Observe any respiratory distress, the level of consciousness, expansion (is it uniform between the two sides?), tachypnea, and so on.

Begin any examination by observing the hands of the patient and work your way up the arms to the head, to the neck, and then down the chest. Remember, for examination of any system follow the sequence: observation (Fig. 10.11), palpation, percussion, and auscultation (Fig. 10.12).

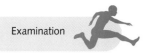

Fig. 10.9 Observation of the eyes for signs associated with metabolic disease.

Observation of the eyes for signs associated with metabolic disease		
Physical examination	**Symptoms and signs**	**Possible diagnosis**
jaundice: observe color of sclerae	yellow discoloration of sclerae is a more sensitive indicator of jaundice than skin color (sclerae turn yellow first)	• liver disease • hemolytic anemia (e.g. due to G6PDH or pyruvate kinase deficiency) (see Chapter 2)
anemia: observe color of conjunctiva (pull down the lower eyelid)	pale/pink color N.B. the best way to look for anemia is by the color of mucous membranes, particularly conjunctiva (also buccal mucosa)	• acute blood loss/infection • iron/B_{12}/folate deficiency • pernicious anemia • hemolytic anemia • hypothyroidism
xanthelasma: look for yellow fatty lumps in skin of eyelids	yellow fatty masses confined to the skin non-tender	• they may or may not indicate dyslipidemia (see Chapter 4)
(arcus senilis) **corneal arcus**	observe white rim around outer edge of iris due to cholesterol deposition sclerosis in cornea	• common in elderly people • significant in patients <35 years old, as it may indicate hyperlipidemia, such as PH or familial combined hyperlipidemia (see Chapter 4)
Kayser-Fleischer rings: examine corneal-sclera junction for ring	green-brown ring due to copper deposition in periphery of cornea	Wilson's disease: copper overload (see Chapter 8)
observe cornea and conjunctiva for dryness and ulceration	• dryness and ulceration: xerophthalmia • white plaques on conjunctiva: Bitot's spots • opaque scar tissue: keratomalacia and cataracts	all due to vitamin A deficiency
progressive deterioration of vision	loss of visual acuity and cataracts →	diabetes mellitus N.B. in neonates, cataracts may be the result of galactosemia (Chapter 2)

Cardiovascular system

As with the respiratory system, few metabolic diseases manifest as cardiovascular signs. However, anemia of any cause can eventually cause shock and heart failure.

Percussion

Percussion may help to diagnose hepatomegaly (e.g., in cardiac failure).

Observation and palpation

Metabolic signs that can be observed during a cardiovascular examination are listed in Fig. 10.13.

Auscultation

Anemia of any cause can lead to an innocent ejection systolic murmur. For heart failure, you may hear a third heart sound. Checklist for auscultation:

- Always begin at the apex.
- Are there two heart sounds present? The first heart sound is due to the closure of the mitral and tricuspid valves. The second heart sound is due to the closure of the aortic and pulmonary valves. Listen over all four areas (mitral, triscupid, aortic, and pulmonary).
- Listen for extra third and fourth heart sounds.

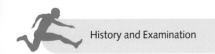
Observation of the mouth and tongue for signs associated with metabolic disease		
Physical examination	**Symptoms and signs**	**Possible diagnosis**
observe color of lips and tongue	central cyanosis: purple-blue color because of excess methemoglobin in the tissues	• inadequate perfusion of tissues, methemoglobinemia • since methemoglobin cannot carry oxygen, this leads to poor perfusion of tissues and cyanosis (see Chapter 3)
observe color of tongue and atrophic changes	glossitis (red, smooth, sore tongue), loss of filiform papillae	• iron/folate/B_{12} deficiency • other B vitamin deficiencies: niacin, B_6 (pyridoxine)
angular stomatitis: observe corners of mouth for cuts and infection	angular stomatitis: inflamed, cracked corners of mouth cracks may become infected with *Candida albicans*	common in elderly due to iron deficiency or deficiency of B-group vitamins

Fig. 10.10 Observation of the mouth and tongue for signs associated with metabolic disease.

- Listen for murmurs. Murmurs are caused by turbulent blood flow. They are classified into systolic, diastolic or continuous, depending on their timing with the cardiac cycle.
- Listen over the carotid, renal, and femoral arteries for bruits. These indicate turbulent blood flow caused by stenosis of arteries; they are heard in patients with disseminated atherosclerosis.

Abdomen

Most metabolic diseases that produce clinical signs in the abdomen do so as a result of excessive deposition of a metabolite or nutrient in organs such as the liver, or in arteries or the skin. This interferes with the correct functioning of the organ. For example:

- In hemochromatosis, iron is deposited in the liver, leading to liver cirrhosis.
- In glycogen storage diseases, the deposition of glycogen in the liver causes hepatomegaly.
- In atherosclerotic disease, the deposition of fat in the walls of arteries leads to atherosclerotic plaque formation: bruits may be heard over carotid or renal arteries. Aortic aneurysm may cause pulsation in the abdomen and peripheral vascular disease.

Useful points for the examination of the abdomen

When examining the abdomen:

- The patient should be lying as flat as possible, with arms by his or her sides.
- The patient should be exposed from the nipples to the knees; however, in the interest of privacy, it is best to expose in stages, beginning with xiphisternum to pubis.
- Kneel beside the bed so that you are at the same level as the patient.
- As with any system of the body, go through the sequence of observation, palpation, percussion, and auscultation.

Observation

Observe the general symmetry and shape of the abdomen. The clinical signs that can be observed during an abdominal examination, and their underlying metabolic causes, are listed in Fig. 10.14.

Palpation

Points to remember when palpating the abdomen:
- Before you start, ask the patient. "Have you any pain anywhere in your abdomen?" If the answer is "yes," begin your palpation furthest from the pain.
- The abdomen is divided either into nine areas or simply into quadrants (Fig. 10.15).

The clinical signs with their underlying metabolic causes that can be detected on palpation of the abdomen are listed in Fig. 10.16.

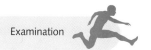
Fig. 10.11 Examination of the respiratory system in metabolic disease.

Examination of the respiratory system in metabolic disease		
Physical examination	**Symptoms and signs**	**Possible diagnosis**
signs of respiratory distress	e.g. tachypnea, use of accessory muscles of respiration, nasal flare and sternal recession	in starvation, severe muscle wasting can eventually cause wasting of the diaphragm, leading to respiratory distress and death
shape of chest wall	• pigeon chest, *pectus carinatum*: prominent sternum often accompanied by indrawing of softened ribs along attachment of diaphragm; Harrison's sulcus • rickety rosary: expansion or swelling of ribs at costochondral junctions	rickets in children
cyanosis	• central cyanosis: observe purple-blue color of lips • peripheral cyanosis: observe purple-blue color of extremities (fingers and toes) caused by increased level of deoxygenated blood	methemoglobinemia (see Fig. 10.10) inadequate perfusion of tissues caused by peripheral vascular disease may be seen in diabetics and dyslipidemias
respiratory rate: count rate for about a minute fast or labored? normal 15–20/min	• hyperventilation • deep Kussmaul respiration • breath smells of acetone • severe dehydration	• metabolic acidosis leading to diabetic ketoacidosis • respiratory compensation of metabolic acidosis results in hyperventilation

Fig. 10.12 Auscultation of the respiratory system: metabolic signs.

Auscultation of the respiratory system		
Physical examination	**Symptoms and signs**	**Possible diagnosis**
breath sounds	↓ breath sounds	in obese people these may be difficult to hear
crepitations/crackles	pulmonary edema often due to heart failure	heart failure may be secondary to: • anemia from iron/folate/B_{12}/vitamin C deficiency • kwashiorkor

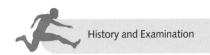

Clinical signs that can be observed during cardiovascular examination		
Physical examination	**Symptoms and signs**	**Possible diagnosis**
signs of shock and heart failure	pallor, tachycardia, heart murmur, and cardiac enlargement untreated progresses to heart failure	severe anemia [hemoglobin <8 g/dL] causes: • blood loss • iron/folate/B_{12} deficiency • acute hemolytic crisis • hypothyroidism
apex beat	visible on inspection	thin, wasted individuals
impalpable apex beat	normally felt fifth intercostal space, mid-clavicular line	obesity
displaced apex beat	heart failure → cardiomegaly	anemia of any cause kwashiorkor hypercalcemia

Fig. 10.13 Clinical signs that may be observed during a cardiovascular examination.

Clinical signs and the underlying metabolic causes that can be observed during an abdominal examination		
Physical examination	**Symptoms and signs**	**Possible diagnosis**
abdominal distension: note shape, symmetry, size of any bulge or mass	general/localized swelling	obesity; pregnancy ascites; kwashiorkor
	asymmetrical enlargement	e.g. liver enlargement due to glycogen storage disorders, dyslipidemias, kwashiorkor
striae (stretch marks)	purple abdominal striae	Cushing's syndrome obesity
spider naevi	single, central arteriole feeding a number of small branches in a radial manner, with blanching (turning white) on pressure	chronic liver failure and cirrhosis in: • alcoholics • hemochromatosis • Wilson's disease (copper overload) • vitamin A toxicity (see Chapter 8)
pigmentation	slate-grey color	iron overload

Fig. 10.14 Clinical signs that can be observed during an abdominal examination and their underlying metabolic causes.

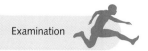

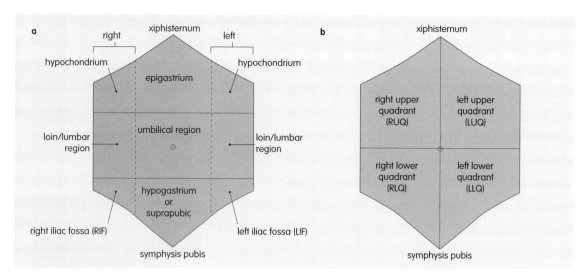

Fig. 10.15 Examination of the abdomen. **a.** A schematic representation of the abdomen showing nine areas. **b.** The four abdominal quadrants simplified.

Fig. 10.16 Clinical signs that can be detected on palpation of the abdomen with their underlying metabolic causes.

Clinical signs with the underlying metabolic causes that can be detected on palpation of the abdomen		
Physical examination	**Symptoms and signs**	**Possible diagnosis**
abdominal pain: determine site, position, radiation, onset, timing, etc.	acute, severe upper abdominal pain ± guarding and rebound tenderness	• acute pancreatitis seen in type I familial lipoprotein lipase deficiency or apoC-II hyperlipidemia (see Chapter 4) • acute porphyria (see Chapter 6)
liver enlargement (hepatomegaly)	• liver edge is not normally palpable below costal margin • gross hepatomegaly can fill whole abdomen	causes: • heart failure • alcohol-induced liver disease • hemolytic anemia, e.g. G6PDH deficiency • porphyria • iron overload: hemochromatosis • glycogen storage disorders (see Fig. 2.36) • galactosemia (see Chapter 2)
spleen enlargement (splenomegaly)	spleen supposedly has a palpable notch on its medial side but it is very difficult to feel	causes: • pernicious anemia • galactosemia • hemolytic anemia
kidneys	they are usually impalpable	• lower pole of right kidney can be felt in very thin or wasted people • renal disease and stones are associated with gout

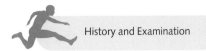

Percussion

Abdominal percussion has two main roles:

- To outline the liver. The liver is "dull" to percussion; therefore, it is useful in determining the degree of hepatomegaly.
- In the presence of abdominal distention, to determine whether it is due to solid, gas, or free fluid (ascites) in the abdomen.

Ascites is seen in congestive heart failure, liver cirrhosis, and secondary to wet beriberi and kwashiorkor.

Auscultation

The clinical signs that can be detected on auscultation of the abdomen, with their underlying metabolic causes, are listed in Fig. 10.17.

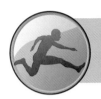 Remember to check the patient's urine for glucose and protein and traces of blood.

Clinical signs with the underlying metabolic causes that can be detected on auscultation of the abdomen		
Physical examination	**Symptoms and signs**	**Possible diagnosis**
bowel sounds	absent if there is mechanical obstruction	• paralytic ileus • gallstones
bruits	listen along course of aorta, usually over femoral and renal arteries	• aortic aneurysm • renal artery stenosis • peripheral vascular disease, e.g. patients with diabetes or dyslipidemias

Fig. 10.17 Clinical signs that can be detected on auscultation of the abdomen and their underlying metabolic causes.

- Name three clinical signs observed on the hands and nails and their possible metabolic causes.
- Name four main metabolic diseases that result in skin or joint lesions in the limbs. Describe the types of lesions produced.
- Describe the characteristics of peripheral ulcers seen in chronic diabetes.
- What symptoms and signs are characteristic of gouty tophi?
- List the main symptoms and signs you might expect in diabetic ketoacidosis
- Name the clinical signs you would expect in a patient with a hemoglobin of 7 g/dL.
- What criteria do you assess when examining a lump?
- Describe the metabolic causes of respiratory distress and cyanosis.
- Give a general outline of examination of the abdomen
- Describe the metabolic causes of spider nevi.

11. Further Investigations

Routine investigations

Like the clinical assessment chapter, this chapter describes only selected aspects of clinical investigation relevant to metabolic disease. It is not a comprehensive description of laboratory tests used in clinical practice.

The main tests used every day to assess metabolic function can be divided conveniently into:

- "First-line" tests; that is, the tests most frequently requested.
- "Second-line" tests and specialist tests.

Please note that clinical biochemistry and hematology tests should not be interpreted separately (e.g., in the diagnosis of anemia); they are all part of the comprehensive patient assessment.

Hematology
The simplest, first-line hematology test is the complete blood count (CBC). This measures red cell count and indices, white cell count (increased in infection), and platelets. The second-line tests include clotting studies and assessment of serum iron status and bone marrow iron stores (Fig. 11.1).

Clinical chemistry
First-line tests include urea and electrolytes (abbreviated in the clinical jargon as U and E), blood glucose, and liver function tests (LFTs) (Fig. 11.2). Second-line tests include thyroid function tests, glycated hemoglobin, serum magnesium, ferritin, folate, and lipid profile, as well as more specialized tests, such as the measurements of vitamin and trace elements levels performed in patients who receive total parenteral nutrition, or the specific diagnosis of genetic metabolic defects in pediatrics (Fig. 11.3). The measurement of hormone levels in blood is a substantial part of specialized biochemistry testing. The measurement of C-reactive protein is important in the diagnosis and monitoring of infection.

Figs 11.1–11.3 are included for reference. You do not need to learn all the values for different enzymes. In any exam or for any set of blood test results, either the abnormal results are highlighted or the normal ranges are quoted.

Urine
Urine is commonly tested for glucose, protein and ketones (dipstick tests). Although not as sensitive as blood tests, urine tests provide a quick and easy method of investigation (Fig. 11.4). Note that urinary ketones are important in the diagnosis of diabetic ketoacidosis.

Histopathology
These tests are only performed to confirm a diagnosis, usually after simpler biochemical tests have been done (Fig. 11.5), and are often performed together with medical imaging tests.

Immunopathology
Some examples of immunopathological investigations are listed in Fig. 11.6.

Medical imaging
There are many medical imaging tests used, from simple radiographs and ultrasound to magnetic resonance imaging and positron emission tomography scanning. Fig. 11.7 illustrates some examples.

Remember: any patient presenting to the emergency department will probably require a combination of first-line tests. For example:

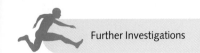

Hematologic investigations		
Test	**Normal range**	**Low/high**
Full blood count (FBC)		
hemoglobin g/dL	men 13–18 women 11.5–16	low: anemia high: polycythemia
red cell count (×10^{12}/L)	men 4.5–6.5 women 3.9–5.6	high: polycythemia low: anemia
mean cell volume (MCV)	76–96 fL	low: "microcytic RBC" in iron deficiency anemia high: macrocylic RBC in B$_{12}$/folate deficiency
mean cell hemoglobin (MCH)	27–32 pg	low: iron deficiency high: B$_{12}$/folate deficiency
reticulocyte count	0.8–2%	low: iron/B$_{12}$/folate deficiency anemia thalassemia high: hemolytic anemia
bone marrow iron stores		low: iron deficiency high: thalassemia sideroblastic anemia
clotting studies:		
• prothrombin time	10–14 s	both high—vitamin K deficiency
• activated partial thromboplastin time (APTT)	35–45 s	prothrombin time is a good indicator of liver function (protein synthetic capacity)
blood film	normocytic, normochromic red blood cells (RBC)	microcytic, hypochromic: iron deficiency macrocytic: B$_{12}$/folate deficiency sickle cells: sickle cell anemia irregular "blister" cells: G6PDH deficiency (very rare)

Fig. 11.1 Hematologic investigations.

- Complete blood count.
- Urea and electrolytes.
- Blood glucose. Bedside blood glucose can be life saving if a patient comes in unconscious or confused: he or she may be drunk or severely hypoglycemic.
- Liver function tests.
- If there are obvious signs of infection, blood and urine must be taken for culture, and the measurement of C-reactive protein is useful.
- Electrocardiogram and chest radiograph if necessary.

Investigation of glucose homeostasis

Measurement of blood glucose

Use
The measurement of blood glucose is used to confirm or reject a diagnosis of diabetes mellitus or impaired glucose tolerance and to monitor the control of blood glucose in diabetic patients.

Reference ranges for blood glucose levels are shown in Fig. 11.8.

Test
The estimation of blood glucose uses the glucose oxidase and peroxidase reaction.

Method
The test is based on the reaction catalyzed by the enzymes glucose oxidase and peroxidase, and a peroxidase substrate (a dye). Glucose oxidase oxidizes glucose present in a deproteinized blood sample to gluconolactone and hydrogen peroxide. The hydrogen peroxide reacts with a dye to form a colored complex, absorbance of which is read in a spectrophotometer. Under standard conditions, the amount of glucose in the unknown blood sample is equal to the amount of colored product formed. Standardized solutions of glucose are processed at the same time in order to construct a calibration curve. Therefore, the amount of glucose in the unknown blood sample can be read from the curve.

Advantages
The test is specific for glucose. A similar enzyme reaction is found in commercially available self-monitoring reagent strips: the Dextrostix/Glucometer system (and many other systems) is commonly used at home by patients with type 1 diabetes.

First-line biochemical investigations on blood or serum		
Test	Normal range	Low/high
fasting blood glucose	2.5–5.9 mmol/L	low: hypoglycemia high: hyperglycemia → diabetes
liver function tests		
AST ALT	<35 U/L <55 U/L	high: hepatocellular damage, e.g. hepatitis cirrhosis fatty liver
alkaline phosphatase (ALP)	<120 U/L (different isoenzymes present in liver, bone, placenta and intestine)	high: obstruction of biliary tract or intrahepatic cholestasis: cirrhosis
γ-glutamyl transferase (GGT)	<80 U/L	high: alcohol abuse obstructive liver disease carcinoma of head of the pancreas (fairly non-specific test of liver function)
serum total bilirubin	<22 μmol/L	high: liver disease hemolytic anemia anemia
Urea and electrolytes (U and Es)		
sodium	135–145 mmol/L	high: dehydration low: extracellular water excess
potassium	3.5–5.0 mmol/L	high: diabetic ketoacidosis renal failure potassium-sparing diuretics low: renal or intestinal loss surgical drainage of the bowel, vomiting insulin treatment of diabetic ketoacidosis hyperaldosteronism, diuretics
bicarbonate	22–32 mmol/L	high: metabolic alkalosis low: metabolic acidosis
urea	2.5–6.7 mmol/L	high: renal disease catabolic state
creatinine	70 to ≤150 μmol/L	high: renal damage and failure increased muscle bulk, e.g. athletes
(U and E profile also includes chloride)		
total protein	60–80 g/L	high: myeloma
albumin	35–50 g/L	low: chronic liver disease
calcium	2.12–2.65 mmol/L	low: vitamin D deficiency high: hypercalcemia
free T_4 (thyroxine)	9–22 pmol/L	high: hyperthyroidism
free T_3 (triiodothyronine)	5–10.2 pmol/L	low: hypothyroidism
thyroid stimulating hormone (TSH)	0.5–5.7 mU/L	low: hyperthyroidism high: hypothyroidism

Fig. 11.2 First-line biochemical investigations on blood or serum. AST, aspartate aminotransferase; ALT, alanine aminotransferase.

211

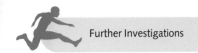

Second-line biochemical investigations on blood or serum		
Test	**Normal range**	**Low/high**
serum iron	13–32 µmol/L	low: iron deficiency high: hemochromatosis thalassemia
total iron binding capacity (TIBC)	42–80 µmol/L	low: iron deficiency
serum B₁₂	160–925 ng/L	low: pernicious anemia
folate	4–18 µg/L	low: pregnancy, cancer, drugs, e.g. methotrexate
serum urate	<0.48 mmol/L	high: hyperuricemia and gout
lipid profile: total cholesterol triacylglycerol (triglycerides) HDL-cholesterol	<5.0 mmol/L 2.0 mmol/L >1.0 mmol/L	high: dyslipidemias chronic liver disease
vitamin D: 25-hydroxyCC 1,25-dihydroxyCC	37–200 nmol/L 60–108 pmol/L	low: rickets or osteomalacia
copper ceruloplasmin	12–25 µmol/L 0.20–0.45 g/L	high: Wilson's disease

Fig. 11.3 Second-line biochemical investigations on blood or serum. CC, cholecalciferol.

Examples of histopathology investigations	
Test	**Results in metabolic disease**
liver biopsy	Wilson's disease: increased copper deposition leading to liver cirrhosis hemochromatosis: iron deposition may cause cirrhosis which may progress to hepatocellular carcinoma
synovial joint fluid analysis	gout: the presence of yellow, needle-shaped negatively birefringent monosodium unate crystals

Fig. 11.5 Examples of histopathology investigations.

Examples of urine tests	
Test	**Results**
glycosuria	high: diabetes, pregnancy, renal tubular damage lowered renal threshold for glucose
ketones	high: diabetic ketoacidosis and starvation
proteinuria	high: renal damage urinary tract infections
porphobilinogen (PBG) and δ-aminolevulinic acid (ALA)	high: acute porphyrias (see Chapter 6)
bilirubin	high: hepatocellular or obstructive jaundice, hemolytic anemia
urobilinogen	high: hemolytic or hepatocellular jaundice low: obstructive jaundice

Fig. 11.4 Examples of urine tests.

Examples of immunopathology investigations		
Test	**Normal result**	**Result**
Schilling test: patient given radioactive B₁₂ and its excretion is monitored (see Chapter 8)	excretion >10% radioactive B₁₂	<10% excretion is indicative of B₁₂ deficiency; if the test is repeated with intrinsic factor and excretion remains within normal range, the diagnosis of pernicious anemia is confirmed
Direct Coombs' test (detection of antibodies to red blood cells)	usually no antibodies are present and therefore there is no agglutination of RBCs	positive test = agglutination of RBCs, e.g. in hemolytic disease of the newborn or in autoimmune hemolytic anemia

Fig. 11.6 Examples of immunopathology investigations.

Examples of medical imaging investigations

Test	Examples of diagnostic utility
chest X-ray (CXR)	diagnosis of heart failure: anemia of any cause, ischemic heart disease, hypercalcemia, or iron overload, can all result in heart failure; on X-ray this can show up as: • an enlarged heart (cardiomegaly) • pleural effusion • increased perihilar shadowing (bat wings) due to edema • prominent upper lobe veins • Kerley B lines
radiological changes in bone structure	defective bone mineralization: in rickets and osteomalacia: defective mineralization seen in pelvis, long bones and ribs in the early stages → see soft tissue swelling late stages → well-defined "punched out" lesions in juxta-articular bone
electrocardiogram (ECG)	abnormalities of ECG pattern can be related to: • ischemic damage and myocardial infarction • conduction defects (heart blocks) • arrythmias • some electrolyte disturbances • congenital heart defects
CT scan	used to identify abnormalities and to exclude focal lesions due to tumors or infection; essential tool in the diagnosis of space-occupying lesions

Fig. 11.7 Examples of medical imaging investigations.

Diagnostic criteria for diabetes mellitus and impaired glucose tolerance

	Normal (mmol/L)	IGT (mmol/L)	Diabetes (mmol/L)
fasting plasma glucose	<7.0	<7.8	>7.8
2h post-load blood glucose	<7.8	7.8–11.1	>11.1

IGT = impaired glucose tolerance

Fig. 11.8 Diagnostic concentrations of plasma glucose.

Results of oral glucose tolerance test

Result	Reference range
normal	returns to fasting level
impaired glucose tolerance (IGT)	fasting plasma glucose <7.0 mmol/L and 2h value between 7.8 and 11.1 mmol/L in an OGTT
impaired fasting glucose	fasting plasma glucose 6–7 mmol/L
diabetic	fasting blood glucose ≥7.0 mmol/L and/or 2h value >11.1 mmol/L in an OGTT

Fig. 11.9 Results of an oral glucose tolerance test (OGTT).

Oral glucose tolerance test
Use
The oral glucose tolerance test (OGTT) is a reference method to diagnose disturbances in glucose homeostasis. However, fasting blood glucose provides very similar information and should be used first. The use of OGTT is restricted to the detection of borderline cases.

Method
Patients should make sure that they eat a normal diet, containing adequate carbohydrate, for the preceding 3 days. This ensures that the enzymes involved in glucose metabolism are present at normal levels. After an overnight fast, an initial basal blood sample is taken and the blood glucose concentration is determined. A drink containing 75 g of glucose in 250–300 mL of water is drunk, and the blood glucose is measured every 30 min for the next 2 h. The blood glucose concentration is determined by the glucose oxidase method. Patients must sit comfortably during the test because stress can lead to cortisol release, which increases blood glucose concentration. Figs 11.9 and 11.10 illustrate the results of an OGTT.

Assessment of glycemic control: glycosylated hemoglobin
Use
The concentration of glycosylated hemoglobin (HbA_1 or HbA_{1c}) provides a measure of the average blood glucose concentration over the preceding 6–8 weeks, that is, the lifetime of a hemoglobin molecule. This is useful for patients with diabetes, to show how well their blood glucose concentration is

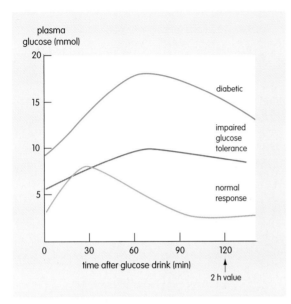

Fig. 11.10 Oral glucose tolerance test. Please note that persons with impaired glucose tolerance can have a normal fasting glucose concentration.

Reference values	
Result	**Reference values for HbA$_{1c}$**
normal	4–8%
poorly controlled	>10%

Fig. 11.11 Reference values for HbA$_{1c}$ expressed as a percentage of total hemoglobin.

being controlled over a period of time. The value is high in poorly controlled diabetics.

Method

Glucose attaches nonenzymatically to adult hemoglobin (HbA) over the lifetime of a RBC. The extent to which this occurs is proportional to the blood glucose concentration. The amount of glycosylated hemoglobin (HbA$_{1c}$) present in blood can be measured by a number of methods, including high-pressure liquid chromatography, electrophoresis or immunoassay. It is presently expressed as a percentage of total hemoglobin (Fig. 11.11).

Assessment of glycemic control: serum fructosamine concentration
Use

The serum fructosamine concentration is a measure of glycemic control over the previous 2 weeks but is now very rarely used.

Enzyme assays
Glucose-6-phosphate dehydrogenase
Use

An enzyme assay is used for the diagnosis of glucose-6-phosphate dehydrogenase deficiency, the most common RBC enzyme defect (see Chapter 3). It

allows patients with glucose-6-phosphate dehydrogenase deficiency to be detected between hemolytic attacks, such that diagnosis is not just dependent on the blood picture during an attack. An enzyme activity of <2% of the normal level may be seen in very severe cases.

Pyruvate kinase assay
Use

Pyruvate kinase assay is used for the diagnosis of RBC pyruvate kinase deficiency (see Chapter 2).

Test

The production of pyruvate is coupled to the reduction of a dye, with the color change monitored spectrophotometrically. A decreased production of ATP can also be measured when radioactively labeled ^{32}P is added to RBCs and its incorporation into ATP is monitored.

Reference values

Patients typically need to have an enzyme level of 5–25% of the normal level to show clinical features.

Galactose and fructose

Both galactose and fructose are reducing sugars and are detected in the urine of patients, using alkaline copper (II) reagents, such as Benedict's reagent.

Galactosemia

Galactosemia is usually caused by a deficiency of the enzyme galactose-1-phosphate uridyl transferase.

Tests

Screening tests are performed in infants with suspicious symptoms:

- Test for galactosuria: Clinitest tablets or reagent strips contain copper citrate, which is reduced by galactose. The color change observed is clear blue to green to brown to a brick red precipitate if the reduction is complete. The presence of galactose

in the urine and positive symptoms lead to the withdrawal of galactose and lactose from the diet until a diagnostic test can be performed.
- Diagnostic test: assay RBCs for decreased galactose-1-phosphate uridyl transferase activity.

Fructokinase deficiency: essential fructosuria

The absence of fructokinase leads to a combination of a high fructose concentration in the blood and fructose accumulation in the urine. Both must be present to form a diagnosis. Fructose, like galactose, is a reducing sugar and its presence in urine can be detected with Clinitest tablets. Bear in mind that this is a rare diagnosis, virtually exclusively seen in pediatric practice.

Investigation of lipid metabolism
Cholesterol and triacylglycerol concentration
Uses

Coronary heart disease is a major cause of death in the U.S. Therefore, cholesterol levels are monitored routinely in at-risk groups and when necessary in the rest of the population. At-risk groups include:
- Patients with coronary heart disease (angina, post-myocardial infarction, post-angioplasty or coronary artery bypass graft) and patients with peripheral or cerebrovascular disease.
- Patients with hyperlipidemias and their families and patients with a family history of premature cardiovascular disease.
- Patients with multiple risk factors; for example, patients with diabetes, high blood pressure, or high cholesterol (a full list of risk factors can be found in Chapter 4).

Investigations

Screening for cholesterol levels can be done on a nonfasting sample. If a raised cholesterol is found, a full lipid profile may be performed, which measures the total cholesterol, high-density lipoprotein (HDL)-cholesterol, and triacylglycerol (triglycerides). Blood taken for lipid studies is obtained after an overnight fast. Reference values for fasting plasma lipid concentrations are shown in Fig. 11.12.

Low-density lipoprotein (LDL) cholesterol levels can also be obtained by calculation using the Friedewald equation. This is only valid if triacylglycerol levels are less than 4.5 mmol/L.

Desirable values for fasting plasma lipid concentrations

Lipid	Plasma concentration (mmol/L)
total cholesterol	<5.0
LDL-cholesterol	<3.0
HDL-cholesterol	>1.0
triacylglycerol (triglyceride)	<2.0

Fig. 11.12 Desirable fasting plasma lipid concentrations.

$$LDL\,(mmol/L) = total\ cholesterol - HDL - (triacylglycerol/2.2)$$

$$LDL\,(mg/dL) = total\ cholesterol - HDL - (triacylglycerol/5)$$

Triacylglycerol levels of greater than 10 mmol/L are associated with an increased risk of pancreatitis.

Other investigations
Urine porphobilinogen in acute porphyries
Use

Porphobilinogen can be detected in the urine during acute attack of porphyria; for example, in acute intermittent, variegate and hereditary coproporphyrias, discussed in Chapter 6. In unexplained acute abdominal pain, peripheral neuropathy and neuropsychiatric symptoms, especially if there is a family history of porphyria, urine should be tested for porphobilinogen by a simple screening test.

Test

Porphobilinogen in urine is detected by adding one part Ehrlich's aldehyde reagent to one part urine, which causes a pink–red color to appear. If very high levels of porphobilinogen are present, the pink color persists on the addition of two parts chloroform. In the presence of excess porphobilinogen, urine will darken on standing, "auto-oxidizing" to a red color without the addition of Ehrlich's reagent. This is only a screening test because porphobilinogen is only present in urine during acute attacks. Accurate diagnosis depends on the measurement of defective enzyme levels and on genetic diagnosis.

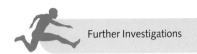

Diagnosis of phenylketonuria

Every neonate is now screened for phenylketonuria as part of the Guthrie test. Diagnosis is based on a high concentration of phenylalanine in the blood (see Chapter 5 for a full discussion).

Screening test

A sample of capillary blood is taken from a heel-prick at 5–10 days after birth. The delay allows sufficient time for feeding and, therefore, for protein intake to be established and for the effect of the mother's metabolism to subside. This test used to be based on a microbiological technique, using a strain of *Bacillus subtilis* which only grows if excess phenylalanine is present. However, it is now based on chromatography. Increased plasma phenylalanine levels are indicative of phenylketonuria. The neonatal screening also includes the measurement of thyroid stimulating hormone (TSH), to screen babies for hypothyroidism.

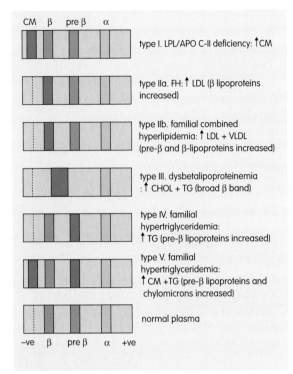

Lipoproteins in the blood can be separated by electrophoresis (Fig. 11.13). Electrophoresis is now rarely used in the detection of hyperlipidemias.

Know about the criteria for the diagnosis of diabetes and glucose intolerance.

Assessment of nutritional status

For any individual, adequate nutrition is essential to maintain growth and development and recovery from illness. It is especially important in newborn babies, infants and during pregnancy, when nutritional deficiency can lead to wasting, severe mental retardation and even death. Malnutrition must be recognized and assessed accurately, to enable decisions to be made about treatment and re-feeding methods. Assessment is divided into:
• Dietary history.
• Anthropometry.

Fig. 11.13 Electrophoretic patterns of hyperlipidemias. Lipoproteins in the blood can be separated by electrophoresis. Each hyperlipidemia gives a characteristic separation pattern. (APO C-II, apolipoprotein C-II; CHOL, cholesterol; CM, chylomicron; FH, familial hypercholesterolemia; LDL, low-density lipoprotein; TG, triacylglycerol; VLDL, very-low-density lipoprotein.) Lipid electrophoresis is now rarely used in clinical practice.

• Physical examination.
• Laboratory tests.

Medical, social, and dietary history

The main aspect of this is the dietary history, but often weight loss and poor nutrition are related to medical, psychological or financial factors (see Fig. 9.2).

Medical history

Ask specifically about:
• Loss of appetite.
• How much weight loss or gain? The time course of the weight change.
• Dysphagia, nausea, vomiting.
• Periods of weight loss and gain in the past; use of laxatives.

- Symptoms of hyperthyroidism: weight loss, increased appetite, irritability, preference for hot or cold temperature, and so on.
- Psychiatric history, especially if there is the possibility of depression or an eating disorder (e.g. anorexia nervosa).

Social history
In developed countries:
- Malnutrition may be related to the poor socioeconomic status of a family.
- Inquire about housing, social support and income support.

In developed countries, nutritional deficiency is particularly seen in:
- Elderly people ("tea and biscuit brigade") living alone who are unable to cook or shop.
- Young pregnant mothers who live off a staple diet of chips, pizzas, and so on.
- Chronic alcoholics.

In developing countries, nutritional deficiency may be related to war, poor crops, and the poor socioeconomic status of the entire country.

Dietary history
Dietary recall
Ask specifically:
- What do you eat in a typical day?
- What do you like and dislike eating? (important in children).
- Access to food or presence of financial problems?
- Do you watch what you eat? Are you on any particular diet?
- Ask specifically about alcohol intake.

Patients are often asked to keep a food diary. This is usually more accurate than simply questioning the patient, although it relies on the patient's compliance to fill the diary in and also on the patient's willingness to provide accurate information (patients with eating disorders are not usually willing to do so).

Anthropometric measurements
The basic anthropometric measurements are:
- Height.
- Weight.
- Calculation of the body mass index (BMI): weight (kg)/height (m)^2.

- Midarm circumference: a measure of skeletal muscle mass (less frequently used).
- Skinfold thickness. This helps to assess the amount of subcutaneous fat stores (less frequently used).

The reason for weight loss or poor nutrition is often not as simple as "not eating enough." You must eliminate serious underlying illnesses such as cancer before you move on to diagnoses of psychiatric illness (depression or anorexia nervosa) or poor socioeconomic status.

For infants, it is difficult to measure skin-fold thickness accurately, and this measurement is therefore of little value. The World Health Organization recommends that nutritional status be expressed as:
- % Weight/height: a measure of wasting as an index of acute malnutrition.
- % Height/age: a measure of growth retardation as an index of chronic malnutrition.

In infants, regular growth measurements are very valuable in assessing their nutritional status. Therefore, all infants have their height and weight plotted on a growth chart (Fig. 11.14), which allows a decrease in the rate of growth to be easily recognized and monitored as an early sign of malnutrition.

Physical clinical examination
Physical examination is a nonspecific method useful in severe malnutrition; for example, marasmus or kwashiorkor, when obvious signs are present. However, it only detects about 25% of moderate cases of malnutrition.

Clinical signs
These can be a combination of any of the following:
- Wasting or cachexia.
- Pallor, which indicates anemia, possibly caused by an iron, vitamin B$_{12}$ or folate deficiency.

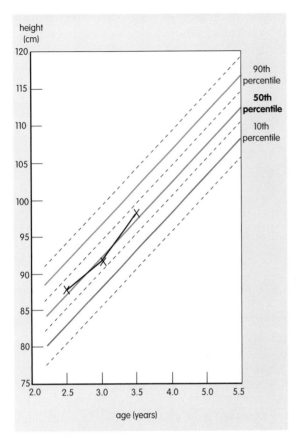

Fig. 11.14 Example of a growth chart often used to help in assessment of nutritional status in children. The line plotted shows that the patient's height lies along the 50th centile, i.e., average height.

- Specific effects of vitamin deficiency; for example, deficiency of vitamin A, causing Bitot's spots on the eyes, or of vitamin D and calcium, causing rickets.
- Edema.
- Bruising, for example in vitamin D or K deficiency.

Biochemical tests

Biochemical tests are useful in the detection of early or mild to moderate malnutrition, that is, before clinical signs become evident. The tests for individual nutrients, vitamins and minerals are dealt with in Chapter 8. Here, the different types of tests are considered.

Types of biochemical tests
Direct measurement

Direct measurement of the concentration of a nutrient or a metabolite in the body fluid, usually in the serum or urine.

Such measurements can be made exploiting the activation of an enzyme by a vitamin. For example, thiamin is a cofactor for RBC transketolase. In thiamin deficiency, the RBC enzyme activity can be measured before and after the addition of thiamine pyrophosphate (the active form of thiamin). Addition of thiamine pyrophosphate to RBCs should lead to an increase in enzyme activity, proving thiamin deficiency.

Measurement of stores

The best way to measure the level of a nutrient is to measure its stores because:

- A decrease in the dietary intake of a nutrient leads to the mobilization of that nutrient from its stores to maintain a normal plasma concentration.
- Usually, only in severe deficiency does the plasma concentration drop significantly.
- Therefore, by measuring a decrease in the body stores we can detect a deficiency earlier.

For example, the best way to assess iron deficiency is to measure a decrease in bone marrow iron stores (serum ferritin reflects iron stores and is low; serum transferrin binds circulating iron and so its iron binding capacity is high), and the best way to assess vitamin C deficiency is to measure a decrease in white cell vitamin C content (Fig. 11.15).

A plasma albumin of less than 30 g/L is often used as an index of malnutrition. However, albumin level is severely affected by fluid and electrolyte disorders, and in these patients albumin is not an accurate index of nutritional status. The diagnosis of severe malnutrition is usually made on clinical assessment.

Parenteral nutrition

Nutritional support is provided for all patients who are severely malnourished or are unable to eat because of physical illness. Whenever possible, enteral nutrition is used; that is, via a nasogastric tube, because it is more natural, cheaper and far less hazardous in terms of the effects on fluid and electrolyte balance than parenteral nutrition. Enteral

Some biochemical tests related to nutritional status	
Nutrient	Tests
protein	serum protein, albumin, prealbumin
fat	total cholesterol and triglycerides
carbohydrate	blood glucose
vitamin A	plasma vitamin A, retinol binding protein
vitamin D	↓calcium, ↓phosphate, ↑alkaline phosphatase measure vitamin D levels and parathyroid hormone
vitamin K	↑prothrombin time
vitamin C	white cell vitamin C content (storage site)
B_1 (thiamin)	red blood cell (RBC) thiamin
B_{12}	FBC, serum B_{12}, MCV
folate	serum and RBC folate
iron	FBC, ferritin, MCV etc., serum transferrin best estimate is a fall in bone marrow iron stores

Fig. 11.15 Some biochemical tests for nutrients (FBC, full blood count; MCV, mean cell volume).

Complications of total parenteral nutrition

- infection and sepsis associated with the central catheter (the most common complication)
- hyperglycemia
- hypokalemia, hyperkalemia, hyponatremia, hypomagnesemia
- hypophosphatemia
- abnormal liver function
- long-term: metabolic bone disease, vitamin deficiencies, trace metal deficiencies

Fig. 11.16 Complications of total parenteral nutrition.

into a peripheral vein. It involves the intravenous infusion of a mixture of high-concentration glucose, fat emulsion, amino acids, vitamins, electrolytes, and trace elements.

Monitoring the patient

The most frequent complication of TPN is infection of the line; therefore, a meticulous aseptic technique is essential. Also, these patients require careful daily clinical monitoring to avoid complications (Fig. 11.16).

- Fluid balance. The patient requires a daily fluid balance chart.
- Plasma electrolytes (sodium, potassium, chloride, bicarbonate, urea, creatinine) are monitored daily; glucose is checked even more often if required.
- Glucose intolerance and hyperglycemia are common side effects.
- Regular hematological measurements (full blood count and so on) are necessary, as is the monitoring of iron, vitamin B_{12} or folate deficiencies.
- In a patient with stable renal function, 24h urinary urea excretion can provide an index of the body's protein status.
- Liver function tests should be checked about three times a week.
- Patients on long-term TPN require periodical assessment of vitamins and trace elements.

nutrition is always given in preference if the gastrointestinal tract is functional. Feeding through a gastrostomy tube is also an option to be considered before total parenteral nutrition (TPN).

Indications for parenteral nutrition

Indicators for parental nutrition include:
- Intestinal failure, either as the result of surgery (gut resection) or because of a fistula or GI tract obstruction by tumor.
- Patients with a very high energy requirement (i.e., hypercatabolic state); for example, patients with severe trauma or burns and patients unable to eat.

Administration

Administration is usually via a central venous catheter into the superior vena cava, or sometimes

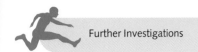
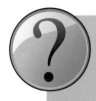

- Name the important first-line hematological and clinical chemistry tests that are performed routinely, and describe why they are used.
- How can the results obtained in patients with metabolic disease vary?
- Describe the Schilling test and its diagnostic use in pernicious anemia.
- Explain the significance of a blood glucose level of 10 mmol/L after 60 min during an oral glucose tolerance test.
- Describe the methods of determining averaged blood concentration in diabetic patients.
- What are the classic radiological changes associated with heart failure?
- How are hematologic investigations affected in vitamin K deficiency?
- Explain how mean cell volume is useful in determining different types of anemia.
- Give four methods for assessing nutritional status. For each know the main principles involved, the uses, and any limitations.
- Describe the indications for parenteral nutrition and its main complications.

Index

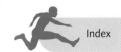

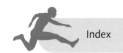

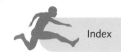

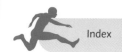

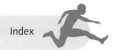

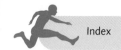

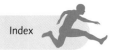

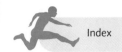

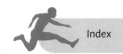

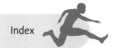

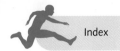